OLD AND RARE BOOKS ON

MATERIA MEDICA

The 'Double-Pelican' on the front cover

The vignette on the front cover depicts a vessel used for distillation and sublimation. The forms of the vessels used in practical operations were supposed to exert a mystical influence upon the character of the product. The 'double-pelican', an intercourse of two distilling vessels, appears as an image of copulation. It is an example of the rich imaginative activity unfolded by the alchemists during their chemical work.

Hand-coloured woodcut reproduced in natural size from the pocket edition of Ulstadius' *Coelum Philosophorum*, Lyon, 1557 (see p. 49).

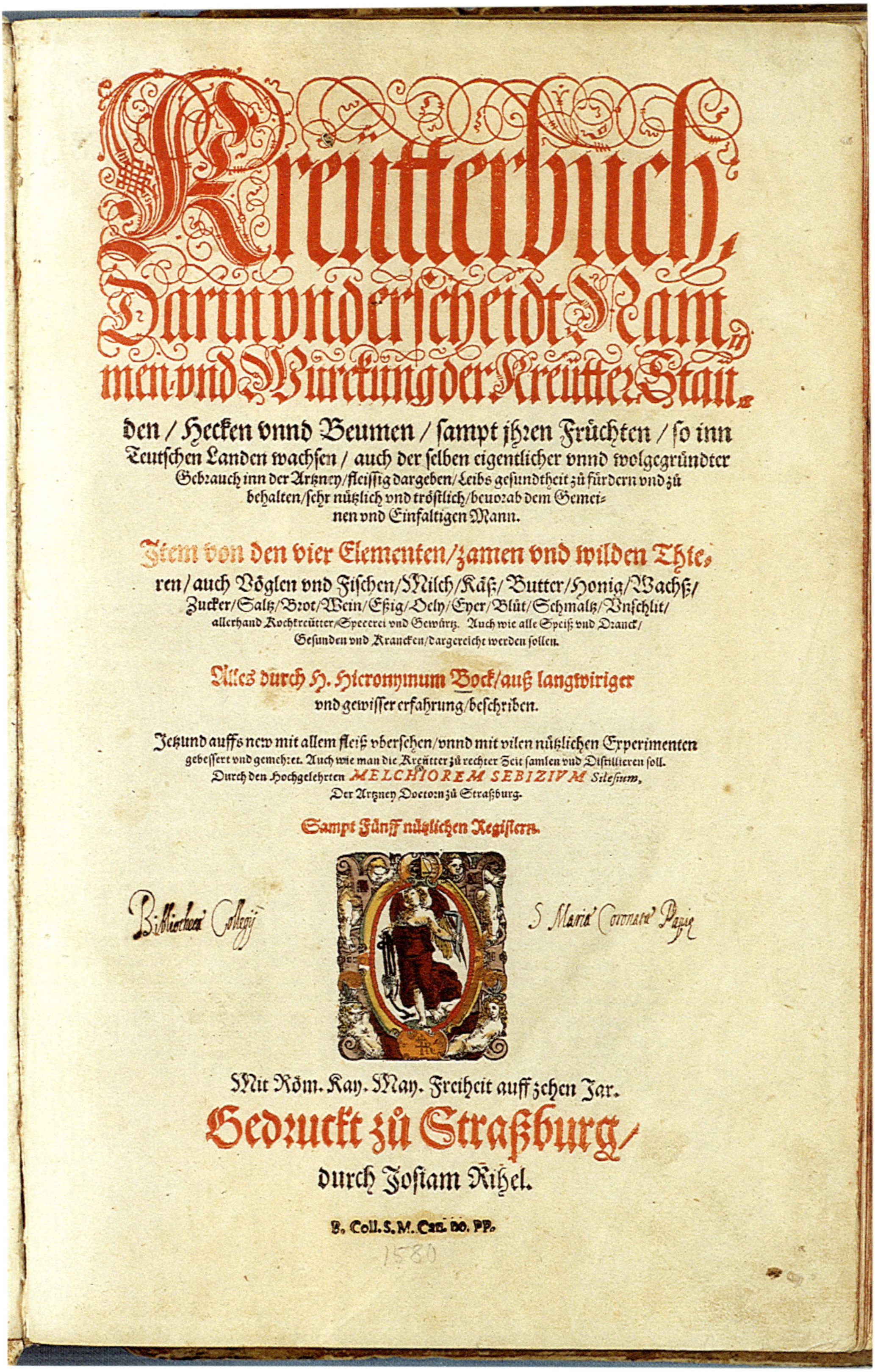

Kreütterbuch/

Darin underscheidt/ Nammen und Würckung der Kreütter/ Stauden/ Hecken unnd Beumen/ sampt jhren Früchten/ so inn Teutschen Landen wachsen/ auch der selben eigentlicher unnd wolgegründter Gebrauch inn der Artzney/ fleissig dargeben/ Leibs gesundtheit zů fürdern und zů behalten/ sehr nützlich und tröstlich/ bevorab dem Gemeinen und Einfaltigen Mann.

Item von den vier Elementen/ zamen und wilden Thieren/ auch Vöglen und Fischen/ Milch/ Käß/ Butter/ Honig/ Wachß/ Zucker/ Saltz/ Brot/ Wein/ Eßig/ Oely/ Eyer/ Blůt/ Schmaltz/ Unschlit/ allerhand Kochkreütter/ Speecerei und Gewürtz. Auch wie alle Speiß und Dranck/ Gesunden und Krancken/ dargereicht werden sollen.

Alles durch H. Hieronymum Bock/ auß langwiriger und gewisser erfahrung/ beschriben.

Jetzund auffs new mit allem fleiß ubersehen/ unnd mit vilen nützlichen Experimenten gebessert und gemehret. Auch wie man die Kreütter zů rechter Zeit samlen und Distillieren soll. Durch den Hochgelehrten MELCHIOREM SEBIZIUM Silesium, Der Artzney Doctorn zů Straßburg.

Sampt Fünff nützlichen Registern.

Bibliothecae Collegii S. Mariae Coronatae Papiae

Mit Röm. Kay. May. Freiheit auff zehen Jar.

Gedruckt zů Straßburg/ durch Josiam Rihel.

Hieronymus Bock, *Kreütterbuch* (Strassburg, 1580)
see pages 78-81

OLD AND RARE BOOKS ON

MATERIA MEDICA

IN THE LIBRARY OF
THE SWEDISH PHARMACEUTICAL SOCIETY
[APOTEKARSOCIETETEN]

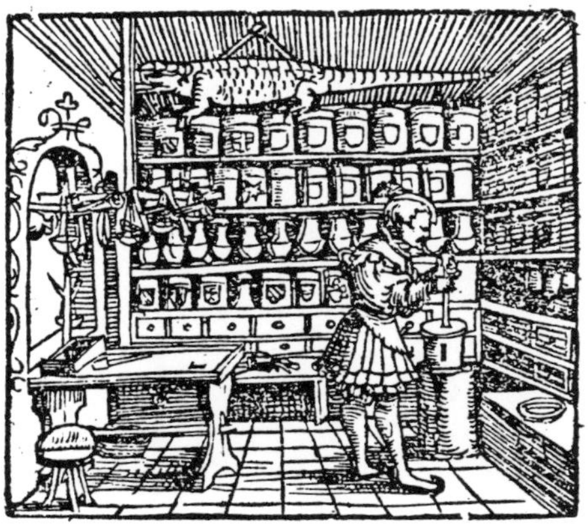

AN ILLUSTRATED AND ANNOTATED

CATALOGUE

compiled by
OVE HAGELIN

STOCKHOLM . SWEDISH PHARMACEUTICAL PRESS . MCM XCVII

This catalogue is produced by
HAGELIN RARE BOOKS AB
P.O. BOX 3321 · S-10366 STOCKHOLM

Photo by
OVE HALLIN STUDIO · LUND

Printed by
HAMMAR OFFSET AB · ALINGSÅS

Bound by
WICKSTRÖMS BOKBINDERI AB · UDDEVALLA

Stockholm 1997

ISBN 91 86274 68 6

Publisher
THE SWEDISH PHARMACEUTICAL PRESS
P.O. BOX 1136 · S-111 81 STOCKHOLM · SWEDEN

LIST OF CONTENTS IN CHRONOLOGICAL ORDER

☛

LIST OF CONTENTS IN CHRONOLOGICAL ORDER

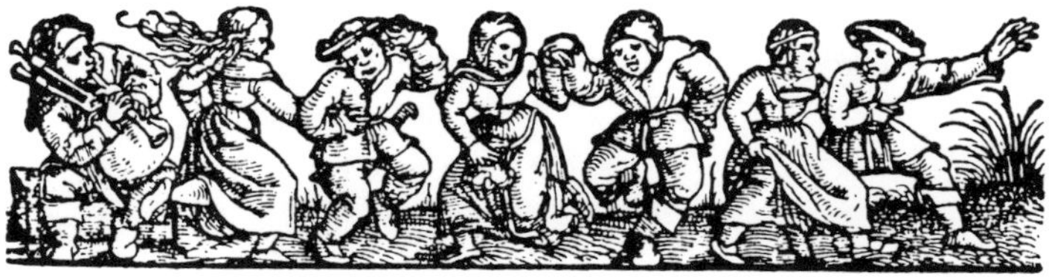

F O R E W O R D

The present catalogue of old and rare books in the library of the Swedish Pharmaceutical Society is the fifth in a series, the purpose of which is to present a selection of important and interesting books that have for long been stored in various medical libraries in Stockholm without having been fully appreciated from a bibliophilistic or historical point of view. My excavations among the shelves in the old stacks in the libraries of the Swedish Society of Medicine and the Karolinska Institute, described in the first three catalogues in the series, have now resulted in their old collections having been at last safely assembled under one roof in a new separate library on the Karolinska Institute campus. This new library, which more correctly should be designated a medical book museum, will comprise some twenty thousand items, and has received the name of *Hagströmer Biblioteket* (The Hagströmer Medico-Historical Library) in honour of Anders Johan Hagströmer, who in 1825 published the first catalogue of the books in the Karolinska Institute Library, the majority of which derived from his own private library. A great part of these old holdings, which has in time come to represent a not insignificant historical and economic value, has routinely been handled as mere literature rather than valuable books. An original edition of an epoch-making work should be handled as a museum piece, an exquisite piece of handicraft, and if preserved in its original state, it is a precious relic, bearing in a hundred hidden ways the whole tale of its history. Without collectors very few old books would be found in these libraries and there would be no special collections at all. The library of the Swedish Pharmaceutical Society is no exception in this respect. Thanks to the generosity of private collectors, and here primarily to two particular pharmacists, the Society has an interesting and representative collection of rare and important pharmaceutical books well worth being presented to a wider public.

The history of pharmacy covers an enormous and fascinating field, of interest not only to specialists. It deals with the history of drugs, their use in the treatment of diseases and our knowledge of their action. The earliest medical practitioners were the herbalists, who came to acquire knowledge of the healing properties of plants. From experiments and from accidents, with both happy and fatal results, they gradually acquired empiric learning and soon began to prepare their remedies so as to make them easier to take or apply, making infusions, decoctions, and ointments. Realizing that their skill and services had a marked value, they kept their knowledge secret and surrounded by mystery. Commercialism has always been a dominating factor, which in the present era has reached astronomical proportions. 'The records of this art and mystery go back to the remotest periods of human history. In the course of ages they become associated with magic, with theology, with alchemy, with crimes and conscious frauds, with the strangest fancies, and dogmas, and delusions, and with the severest science. Deities, kings, and quacks, philosophers, priests, and poisoners, dreamers, seers, and scientific chemists, have helped to build the fabric of pharmacy', says Wootton in the preface to his *Chronicles*. It is my hope that you will find some feautures of their work imperfectly reflected in the following pages. By presenting a panorama of books on *Materia Medica*, from Dioscorides two thousand years ago up to the nineteenth century, in their original or early editions, this should be seen as an attempt to popularise the history of pharmacy as well as to stimulate interest for the book as a collector's item. With the help of illustrations and shorter commentaries compiled from various indicated sources I hope this catalogue will provide a glimpse of some of the book treasures in the library of the Swedish Pharmaceutical Society.

During the early period of the *Apotekare Societeten*, the existence of which was first mentioned in 1675, there was as far as we know no library. In 1782 Georg Eberhard Georgii was appointed librarian of the Society in spite of there being no books. According to the first list of books, dated 1821, the library comprised 22 books and 12 duplicates. One of the first books seems to have been Erik Rydbäck's Swedish translation of the second edition of the *Pharmacopoea Svecica*, the whole edition of which, except for some 20 copies, was confiscated and burnt by the Society (page 196). By the 1880s the number of volumes had increased to over 1000, consisting mainly of gifts from pharmacists. Among the early donators we find both Hagströmer and Berzelius.

One of the most interesting acquisitions of the past, in my opinion, is the Hyltén-Cavallius collection, rich in chemistry, alchemy and practical handbooks. These books seem to have been included in the Cavalli purchase of 1910. Carl Erngisel Hyltén-Cavallius (1817–1853) was a pharmacist and proprietor of the pharmacy in Kungälv, which he sold to his relative Johan Gustaf Cavalli in 1849 when he became a teacher of chemistry at the Chalmer Technological High School in Gothenburg. He was also the author of a comprehensive textbook on inorganic chemistry (1854). His books, many of which bear his signature and the date 1843, are distinguishable on the shelves due to their nice bindings, probably the work of Hyltén-Cavallius himself. They are bound in stiff paper boards, painted in dark ink to resemble leather (he was a pioneer in the technique of tanning) with gilt title spine labels in various bright colours, such as orange, blue or green, indicating subject. These volumes, even though rebound, are very pleasant and in good condition, a judgement that unfortunately cannot be passed on the older books in the great collection of over 1600 volumes assembled by Thor Ekecrantz (1856–1939), professor of chemistry at the Pharmaceutical Institute in Stockholm.

The Ekecrantz collection was a gift to the Society in 1921 after having been purchased by twenty-five of its members. This collection has ever since been considered a particularly well-conditioned and beautiful run of volumes, uniformly bound (regardless of the period in which they were printed) in half leather. Especially appreciated was his collection of Linnaeus items, whose richly gilt spines 'enchant the eye through their brilliance'. However, he had unfortunately all copies rebound and many were cropped by the bookbinder's knife. The quality of the leather has by time been proven to be of poor quality. After having been housed on the library's balcony, near the ceiling in a dry and hot central heating climate, all leather spines, with their elaborate gilding, have fallen apart and the rest has been transmuted into something similar to cocoa. The few of the Ekecrantz eighteenth-century books that escaped rebinding were those in fine contemporary full calf, which he had lacquered to acquire an even brighter shine. My late colleague, Eric Österlund, recounts in his memoir *Bokvandringar* that the professor was a sedulous visitor at the Stockholm Book Auctions and that he rather looked for bargains than for copies in good condition. One day he showed Österlund a fairly rare book (there are several in his collection), but dirty, spotted and in a damaged binding. He nonetheless seemed most content, and Österlund agreed that it was indeed a bargain – but what a poor copy! Ekecrantz replied that, when he had had it cleaned and rebound, it would be in excellent condition. In his laboratory at the Institute the professor had developed a method for cleaning books. The process included soaking them in 70° hot water to dissolve the spine glue, and later washing the sheets in a bleaching liquor, consisting of a hydrogen peroxide solution and a potassium solution. The paper is now chalk-white, limp and soft, having been insufficiently re-sized after treatment. This sad story may at least serve as an instructive example of how well-intended book care may have fatal consequences.

In the Rare Book Room the Society is also proud to house an antique bookcase with glass doors, containing one of the most complete Scheele collections in existence, gathered by Gustaf H.J. Dahl (1877–1942), apothecary in Delsbo in the province of Hälsingland, and in Örebro. This great collection comprises the original editions of Scheele's works and most of his contributions in various scientific periodicals, as well as translations, books and articles about Scheele, all of which are listed by Dahl himself in a typed catalogue. He also wrote 'Scheeleiana' published in *Svensk Farmaceutisk Tidskrift*, 17-21 (1935) and 18 (1938). The remaining part of his library, consisting of 1543 items of Swedish books on botany, medicine and chemistry, was sold at the Stockholm Book Auctions in 1943. His steel-engraved book-plate, depicting his parental home, is one of the most delightful I have ever seen.

Axel Kockum (1869–1958), author of a comprehensive work of 368 pages on the history of medicine and pharmacy during the sixteenth century in Sweden, *Läkare och Apotekare vid Gustav Vasas och hans söners hov* (1949), has also contributed to the Society's library with important books, including some old illustrated herbals.

As compared to the Hagströmer Library the library of the Swedish Pharmaceutical Society is relatively small. This scant quantity is, however, more than adequately compensated by quality, due to the two substantial collections that were acquired in recent times. In 1955 the heirs of Ernst Matérn donated the major part of their father's library and ten years later the great C.D. Carlsson collection was bequeathed by him to the Society. Ernst Matérn (1879–1954), proprietor of the Reindeer Pharmacy (*Renen*) in Stockholm (1935–46) and Divisional Head of the Swedish Board of Health during the 1930s, and Carl David Carlsson (1875–1965), were both keen collectors of all aspects of pharmacy during a period when they had to compete with the greatest collector of medical books in modern times, Dr. Erik Waller, who by no means left out pharmacology and pharmacopoeias from his realm. The two pharmacists did apparently manage to snatch some real rare and important items from under the nose of the voracious Dr. Waller, who otherwise seems to have been quicker than most of his international competitors in ordering from the once so comprehensive catalogues of scholarly booksellers specialized in medicine and science in the 1920s and 1930s. One of Matérn's daughters has told me that, when a visit from Dr. Waller was expected, her father removed from the shelves those books he knew the doctor would find desirable. Matérn succeeded in building up a quite respectable collection of pharmacopoeias, including nearly all editions and translations of the very first, although unofficial, European pharmacopoeia: the famous *Ricettario Fiorentino* (pages 82-4). Of the first official pharmacopoeias he never found, or could not afford, the notoriously rare first edition of Valerius Cordus' *Dispensatorium* (Nuremberg, c. 1546) or the first edition of the Augsburg *Enchiridion*, 1564, but he succeeded in acquiring the equally rare first edition of the Cologne pharmacopoiea of 1565 (page 100) as well as all the successive editions of the *Pharmacopoeia Augustana* up to 1734 (pages 94-9). In the Matérn family is preserved a notebook in which he registered every book purchase with the date when he bought it, from whom it was bought and which price he paid. From this we can learn that whole lots of books were purchased from a certain Mr Rincklake, who among other things was commissioned to restore the holdings of the library of the University of Louvain, that was destroyed by the Germans during World War I.

C.D. Carlsson (1875–1965), always referred to as 'C D', was born in Lommaryd in the province of Småland. In 1905 he qualified as a pharmaceutical chemist and from then on worked in several pharmacies in Gothenburg, his longest tenures being at *Svanen* (the Swan Pharmacy, 1908-23), *Enhörningen* (The Unicorn Pharmacy, 1924-32), and at his own pharmacy *Måsen* (The Gull) during the years 1932-42. One of the attributes on his book-plate is a gull. 'C D' lived unmarried with a housekeeper. His appearance was that of a cultivated and well-dressed gentleman. He was an appreciated member of the Freemasons and his gentlemen's goose dinners were held in high esteem. More famous perhaps than his pharmaceutical books was his collection of some 500 pen-and-ink drawings by the celebrated Swedish artist and author, Albert Engström, which he donated to a museum opened in 1963 in the small town of Eksjö, the home of both Engström and 'C D'. Where Matérn concentrated on pharmacopoeias, 'C D' seems to have had a more general taste, not hesitating to acquire the more expensive items, including early illustrated herbals and two incunabula. The majority of the books described in the present catalogue derives from 'C D':s collection (see list on pages 210-11). His valuable donation also includes some eighty old apothecary jars, eight of which are Chinese, bought on his 'vacation-tour' to China on the Trans-Siberian

Railway in 1926. These beautiful ceramic jars now adorn the shelves in the library and the pharmacy museum. The two colleagues, Matérn and 'C D', travelled together on the Continent, where they may also have visited antiquarian booksellers.

The works, or rather the unique copies of certain editions of more or less famous pharmaceutical books, which you will find described in the present catalogue, should not be seen as a panorama of the most significant works within the history of pharmacy. They are just a subjective selection of some of the 1200 books I have chosen to move from the open library to the Rare Book Room, in which they will with hope be taken care of adequately and responsibly for the enjoyment of coming generations. The reference works and bibliographies quoted or consulted are given for each entry, often in abbreviated form, but all the principal references are listed in full at the end of the catalogue. The arrangement of the catalogue is chronological, but all names, except for trivial ones, and a few subjects, are also found listed in alphabetical order in the *Index*, where the authors of books described in the catalogue are in bold face. There is also a list of donators and significant provenances and finally a concordance to the *Bibliotheca Walleriana*.

With this illustrated and annotated catalogue I hope to have paid a just tribute to givers and donators, and primarily to the late C.D. Carlsson and to the heirs of Ernst Matérn, whose generosity has so greatly enriched the library of the Swedish Pharmaceutical Society.

Ove Hagelin

ACKNOWLEDGEMENTS

The Swedish Pharmaceutical Society (Apotekarsocieteten) is today a non-profit organisation of people engaged in the field of medicinal drugs. The aim of the Society is to further developments in pharmaceutical research, and to promote high professional pharmaceutical standards. The Society is in actual fact one of the oldest Swedish scientific organisations still in existence: the *Apotekare Societeten* was first mentioned in 1675 as a guild, formed by the apothecaries in Stockholm. A Museum of Pharmacy has been founded on our premises in central Stockholm, the first and largest of its kind in Sweden. In addition there is an extensive library of some ten thousand volumes, covering the fields of Pharmacy, Chemistry, Medicine, and allied sciences.

This library has gradually been built up over the years through gifts and purchases of single items and whole collections; but by far the most important and valuable parts, are those donations of books brought together by knowledgeable individuals, the book collectors, who combined their profession as pharmacists with historical interests within their field. Thus the number of books has accumulated steadily during the last one hundred and fifty years. From time to time over the years, mainly during periods of re-organisation, there have been some lapses in historical interest, resulting in certain books being forgotten, only to be rediscovered later. It cannot be said, however, that the books in our library have really been neglected – they have always rested in the hands of librarians, and people dedicated to the history of pharmacy – but to the uninitiated, the treasure has been virtually unknown.

During the 1980s the library and its books became a subject for lenghty discussions within the Society. Representatives for the History of Pharmacy Section and my predecessor, Lars-Einar Fryklöf, advocated a re-appraisal of our old book collection. In connection with the restoration of our premises in 1992 it was decided to reorganise, catalogue, and document the contents of the library. Ove Hagelin was contacted and later contracted to carry out this task. The major part of about 6500 volumes was sorted out and put in order, and from this portion some 1200 of the most valuable books were put aside to form a historical section, now preserved in a secure Rare Book Room. These old and rare books have all been collated and properly catalogued in a hand-written *Catalogus Librorum Rariorum*. Two hundred of these books are further fully described with bibliographical and historical commentaries. This task having been accomplished, it was a natural decision to ask Ove Hagelin to produce another of his distinctive *Illustrated and Annotated Catalogues of Rare Medical Books*, the fifth in the series.

It is with great pleasure that the Swedish Pharmaceutical Society now presents the fruits of the labour of the experienced and dedicated medical book expert, Ove Hagelin. In my opinion, his presentation of a choice selection from our library is of sterling quality. It is a beautiful piece of work, which, in these times of cyber-space and individualised mass communication, brings back to life the skills of old craftsmen and the splendour of bygone days. While leafing through the pages, one cannot fail to revere our predecessors, and especially those book collecting donators, for their legacy, which emphasises our responsibility to future generations.

This is a reason as good as any to present our catalogue, which we hope will prove a valuable bibliographical reference work, and a useful guide through the mysterious paths of the older literature on *Materia Medica*.

Björn Lindeke, Executive Director,
Swedish Pharmaceutical Society
Swedish Academy of Pharmaceutical Sciences

'. . . Many highly learned philosophers who lay snares for our art will be greatly displeased that a work is now appearing which contains a great many truths hitherto kept secret . . .'

Philipp Ulstad's Dedication to the noble Felix in *Coelum Philosophorum* (Heaven of the Philosophers) written in 1525 (English translation).

The fountainhead of all European herbals

DIOSCORIDES, Pedianos (1st century A.D.)

P. Dioscoridæ Pharmacorum Simplicium, reiq[ue] Medicæ libri VIII. Io. Ruellio interprete. Una cum Herm. Barbari Corollariis, & Marc. Vergilii, in singula Capita ce[n]suris, sive Annotationibus. Adiecto Indice duplici singuloru[m] Simplicium, & difficilium terminorum. Strassburg [Argentorati], Johann Schott, 1529.

Folio – leaf: 300 x 200 mm. 378 leaves: ff. [4], *361,* [13]. *Title printed in red and black, woodcut border with animals and plants. Fine woodcut initials to each of the eight Books. Early 19th century leather-backed marbled boards, new endpapers.*

Book-plate: C.D. Carlsson.

This edition of Dioscorides was edited by Otto Brunfels under the title *Pharmacorum Simplicium* and was published and printed by Johann Schott in Strassburg, who in the following year brought out the first volume of Brunfels' *Herbarum vivae eicones*, the first herbal with 'Living Portraits of Plants'. Brunfels' edition of Dioscorides includes the *De materia medica* (Books I–V), the *De venenis* (Book VI), and the *De venenatis animalibus* (here divided into three chapters, called Books VII–IX in the caption and running titles). The Latin translation is that of Jean de la Ruel (1474–1537) which was first printed in Paris by Henri Estienne in 1516. To each plant is added the *Corollarium Dioscorides* by Ermelao Barbaro (1454–1493), written before 1489 but not published until twenty years after his death in the form of a supplement to Barbaro's Latin version of Dioscorides (Venice, 1516). It also has the annotations by Marcello Virgilio Adriani (1464–1521), whose long Latin version of Dioscorides (1518) had extensive commentaries on the medicinal and other uses of the plants taken chiefly from older physicians and pharmacists.

The modern science of pharmacology can be traced back to Dioscorides' efforts to systematize man's knowledge of the materials of medicine. His only surviving work is the *De materia medica*, known to all botanists and physicians, and the fountainhead of all European herbals.

Of Dioscorides himself very little is known. He flourished about 60 A.D., at which time it is likely that he wrote the *De materia medica,* dedicated to his friend and fellow physician, Areius. He may have served as physician to Nero's armies, or those of Caligula or Claudius. The name by which he was known to his contemporaries was, Pedanus Dioscorides of Anazarbus, a small town near Tarsus in Cilicia (southern Turkey). His native language, in which his books were written, was Greek. The Greek text of the *De materia medica* was translated into Syriac when pagan Greek scholars fled eastward after Constantine's conquest of Byzantium. Later it was translated into Arabic and Persian, and became an important element in the medical knowledge of the Moslem world. In the West it was translated into Latin where it survived until the Renaissance in various forms.

The original Greek manuscript is no longer extant. The oldest known manuscript is of 512 A.D., now preserved in the Austrian National Library in Vienna. It was discovered in Turkey in 1562 by a Flemish antiquarian, Ogier Busbecq, Ambassador of the Holy Roman Empire. The manuscript was then in the possession of the son of Hamon, former physician to the sultan Suleiman the Great, who wanted 100 ducats for it. The sum was paid and in 1569 it entered Vienna and the library of Emperor Maximilian.

The first Latin edition was printed in 1478 at Colle, Tuscany, Italy. The first Greek edition was printed by Aldus Manutius in Venice, in July, 1499. The first illustrated edition was that printed and published by Christian Egenolph in 1543, illustrated with 595 woodcuts. Some thirty editions were published before Mattioli's translation and commentary in the mid-1550s, which became a classic in its own right, running through at least sixty editions.

Durling, 1144; Wellcome, 1783; Greene/Egerton, vol. II, pp. 598-657 (Ruel), pp. 553-68 (Barbaro), pp. 569-83 (Marcello); Anderson, pp. 7-15; Stillwell, 354; Waller 2486.

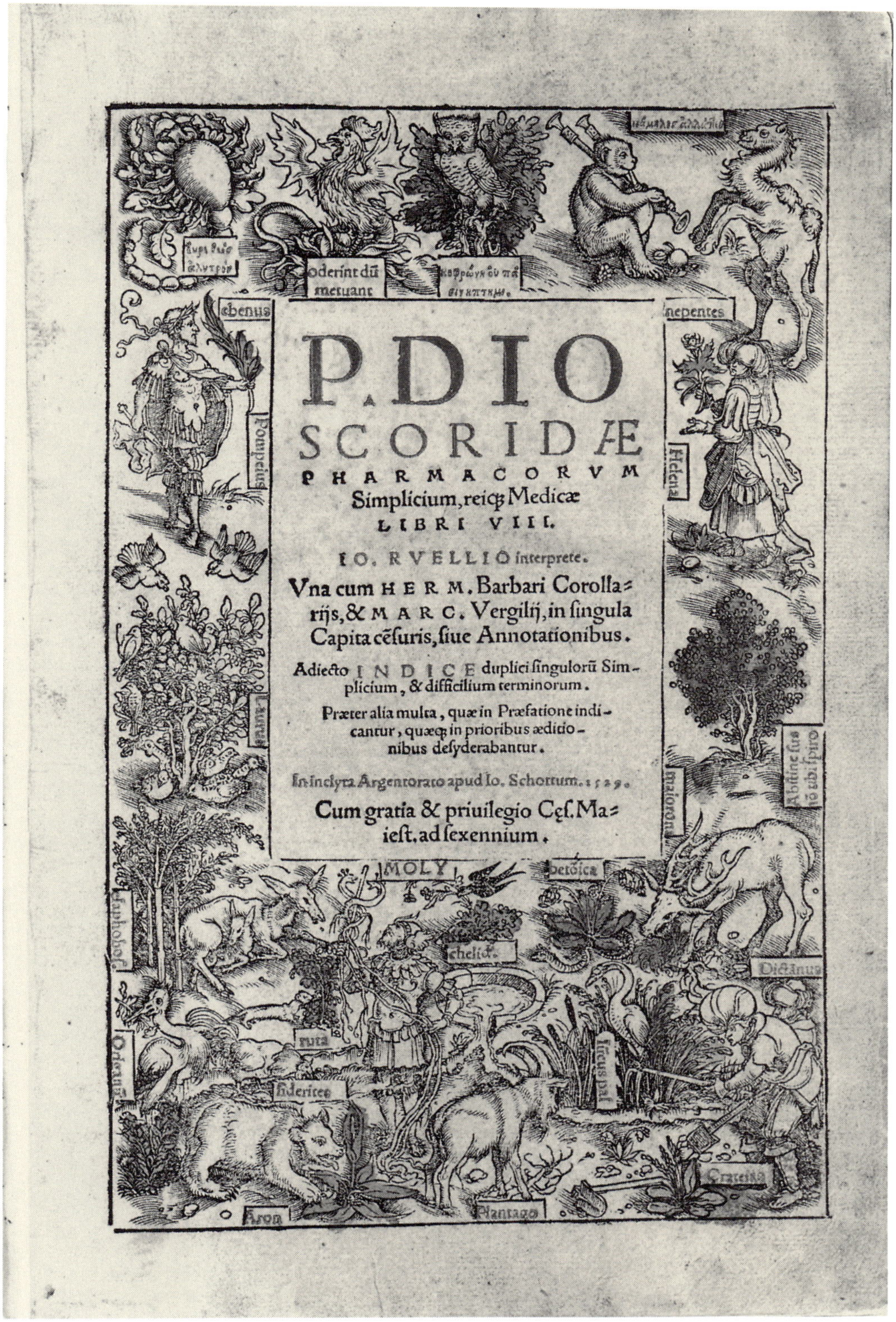

P. DIO
SCORIDÆ
PHARMACORVM
Simplicium, reiq; Medicæ
LIBRI VIII.

IO. RVELLIO interprete.

Vna cum HERM. Barbari Corolla-
rijs, & MARC. Vergilij, in singula
Capita cẽsuris, siue Annotationibus.

Adiecto INDICE duplici singulorũ Sim-
plicium, & difficilium terminorum.

Præter alia multa, quæ in Præfatione indi-
cantur, quæq; in prioribus æditio-
nibus desyderabantur.

In inclyta Argentorato apud Io. Schottum. 1529.

Cum gratia & priuilegio Cæs. Ma-
iest. ad sexennium.

The title page of this esteemed edition of Dioscorides, printed in red and black, has a beautiful woodcut border by Hans Weiditz, who also made the fine pictorial initials to the chapters with scenes from the Bible.

The pharmacological quintessence of Arabian therapeutics

MESUE, the Younger, or Pseudo-Mesue (c.926–1016)

[*Title on* a1]: Textus Mesue noviter Emendatus. [Canones universalis. De simplicibus. Grabadin. Grabadin medicinarum particularium. Petri Apponi medici clarissimi in librum Joannis Mesue additio.] Venice, Jacopo Pencio, 1505.

Octavo – *leaf*: 155 x 105 *mm.* 352 *unnumbered leaves. Sign.*: a-z⁸ (aa)-(cc)⁸ A-C⁸. *Woodcut initials, white on black, guide letters in spaces left for other initials. Modern half vellum, gilt lettering on spine. Copious manuscript annotations in the margins by a contemporary hand.*

From the C.D. Carlsson Collection.

A rare early edition, perhaps the first octavo edition, of the works of Mesue the Younger, Masawaih al-Mardini, supposed to have been a Jacobite Christian from Maradin in Upper Mesopotamia who lived in the 10th century. At the end is added the supplement to Mesue's *Grabadin* by Pietro d'Abano (c.1250–c.1316), with remedies for cardiac and digestive troubles.

Mesue the Younger is not to be confused with Mesue the Elder, Yuhanna ibn Masawaih (c.777–857), an outstanding physician in Bagdad, also called Johannes Damascenus (of Damascus). No Arabic manuscripts of the works of Mesue the Younger have ever been found. Indeed his very existence is doubtful and rests solely on the statements of Leo Africanus. Many think the name was assumed by some Latin compiler of the 13th century who sought recognition for his work by giving it an authority borrowed from a long-dead Arab physician. This indicates the profound and enduring influence of Arab medicine and pharmacy and the high esteem in which Arab contributions were held. A Latin edition of the works of Mesue the Younger was one of the first medical books to be printed (Venice, 1471) and passed through more than thirty editions up to 1581. It was for centuries the authority on the composition of medicaments. The book was not only in use in practically every European pharmacy but also became the basis of the later official pharmacopoeias. The *Grabadin* is, as Sudhoff calls it, 'the pharmacological quintessence of Arabian therapeutics' and contains the entire armamentarium of compounded medicines which we owe to Arabians.

The *De simplicibus* is concerned with the use of purgatives and discusses the characteristics of the numerous purges then in use. The purges are categorized as gentle (tamarinds, figs, prunes, cassia), mild (wormwood, senna, aloes, rhubarb), and drastic, (jalap, scammony, colocynth). The *Grabadin*, from the Arabic term for a formulary, 'aqrabadhin', represents an apothecary's manual, which for centuries remained the standard textbook of pharmacy in the West. The *Liber medicinarium particularum* is a manual of special therapeutics. It remained incomplete, containing only the diseases of the head and chest, breaking off with the treatment of heart diseases.

In our library is also a folio edition of Mesue's works, *Opera de medicamentorum* (Venice, 1589) edited by Giovanni Costeo with commentaries by Mundinus, Christoph de Honestis, Johannes Manardus and Jacob Sylvius. It also has a number of supplementary writings: the *Additio* of Mesue's *Grabadin* by Pietro d'Abano and the *Complementum* to *Grabadin* by Francesco di Piedimonte (d.1319), one of the most complete compendia of practical medicine of the Middle Ages. It also has the *Antidotarium* of Nicolas of Salerno (Nicolaus Praepositos) with the *Glossa* of Joannes Platearius, followed by Joannes de Sancto Amando's *Expositio super Antidotarium Nicolai* (of Salerno), Gentili da Foligno's (d.1348) *De medicinarum solventium compositarum dosi brevi,* the *Liber servitoris liber* XXVII by Abu-l-Quasim Benaberazerin, translated by Simon of Genoa and Abraham ben Shem-ton (Abraham the Jew of Tortosa), and the *Compendium aromaticorum* by Saladino de Asculo, written in the mid-15th century, the first real treatise on pharmacy in a modern sense. In it he treats not only of the kind of examination to which pharmacists should be subjected, but also of all the medicaments described in the famous *Antidotarium* of Nicolas of Salerno. Saladino writes on the weights and the dosage of the drugs, on the way in which the remedy should be prepared, on the plants, flowers, roots, and the way of preserving simples and compounds, and finally gives details for conducting a pharmacy.

Choulant, pp. 351-8 (not listing this edition); Garrison, p. 133; Kremers & Urdang, pp. 21-2; Sarton, I, p. 728; Cowen & Helfand, p. 68; Frank J. Anderson, pp. 36-40; Waller 6523/4 (other eds.).

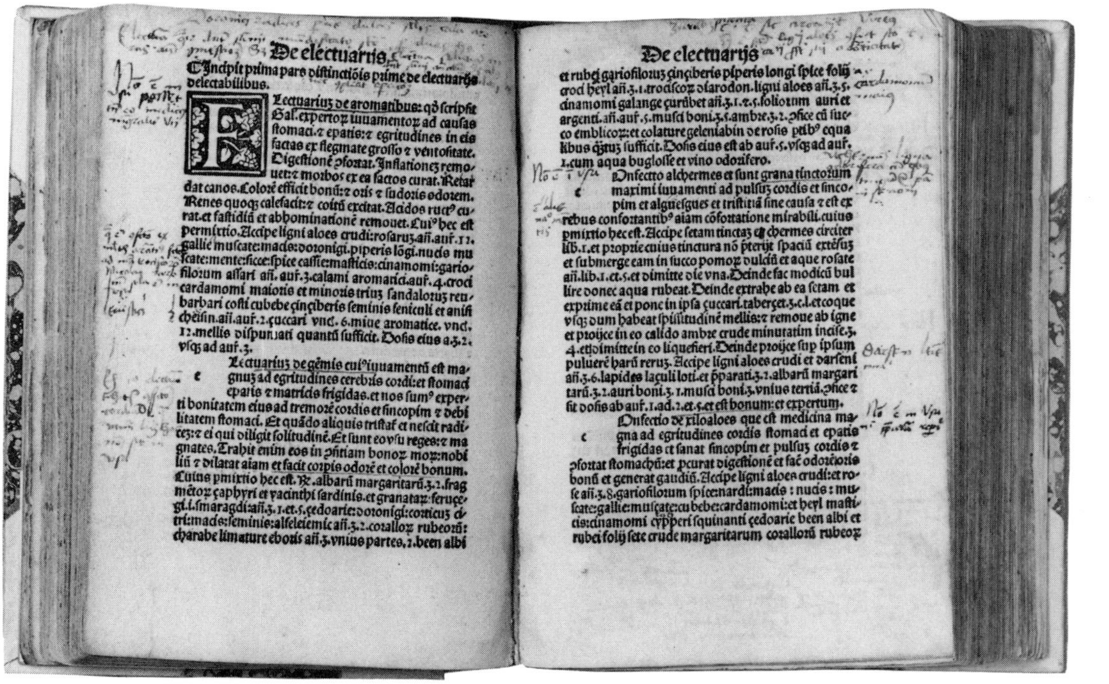
De electuarijs
De electuarijs

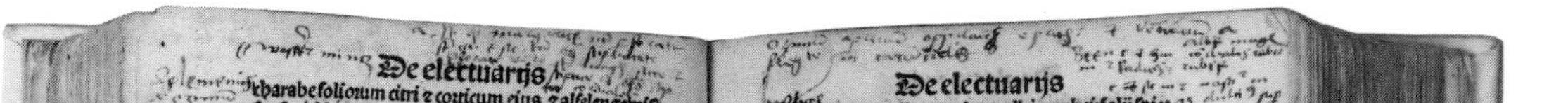
De electuarijs
De electuarijs

Six important medieval pharmacological texts

SERAPION and other writers of the Middle Ages.

Practica Joannis Serapionis aliter breviarium nuncupata. Liber Serap.[ione] de simpli. medi. sumta a plantis . . . Liber Galeni ad Papiam de virtute centauree. Pra.[ctica] Jo. Plateraii . . . liber de simplici medi. eiusdem Plateárii vulgariter circa instans dictus. Thesaurus pauperum ab Jo.[anne] xx. Pon. Max. qui ante Petrus Hispanus . . Cum tabula . . . recenter addita.

Lyon, Jacob [Jacques] Myt, 1525.

Quarto – *leaf:* 250 *x* 180 *mm.* 270 *leaves, numbered* 272 *as two leaves* [03 *and* 04] *are numbered on both recto and verso. Title printed in red and black, fine woodcut border with cherubs and portraits of Serapion, Platearius and Peter Hispanus. Endpapers and blank leaves full of notes by an early owner and pharmaceutical marginalia throughout. Contemporary half-binding, blindstamped pigskin over oak tree covers, two brass clasps. Old and new title labels on the spine.*

Verso of the title with inscription: Foruli Matthaei Stengeli me occupent.
From the Ernst Matérn Collection, *with his book-plate.*

This book is an assembly of six important herbals and pharmacological texts of the Middle Ages including the *Circa instans*, a fundamental work of Western science and the prototype of the modern pharmacopoeia, the *Liber de simplicia* by the spurious Serapion the Younger, and 'The Treasure of the Poor' by Peter of Spain. This early edition is printed in double columns with the *Incipit* (the opening words of a text) for each work printed in red. The beautiful title page is reproduced in Frank J. Anderson, *An Illustrated History of Herbals* (1977) from which most of the commentaries below are quoted and compiled:

I. **SERAPION the Elder**. *Practica sive breviarum.* Fol. 2-112. Serapion the Elder flourished in Damascus in the second half of the 9th century. He wrote two medical encyclopedias, one in twelve books, the other in seven books. The latter one, *Practica sive breviarum,* originally written in Syriac, was translated into Latin by Gerhard of Cremona in the 12th century and had a great influence upon medicine in the the West. The last book deals with antidotes.

II. **SERAPION the Younger.** *Liber de simplicia medicina.* Fol. 113-201. There is considerable doubt about the authorship of this work. The text is often published together with Serapion the Elder, which is why the two are often confused. No Arabic manuscript of his has ever been found, and no writer in any language speaks of him until the time of the translator, Simon of Genoa (13th century), who in his writings claims to have used many manuscripts now lost to the modern world. 'No matter who wrote it, the book did much to spread the advanced medical knowledge of the Arabs throughout Europe. In addition to Greek and Arab sources, it quoted Persian and Indian ones as well. In popularity it surpassed all other Arabic works, including that of the formidable Avicenna . . . Serapion is cited 976 times in the *Herbarius latinus, Gart der Gesundheit*, and the *Hortus Sanitatis*, three of the major early herbals. But despite its popularity, only three editions of Serapion were printed in the incunabula period' (Frank J. Anderson). The first edition appeared in 1473. Serapion's work was usually printed in combination with other pharmaceutical works and herbals, such as in this Lyon edition of 1525. (Sarton, I, p. 608)

III. **GALEN.** *De virtute centaureae.* Fol. 201-02. A pseudo-Galenic tract, known only in this Latin version of Nicholas Rheginus. (Durling, 4776).

IV. **JOANNES PLATEARIUS.** *Practica brevis.* Fol. 203-22. Platearius the Younger was a master of the Golden Period of the Salerno Medical School. He wrote a treatise on urology and this medical compendium, *Practica brevis*, which was first published in 1488 at Ferrara.

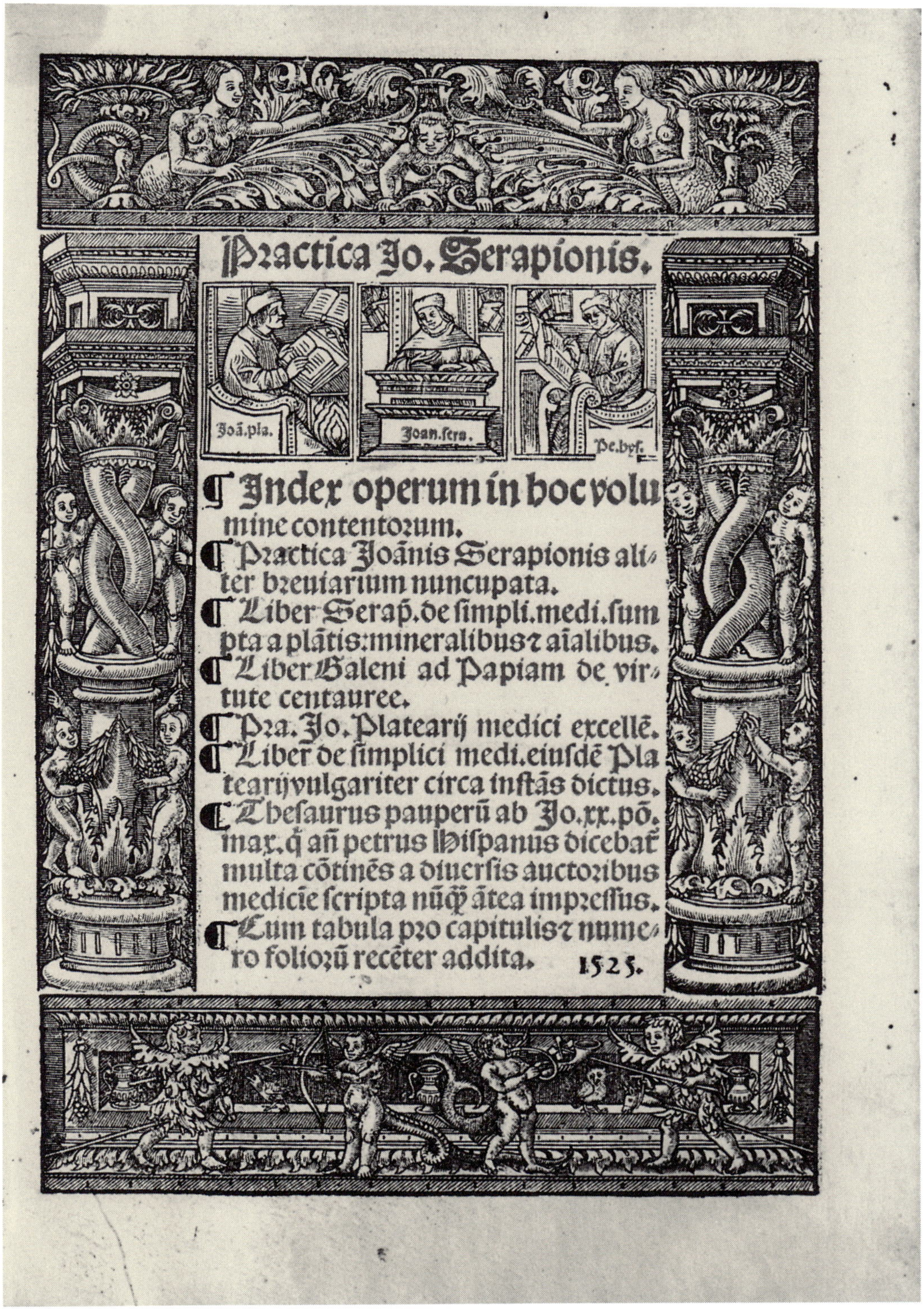
Practica Jo. Serapionis.

¶ Index operum in hoc volumine contentorum.
¶ Practica Joãnis Serapionis aliter breuiarium nuncupata.
¶ Liber Serap. de simpli. medi. sumpta a plãtis: mineralibus & aĩalibus.
¶ Liber Galeni ad Papiam de virtute centauree.
¶ Pra. Jo. Platearij medici excellẽ.
¶ Liber de simplici medi. eiusdẽ Platearij vulgariter circa instãs dictus.
¶ Thesaurus pauperũ ab Jo. xx. põ. max. q̃ añ petrus Hispanus dicebat multa cõtinẽs a diuersis auctoribus medicie scripta nũq̃ ãtea impressus.
¶ Cum tabula pro capitulis & numero foliorũ recẽter addita. 1525.

Title page, printed in red and black, to Serapion's *Practica*, issued together with five other medieval pharmacological texts including Platearius' *Circa instans* (Lyon, 1525).

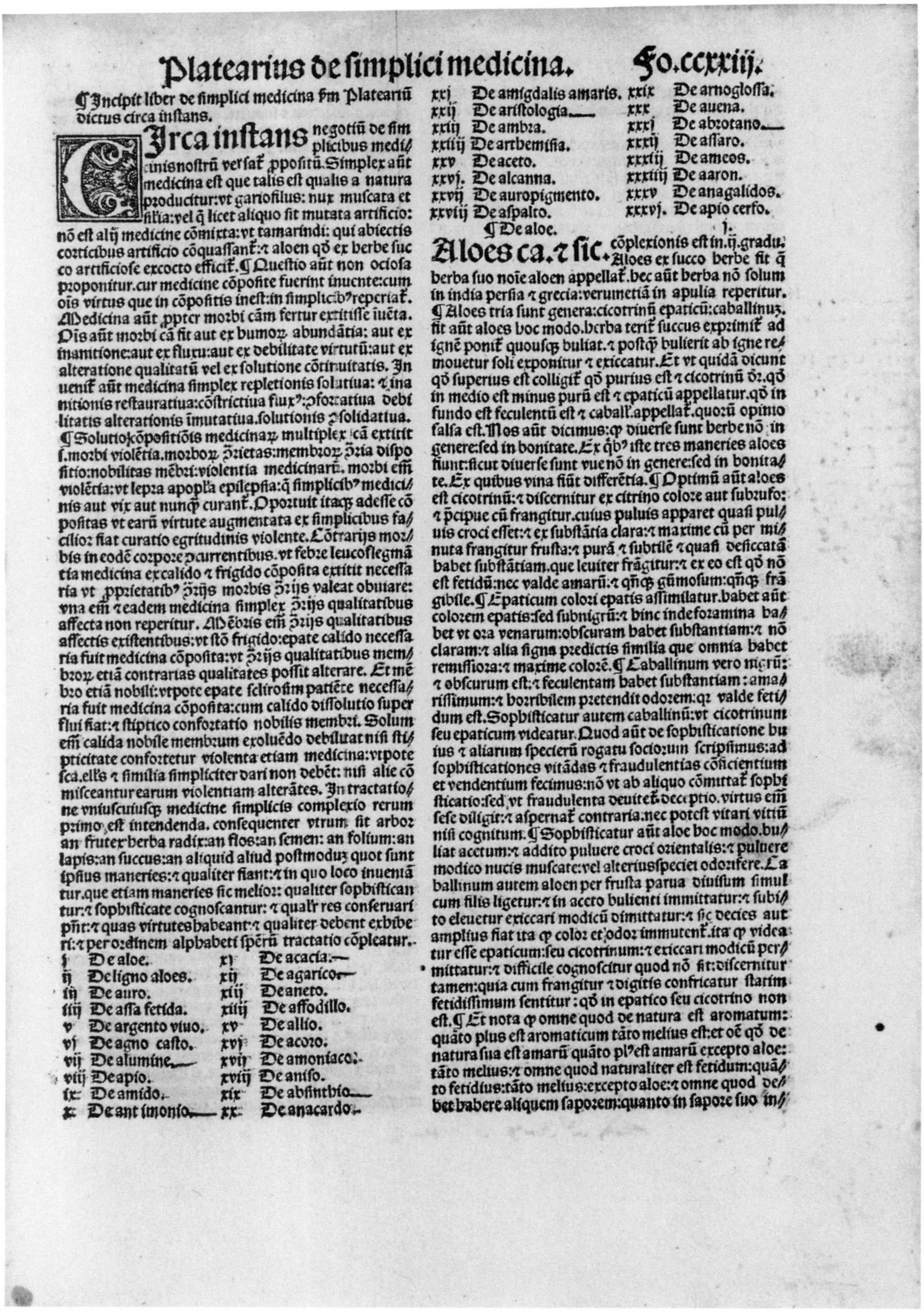

Platearius de simplici medicina. Fo.ccxxiij.

¶ Incipit liber de simplici medicina s'm Plateariū dictus circa instans.

Circa instans negotiū de simplicibus medicinis nostrū versat' ppositū. Simplex aūt medicina est que talis est qualis a natura producitur: vt gariofilus: nux muscata et silia: vel q̄ licet aliquo sit mutata artificio: nō est aliis medicine cōmixta: vt tamarindi: qui abiectis corticibus artificio cōquassant': ⁊ aloen qđ ex herbe succo artificiose excocto efficit'. ¶ Questio aūt non ociosa proponitur. cur medicine cōposite fuerint inuente: cum oīs virtus que in cōpositis inest: in simplicib' reperiat'. Medicina aūt pp̄ter morbi cām fertur extitisse inuēta. Vis aūt morbi cā fit aut ex humor abundātia: aut ex inanitione: aut ex fluxu: aut ex debilitate virtutū: aut ex alteratione qualitatū vel ex solutione cōtinuitatis. Inuenit' aūt medicina simplex repletionis solutiua: ⁊ inanitionis restauratiua: cōstrictiua flux': confortatiua debilitatis alterationis imutatiua. solutionis cōsolidatiua. ¶ Solutio cōpositiōis medicinar multiplex cā extitit s. morbi violētia. morbor cōtrietas: membror cōtria dispositio: nobilitas mēbri: violentia medicinarū. morbi eīm violētia: vt lepra apoplīa epilepsia: q̄ simplicib' medicinis aut vix aut nunq̄ curant'. Oportuit itaq̄ adesse cōpositas vt earū virtute augmentata ex simplicibus facilior fiat curatio egritudinis violente. Cōtrarijs morbis in eodē corpore cōcurrentibus. vt febre leucoflegmātia medicina ex calido ⁊ frigido cōposita extitit necessaria vt pprietatib' cōtrarijs morbis cōtrijs valeat obuiare: vna eīm ⁊ eadem medicina simplex cōtrarijs qualitatibus affecta non reperitur. Mēbris eīm cōtrarijs qualitatibus affectis existentibus: vt stō frigido: epate calido necessaria fuit medicina cōposita: vt cōtrarijs qualitatibus membror etiā contrarias qualitates possit alterare. Et mēbro etiā nobili: vtpote epate sclirosim patiēte necessaria fuit medicina cōposita: cum calido dissolutio superflui fiat: ⁊ stiptico confortatio nobilis membri. Solum eīm calida nobile membrum exoluēdo debilitat nisi stipticitate confortetur violenta etiam medicina: vtpote sca. ell's ⁊ similia simpliciter dari non debēt: nisi alie cō misceantur earum violentiam alterātes. In tractatione vniuscuiusq̄ medicine simplicis complexio rerum primo est intendenda. consequenter vtrum sit arbor an frutex herba radix: an flos: an semen: an folium: an lapis: an succus: an aliquid aliud postmoduz quot sunt ipsius maneries: ⁊ qualiter fiant: ⁊ in quo loco inuentatur. que etiam maneries sic melior: qualiter sophisticantur: ⁊ sophisticate cognoscantur: ⁊ qual'r res conseruari pn̄t: ⁊ quas virtutes habeant: ⁊ qualiter debent exhiberi: ⁊ per ordinem alphabeti sperū tractatio cōpleatur.

j	De aloe.	xj	De acacia.
ij	De ligno aloes.	xij	De agarico.
iij	De auro.	xiij	De aneto.
iiij	De assa fetida.	xiiij	De affodillo.
v	De argento viuo.	xv	De allio.
vj	De agno casto.	xvj	De acoro.
vij	De alumine.	xvij	De amoniaco.
viij	De apio.	xviij	De aniso.
ix	De amido.	xix	De absinthio.
x	De ant imonio.	xx	De anacardo.
xxj	De amigdalis amaris.	xxix	De arnoglossa.
xxij	De aristologia.	xxx	De auena.
xxiij	De ambra.	xxxj	De abrotano.
xxiiij	De arthemisia.	xxxij	De assaro.
xxv	De aceto.	xxxiij	De ameos.
xxvj	De alcanna.	xxxiiij	De aaron.
xxvij	De auropigmento.	xxxv	De anagalidos.
xxviij	De aspalto.	xxxvj	De apio cerfo.

¶ De aloe. j.

Aloes ca. ⁊ sic. cōplexionis est in .ij. gradu. Aloes ex succo herbe fit q̄ herba suo noīe aloen appellat'. hec aūt herba nō solum in india persia ⁊ grecia: verumetiā in apulia reperitur. ¶ Aloes tria sunt genera: cicotrinū epaticū: caballinuz. fit aūt aloes hoc modo. herba terit' succus exprimit' ad ignē ponit' quousq̄ bulliat. ⁊ postq̄ bullierit ab igne remouetur soli exponitur ⁊ exiccatur. Et vt quidā dicunt qđ superius est colligit' qđ purius est ⁊ cicotrinū dr. qđ in medio est minus purū est ⁊ epaticū appellatur. qđ in fundo est feculentū est ⁊ caball'. appellat'. quorū opinio falsa est. Nos aūt dicimus: q̄ diuerse sunt herbe nō in genere: sed in bonitate. Ex qb' iste tres maneries aloes fiunt: sicut diuerse sunt vue nō in genere: sed in bonitate. Ex quibus vina fiūt differētia. ¶ Optimū aūt aloes est cicotrinū: ⁊ discernitur ex citrino colore aut subrufo: ⁊ pcipue cū frangitur. cuius puluis apparet quasi puluis croci esset: ⁊ ex substātia clara: ⁊ maxime cū per minuta frangitur frusta: ⁊ purā ⁊ subtilē ⁊ quasi desiccatā habet substātiam. que leuiter frāgitur: ⁊ ex eo est qđ nō est fetidū: nec valde amarū: ⁊ q̄uis gūmosum: q̄nq̄ frāgibile. ¶ Epaticum colori epatis assimilatur. habet aūt colorem epatis: sed subnigrū: ⁊ hinc inde foramina habet vt ora venarum: obscuram habet substantiam: ⁊ nō claram: ⁊ alia signa predictis similia que omnia habet remissiora: ⁊ maxime colorē. ¶ Caballinum vero nigrū: ⁊ obscurum est: ⁊ feculentam habet substantiam: amarissimum: ⁊ horribilem pretendit odorem: qr valde fetidum est. Sophisticatur autem caballinū: vt cicotrinum seu epaticum videatur. Quod aūt de sophisticatione huius ⁊ aliarum specierū rogatu sociorum scripsimus: ad sophisticationes vitādas ⁊ fraudulentias cōficientium et vendentium fecimus: nō vt ab aliquo cōmittat' sophisticatio: sed vt fraudulenta deuitet'. deceptio. virtus eīm sese diligit: ⁊ aspernat' contraria: nec potest vitari vitiū nisi cognitum. ¶ Sophisticatur aūt aloe hoc modo. bulliat acetum: ⁊ addito puluere croci orientalis: ⁊ puluere modico nucis muscate: vel alterius speciei odorifere. Caballinum autem aloen per frusta parua diuisum simul cum filis ligetur: ⁊ in aceto bulienti immittatur: ⁊ subito eleuetur exiccari modicū dimittatur: ⁊ sic decies aut amplius fiat ita q̄ color et odor immutent'. ita q̄ videatur esse epaticum: seu cicotrinum: ⁊ exiccari modicū permittatur: ⁊ difficile cognoscitur quod nō sit: discernitur tamen: quia cum frangitur ⁊ digitis confricatur statim fetidissimum sentitur: qđ in epatico seu cicotrino non est. ¶ Et nota q̄ omne quod de natura est aromatum: quāto plus est aromaticum tāto melius est: et oē qđ de natura sua est amarū quāto pl' est amarū excepto aloe: tāto melius: ⁊ omne quod naturaliter est fetidum: quāto fetidius: tāto melius: excepto aloe: ⁊ omne quod debet habere aliquem saporem: quanto in sapore suo in

Matthaeus Platearius' *Circa Instans* (the two opening words of the book), is the prototype of the modern Western pharmacopoeia. The first printed edition appeared in Venice, 1497, issued together with Serapion's *Practica*, as in the present edition of 1525. Manuscripts of the *Circa instans* are rare. The earliest surviving illustrated manuscript of this text is in the British Library.

V. **MATTHAEUS PLATEARIUS.** *Circa instans* [*De simplici medicina*]. Fol. 223-52. The *Liber de simplici medicina*, commonly called the *Circa instans*, the two opening words of the book, was very widely distributed and translated into most European languages. It is the prototype of the modern pharmacopoeia, the first attempt to establish nomenclature standards, and the first effort by medieval physicians to create a work that did not echo the past. Although essentially a collective work of the School of Salerno, the leading medical centre of the early Middle Ages, it is attributed by most medical historians to Matthaeus Platearius, one of the School's foremost teaching physicians, who was born at the end of the 11th century and died in 1161. Although the *Circa instans* had been of prime importance until the beginning of the 15th century, its appeal waned with the appearance of the comprehensive printed herbals. They cited it frequently, and may thus have delayed a separate printing. (Frank J. Anderson)

The *Circa instans* has 273 chapters or articles. Each chapter deals with a simple or other drug, and they are arranged in alphabetical order of their Latin names. For each drug we are offered the following information: description, action, mode of application, signs of purity, falsifications, distinctions of various kind. The *Circa instans* is especially important from the botanical point of view. For example, of the 273 chapters, 229 treat of medicinal plants. It marked a progress over Dioscorides and other herbals. During the 13th and 14th centuries it gradually superseded the *Herbarius* ascribed to Apuleius (the first printed illustrated herbal, Rome, c.1481-84), and it became one of the prototypes of our Western pharmacopoeias. (Sarton, II, p. 241).

Garrison & Morton, 1790, list a later edition of *Circa instans* of 1537, in Nicolaus Praepositis *Dispensarium* and call it the first French herbal.

VI. **PETRUS HISPANUS.** *Thesaurus Pauperum.* Fol. 253-72. 'Petrus Hispanus, who finally became Pope John XXI, was born in the early thirteenth century. He studied at the University of Paris at an early age. He was an all-round scholar and specialist in medicine. Pope Gregory X made Peter a cardinal in 1273. He was also an archbishop, and in 1276 the career of the celebrated scholar culminated in his election to the papal see following Gregory's death. The next year Peter met an untimely death from the fall of a ceiling, a catastrophe which according to the gossip of Ptolemy of Lucca occured while he was engaged in a fit of complacent and self-admiring laughter and shortly after he had issued some fulminations against the monks, for whom he had little love. His *Thesaurus pauperum* became perhaps the leading brief medical manual during the remainder of the Middle Ages, as a numerous extant manuscripts and many printed editions bear witness. The work was intended to be a condensed compilation and its title, "The Treasure of the Poor", indicates that it was written especially for the benefit of poor students and medical practitioners, who could not afford many books' (Thorndike).

Among his authorities Peter makes much use of recent works and writers, such as Platearius and the *Antidotarium* of Nicolaus. From Thorndike, who devotes a whole chapter to Petrus Hispanus, we will quote some remedies: 'For toothache is recommended touching the ailing tooth with one from a corpse, holding in the mouth violets cooked in wine, holding a grain of opium between the teeth. Other remedies are vinegar in which a root of jusquiam has been boiled, deer horn burnt until it whitens and dries, and a powder made from dogs' teeth. Cavities may be filled with the brain of a partridge or crow's dung. The latter "breaks the tooth and removes pain". Much use is made of parts of animals. Less nauseating examples are, among many similar parts of animals prescribed for epileptics, the liver of a vulture drunk with its blood for nine days, or the gall still warm from a dog who should have been killed the moment the epileptic fell in the fit . . . Under the caption of remedies for witchcraft and possession by demons are found such procedures as smearing the walls of the house with the blood of a black dog or burying a reed filled with quicksilver under the threshold. A recipe to rescue a patient from infatuation in love produced by sorcery is hardly translatable, . . . It is also stated that wearing the heart of a vulture makes one popular with all men and very wealthy, and that by vivisecting the bird hoopoe and eating its still palpitating heart one may learn the future and all secrets concealed in men's minds' (Thorndike).

Thorndike, II, pp. 488-513; (Petrus Hispanus); Frank J. Anderson, pp. 40-4 (Serapion the Younger), pp. 45-50 (*Circa instans*); Sarton, II, p. 229 (Serapion the Younger), p. 241 (Matthaeus Platearius); Durling 4776; Wellcome 5933; Waller 8868 (Venice, 1530)

The most important materia medica of the Greek Middle Ages

NICOLAUS MYREPSUS (fl. in the 13th century)

Nicolai Myrepsi Alexandrini medicamentorum opus, in sectiones quadraginta octo digestum, hactenus in Germania non visum, omnibus tum Medicis, tum Seplasiarijs mirum in modum utile, à Leonharto Fuchsio . . . Annotationibus illustratum.

Lyon, Balthazar Arnoullet, 1550.

Octavo – *leaf*: 172 *x* 105 *mm. Pp.* [24], 712, [8]. *Contemporary half-binding, blind-stamped pigskin with figures of Justicia, Caritas and Spes, over oak boards, spine with three double bands, two brass clasps.*

Provenance: Christoph Wenzel Graf von Nostitz (1643–1712) *with his signature on the title page. From the* C.D. Carlsson Collection.

This is the octavo edition of Leonhart Fuchs' annotated translation of a Greek manuscript containing an extensive collection of pharmaceutical recipes. It was originally compiled in the late of the 13th or early 14th century by Nicolaus Myrepsus. Fuchs' Latin edition was first published in 1549, a folio printed by Oporinus in Basel, which was followed in the same year by an octavo edition, published by Arnoullet in Lyon, reprinted in 1550.

There has been much confusion as to the mutual relations and the chronology of the pharmacological works ascribed to writers bearing the name of Nicolaus: the anonymous *Antidotarium magnum*, written about 1100, the *Antidotarium Nicolai* (of Salerno), written in the middle of the 13th century, the *Dynameron* [Δυναμερον] by Nicolaus Myrepsus in the early 14th century, and the *Dispensatorium ad aromatarios* by Nicolaus Praepositii (Nicole Prévost) written about 1480.

According to Sarton, Nicolaus Myrepsus (*myrepsus* means 'ointment maker') was a Byzantine physician who flourished at the court of Emperor Johannes III (1222–1254) at Nicaea. He is said to have travelled extensively and may have paid a visit to the old school of medicine at Salerno, and is there to have become acquainted with the *Antidotarium* of Nicolaus. He compiled a large collection of pharmaceutical recipes called *Dynameron* (in Greek), which was completed toward the end of his life. Compared to the c.150 recipes in *Antidotarium Nicolai*, it contains no less than 2656 remedies for all kinds of diseases, classified into 48 groups according to their medical properties. His work was the largest strictly pharmacological work that had as yet appeared, more comprehensive even than any modern pharmacopoeia. Sarton states that the *Dynameron* of Nicolaus Myrespus is the most important medico-botanical work of the Greek Middle Ages. It was largely derived from the Salernian antidotary, but also from Arabic sources, with many mentions of musk, ambergris, camphor and senna. It enjoyed considerable popularity and became a sort of standard book. An abridged Latin translation served as required reading for every master apothecary in Paris up to the middle of the sixteenth century.

The recipes include many superstitious practices and there are also formulas of supposedly religious origin. One of these was for a preparation called the 'Salt of the Holy Apostles', which, when taken morning and evening with meals, would preserve the sense of sight, prevent hair loss, relieve difficulty of breathing, and keep the breath sweet, thus being the first recorded remedy for halitosis. It consisted of a mixture of aromatic herbs ground up with common salt. Another interesting formula was a preparation under the title of *antidotus acharistos*, 'which, literally translated, means "the antidote for which no thanks are given". This title seems to have been bestowed because it cured sufferers so quickly that they did not appreciate how ill they might have been without it and were not sufficiently grateful to the giver' (LaWall).

Leonhart Fuchs, famous for his great herbal, was also the translator of medical texts. When he got hold of the Greek manuscript of Myrepsus he thought he had found the Greek original, from which the very essence of the *Antidotarium Nicolai Praepositus* was derived. It is a tragicomical fate that Fuchs came to translate a Greek text that was largerly derived from the Salernian antidotary and from Arabic sources.

Stübler, Leonhart Fuchs, pp. 183-7; Alfons Lutz, 'Das Dynameron des sog. Nikolaos Myrepsos und das Antidotarium Nicolai' pp. 57-73, in *Veröffentl. d. Intern. Gesellschaft f. Geschichte d. Pharmazie.* N.F., Band 21, Teil 1 (1963); Sarton, *Introduction,* II, pp. 50-1, 1094-5; LaWall, pp. 146-7; Ferguson, II, 123; F.K. Held, *Nicolaus Salernitanus und Nicolaus Myrepsos* (1916), a diss. calling into question Myrepsos' very existence; H. Lehmann, 'Zu Nicolaus Myrepsus', in *Arch. f. Geschichte d. Medizin,* vol. 17 (1925), pp. 299-306, stating that there was but one Nicolaus, he of Salerno, and even this is not entirely certain.

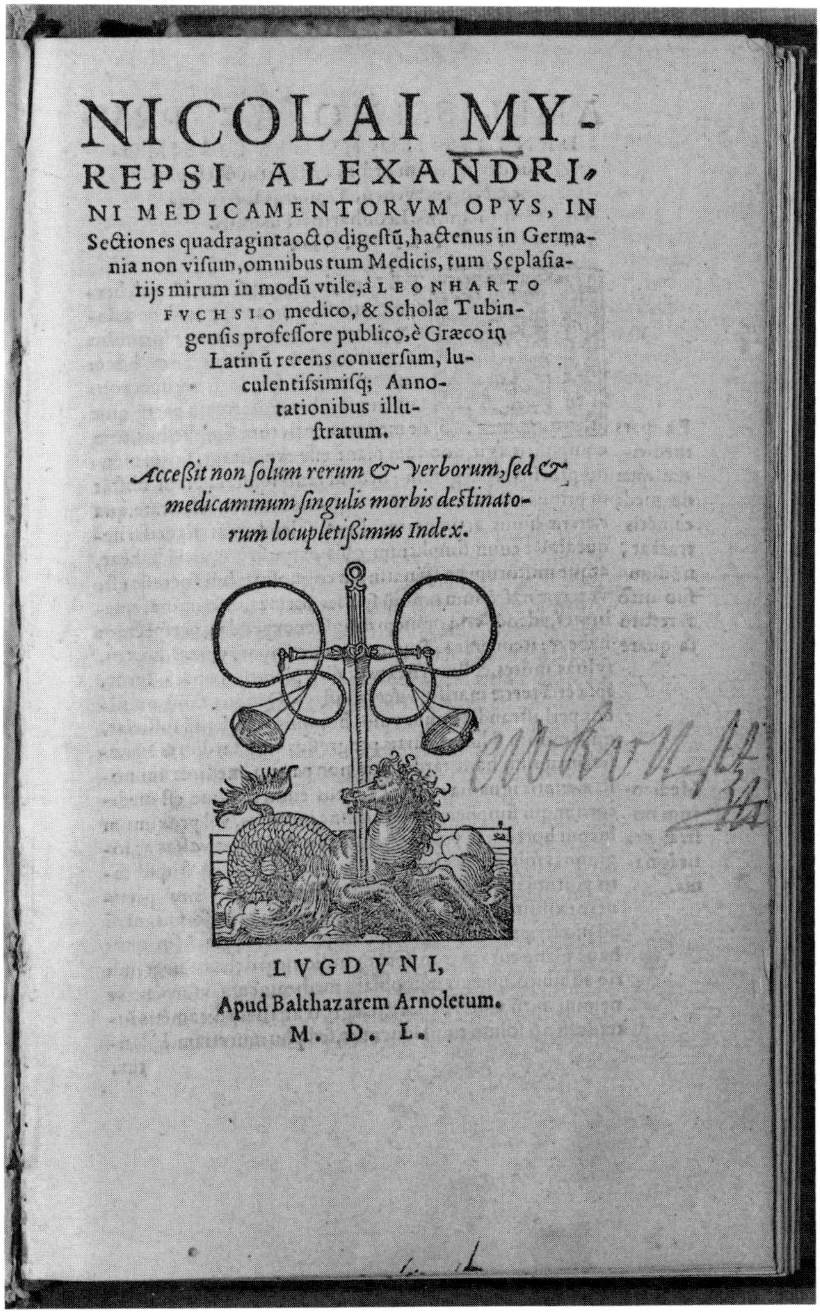

NICOLAI MY-
REPSI ALEXANDRI-
NI MEDICAMENTORVM OPVS, IN
Sectiones quadragintaocto digestũ, hactenus in Germania non visum, omnibus tum Medicis, tum Seplasiariis mirum in modũ vtile, à LEONHARTO FVCHSIO medico, & Scholæ Tubingensis professore publico, è Græco in Latinũ recens conuersum, luculentissimisq; Annotationibus illustratum.

Accessit non solum rerum & verborum, sed & medicaminum singulis morbis destinatorum locupletissimus Index.

LVGDVNI,
Apud Balthazarem Arnoletum.
M. D. L.

The title page of the octavo edition of Leonhart Fuchs' annotated translation of the *Dynameron* of Nicolaus, the ointment maker, adorned with Arnoullet's printing device of a sea-horse with sword and scales. Before the era of modern pharmacopoeias the *Dynameron* of Nicolaus Myrepsus was the standard formulary from which the early dispensatories were largely compiled. The original is said to have been written in barbarous Greek.

ALBERTUS MAGNUS (c.1200–1280)

Doctor Universalis

Summa Phi[losophi]e Naturalis Alberti Magni per Tractat[us] Capitula et Particulas pulcherrime distincta . . .

Leipzig, Martin Landsberg, 1508.

Folio – *leaf*: *265 x 200 mm. 72 leaves, signed* A-M⁶. *Wide margins. Printed in gothic types. Colophon and printer's mark at end. Old vellum, handwritten spine title. Another work has been taken out from the binding. Library stamp on the title:* Duplum Bibl. Reg. Monacensis.

Book-plate: C.D. Carlsson.

Rare early edition of five of Albertus Magnus' philosophical and scientific treatises: 1. *De physicorum*; 2. *De coelo et mundo*; 3. *De generatione*; 4. *De meteoris*; 5. *De anima.*

Albert was born in the family castle near Bollstädt in Swabia, which is why he is often referred to as Count Albrecht of Bollstädt. His birth date could be as early as 1193 or as late as 1206. His family was wealthy and powerful and he received a good education. He studied at Padua and there also entered the Dominican Order in 1222. His life was devoted to teaching, preaching and writing on almost every aspect of theology and philosophy. In c.1241 he taught at the University of Paris and in 1248 went to Cologne to establish a *studium generale*. Among his students was Thomas Aquinas. In 1260 he became bishop of Regensburg. He took part in the Council of Lyons in 1274 and died at Cologne in 1280.

Albert the Great, or Albertus Magnus, was the most eminent naturalist of the thirteenth century and an encyclopaedic writer, who is regarded as probably the most learned man of the Middle Ages. Known as *Doctor Universalis* he was considered a miracle of his century. Albert's principal importance for the history of modern science derives from the role he played in rediscovering Aristotle and introducing Greek and Arab science into the universities in the Middle Ages. His numerous works form a compendium of the writings of Aristotle and are of such comprehensiveness and mass that they constitute a real library.

Thorndike, II, pp. 517-92.

Naturalium Alberti

erit cõsensus rationis prout ẽ cognitiua seu in cognitione. Et sequitur cõsensus voluntatis qui dicit fiat fiat Et dicitur tunc cõnsensus rationis motiue Vterqȝ autem in verum et bonum consensus dicitur liberum arbitrium vel liberi arbitrij consensus ¶ Vnde liberum arbitrium in sua diffinitione comprehendit voluntatem et rationem. Est enim liberum arbitrium rationis facultas et voluntatis qua bonum eligit gratia assistẽte. Et malum fugit gratia deficiente.

Finis summe naturalium Magni Alberti cursorie emendate in almo vniuersitatis Lypzensis gymnasio. per Baccalarium Martinum Lanßperg de Herbipoli ꝛc. Anno incarnationis domini Millesimoquingentesimooctauo.

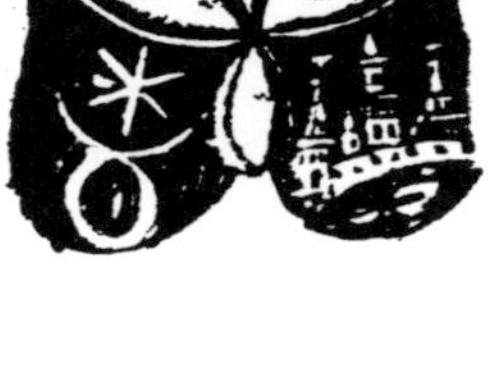

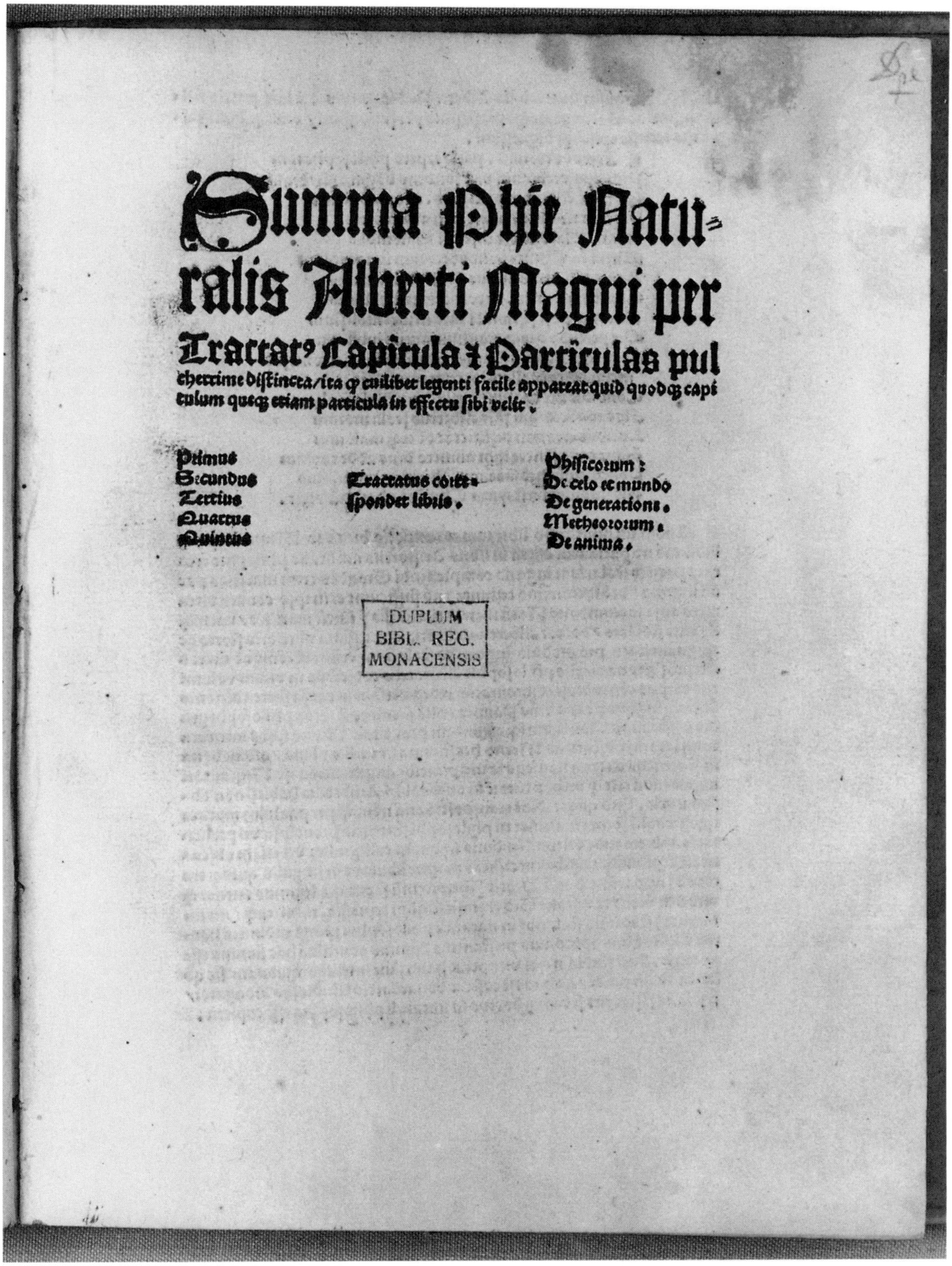

Summa Phie Naturalis Alberti Magni per Tractatꝰ Capitula ⁊ Particulas pulcherrime distincta, ita ꝙ cuilibet legenti facile appareat quid quodqꝫ capitulum queqꝫ etiam particula in effectu sibi velit.

Primus		Phisicorum :
Secundus	Tractatus correspondet libris.	De celo et mundo
Tertius		De generationi.
Quartus		Metheororum.
Quintus		De anima.

ALBERTUS MAGNUS (c.1200–1280)

The Secrets of Women

Tractatus Heinrici de Saxonia Alberti magni discipuli de secretis mulierum.
Augsburg, Antonius Sorg, 1489.

Quarto – *leaf*: 190 *x* 135 *mm.* 76 *leaves, signed*: a-j⁸ k⁴. *Title on* a1, *verso blank. Capital letters painted in red (one in blue), initial strokes painted in red. Marginal notes in an early hand. Early binding, thick wooden boards, rebacked, new endpapers, traces of one clasp.*

Book-plate: C.D. Carlsson.

The *De secretis mulierum* (The Secrets of Women) is one of the most popular works ascribed to Albertus Magnus. The present edition, Augsburg 1489, is in a version of Henry of Saxony, a disciple of Albert. It is only one of about fifty editions printed during the incunabula period, that is before 1501. The text deals with astrological influences during pregnancy and menstruation, common medical facts about sexual life, cosmetic advice and superstitious recipes. The numerous extant manuscripts, chiefly of the thirteenth century, and the steady stream of printed editions since 1476 well up to the seventeenth century, demonstrate how attractive such information was for an immense amount of readers. The book was a best seller for centuries.

Many of the writings ascribed to the legendary Albertus Magnus are of doubtful authenticity. The fame of Albert was so great that many apocrypha were attributed to him. His popular fame was in fact based upon two such apocrypha far more solidly than upon his own publications. These two, indeed far better known than his authentic works, are the *Liber aggregationes*, dealing with the magic properties of plants, stones, and animals, and the *Secreta mulierum* (The Secrets of Women). It was chiefly on account of these two works that Albert obtained his extraordinary fame as a magician, so that *Ars Albertina* came to mean magic, and that numerous chapbooks on 'the white and black art of man and beasts' were peddled under his name for centuries to come. (A Swedish version, *Albertus Magnus Redivivus eller naturhemligheternas bok. En samling af flera hundra, till större delen bepröfwade, sympati- och huskurer, till botande af en mängd sjukdomar och kroppsliga åkommor jemte åtskilliga andra, i forntiden begagnade sympatetiska och magiska konster, . . .* is a typical title, which went through numerous editions well into the 1920s.)

Thorndike gives examples of some of the superstitious recipes in the Secrets of Women: 'To prevent conception for a year women are advised to drink salvia cooked with wine for three days; or to eat a bee, "and she will never conceive". If hairs of menstruating women are buried in rich soil where ordure lies in winter time, the sun's heat will generate a long and strong serpent there the following spring or summer. To tell whether the child will be male or female one should pour a drop of the mother's milk or blood into pure water from a clear spring. If the drop goes to the bottom, the child will be a boy: if it floats on the surface, a girl'.

Klebs, 26:03; Gesamtkatalog 764; Hain, 8434; Sarton, *Introduction*, II:2, p. 941; Thorndike, II, pp. 739-45; Waller 4 & 5 (other inclunabula editions).

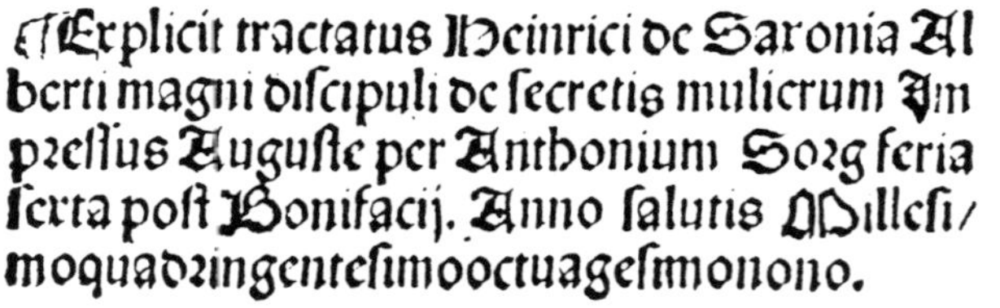
Explicit tractatus Heinrici de Saxonia Al
berti magni discipuli de secretis mulierum Im
pressus Auguste per Anthonium Sorg feria
sexta post Bonifacij. Anno salutis Millesi
moquadringentesimooctuagesimonono.

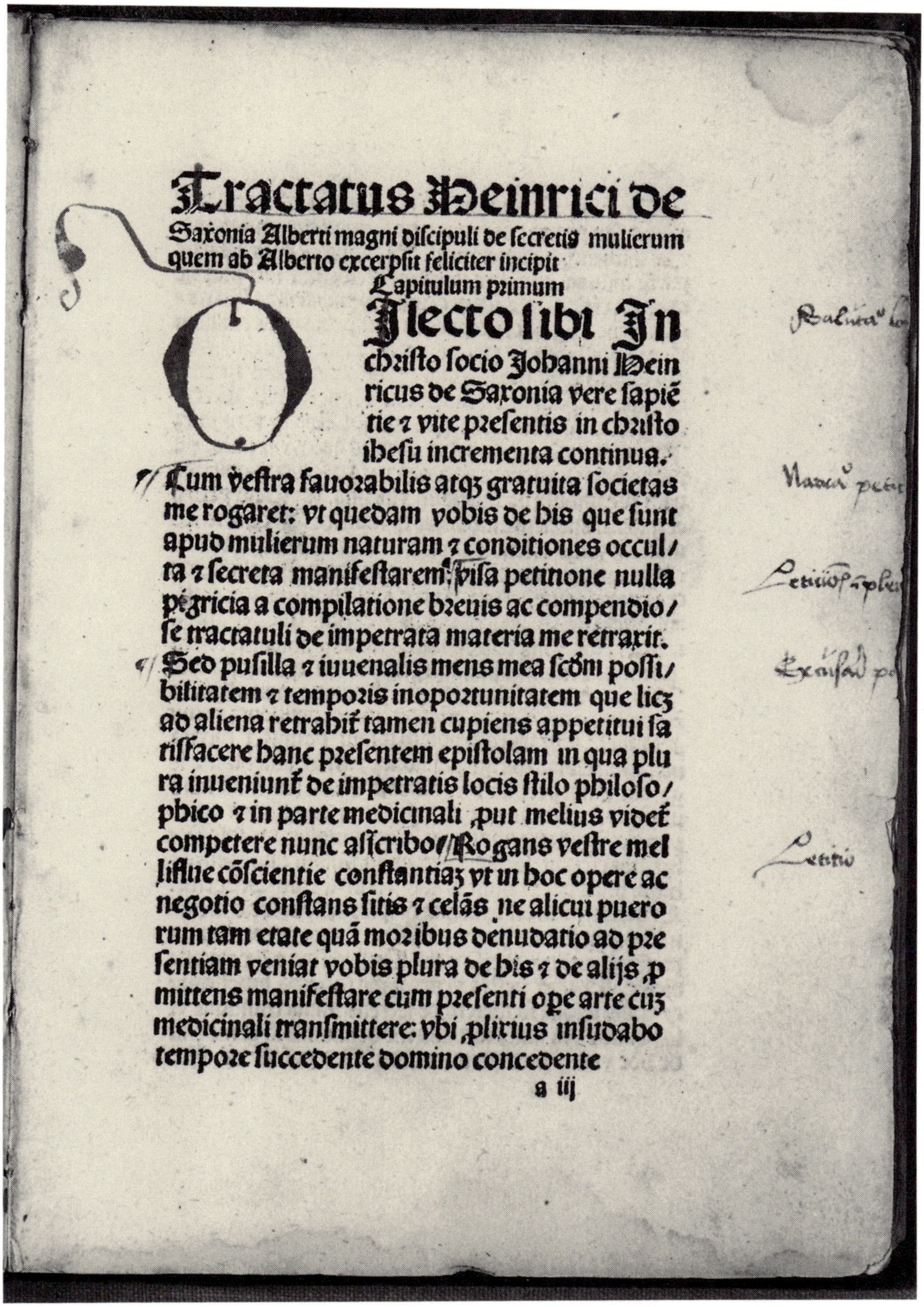
Tractatus Heinrici de
Saxonia Alberti magni discipuli de secretis mulierum
quem ab Alberto excerpsit feliciter incipit
Capitulum primum
Dilecto sibi In
christo socio Johanni Hein
ricus de Saxonia vere sapiē
tie ꝛ vite presentis in christo
ihesu incrementa continua.
Cum vestra fauorabilis atq3 gratuita societas
me rogaret: vt quedam vobis de his que sunt
apud mulierum naturam ꝛ conditiones occul/
ta ꝛ secreta manifestarem. Visa petitione nulla
pigricia a compilatione breuis ac compendio/
se tractatuli de impetrata materia me retraxit.
Sed pusilla ꝛ iuuenalis mens mea scdm possi/
bilitatem ꝛ temporis inopportunitatem que licz
ad aliena retrahit tamen cupiens appetitui sa
tisfacere hanc presentem epistolam in qua plu
ra inueniunt de impetratis locis stilo philoso/
phico ꝛ in parte medicinali prout melius videt
competere nunc ascribo. Rogans vestre mel
liflue cōscientie constantiaz vt in hoc opere ac
negotio constans sitis ꝛ celās ne alicui puero
rum tam etate quā moribus denudatio ad pre
sentiam veniat vobis plura de his ꝛ de alijs p
mittens manifestare cum presenti ope arte cuz
medicinali transmittere: vbi plirius insudabo
tempore succedente domino concedente
a iij

ALBERTUS MAGNUS (c. 1200–1280)

A best seller for centuries

Albertus Magnus, Daraus man alle Heimligkeit dess Weiblichen geschlechts erkennen kan, Dessgleichen von ihr Geburt, sampt mancherley Arztney der Kräuter, auch von tugent der edlen Gestein und der Thier, mit sampt einem bewehrten Regiment für das böse ding. Jtzund [*sic*] aber auffs neuw gebessert, und mit schönen Figuren gezieret, Dergleichen vor nie aussgangen.
Frankfurt am Main, Johann Feyerabend for Sigismund Feyerabend's heirs, 1592.

Small quarto – *leaf*: 190 *x* 150 *mm.* 76 *leaves: ff.* [1], 72, [3]. *Title printed in red and black with woodcut vignette of Adam and Eve and with* 76 *woodcuts in the text. Last leaf with colophon and printer's device. Modern vellum.* C. D. Carlsson Collection.

This is one of numerous popular books published by the famous Feyerabend press in Frankfurt. Its contents is a collection of German abridged versions of works ascribed to the legendary Albert the Great. The book contains the Secrets of Women, the *Liber aggregationes* on the virtues of herbs, stones and animals, a plague tract, followed by a Farmer's Almanac, blood-letting and cupping calendars, a planet-book, etc. The book is richly illustrated with famous woodcuts. Feyerabend had numerous wood blocks in stock and chose to illustrate his Albertus Magnus with woodcuts used in several of his earlier publications. The first part on the Secrets of Women is illustrated with 23 woodcuts by Jost Amman, and the 23 woodcuts of plants and 12 of animals are by Hans Weiditz, whose woodcuts were frequently used in herbals produced in Frankfurt. A series of 17 very charming woodcuts, representing the twelve months and the four seasons, illustrate the Farmer's Almanac, and there is also a woodcut of a blood-letting man.

Jost Amman was the artist of some of the best illustrated German books of the sixteenth century, including the famous *Pfsiter-Bibel,* books on hunting, hippology, cookery, and the *Eygentliche Beschreibung aller Stände auf Erden* with masterly illustrations of the different trades. Feyerabend's edition of Albertus Magnus' *Heimligkeit dess Weiblichen Geschlechts,* first published in 1581, has the same splendid woodcuts as those made by Jost Amman for Feyerabend's edition of Jacob Rueff's *Hebammenbuch* (1580), including the fine title vignette of Adam and Eve standing beside a tree in the shape of a skeleton.

Christmonat hat xxxj. tag.

Darin̄ ist der Tag lang acht Stundt vnd eylff Minuten/ Vnd laufft die Sonn im Steinbock.

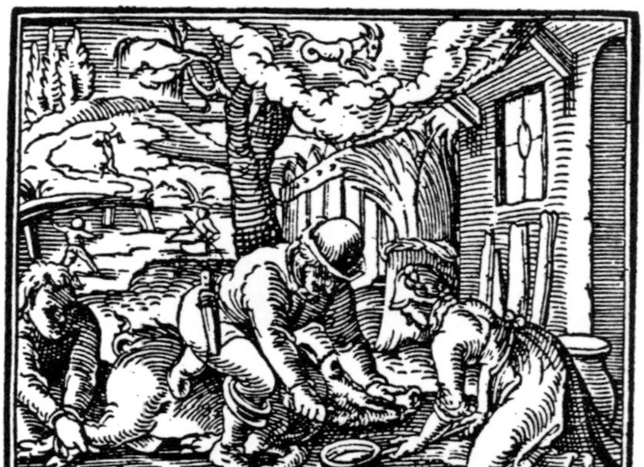

Jn dem Steinbock ist gut Wandern/ neuwe Kleider anziehen/ Kinder zu entwehnen/ säen vnd pflantzen.

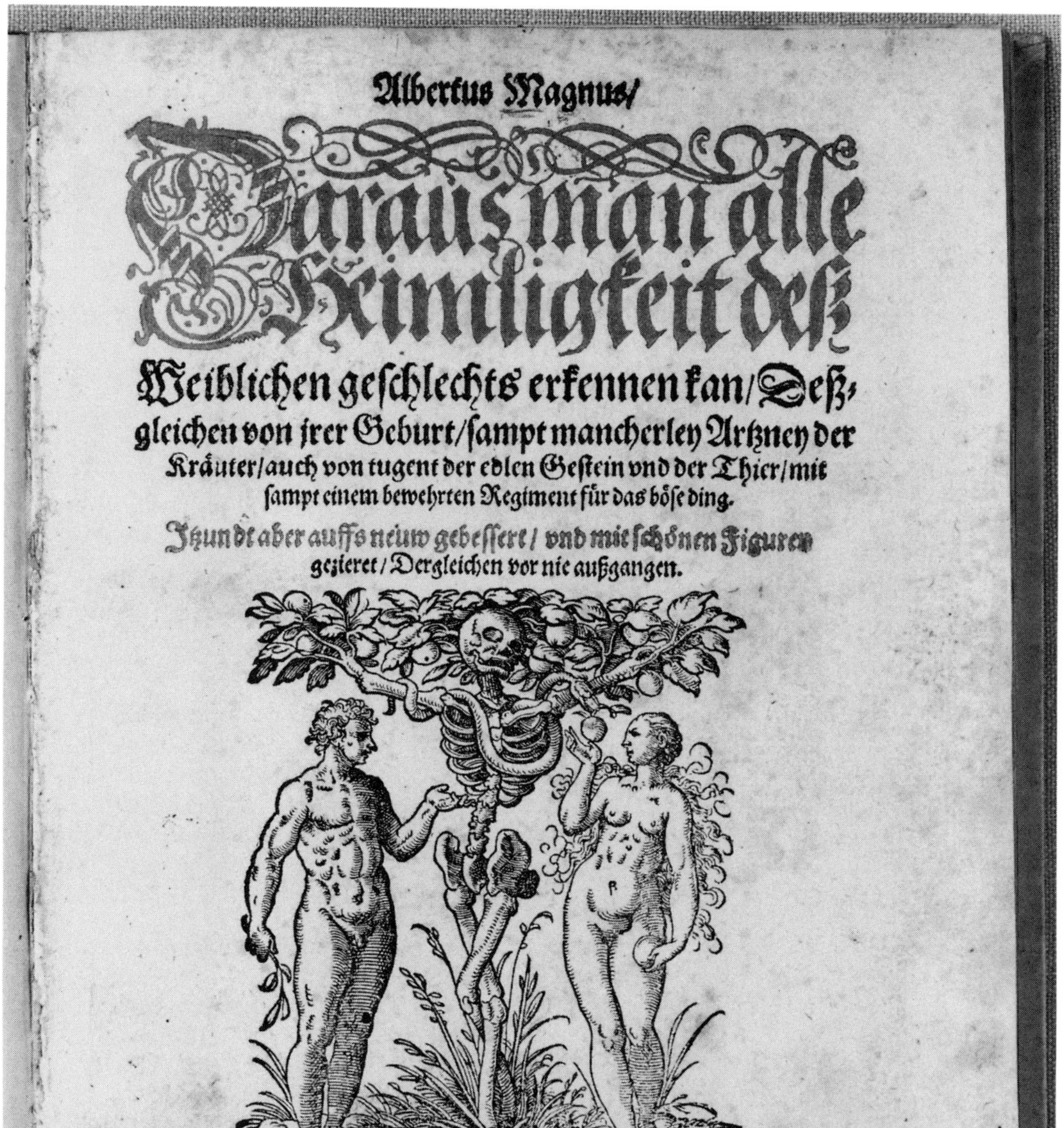

Albertus Magnus/
Daraus man alle Heimligkeit deß
Weiblichen geschlechts erkennen kan/Deß-
gleichen von jrer Geburt/sampt mancherley Artzney der
Kräuter/auch von tugent der edlen Gestein vnd der Thier/mit
sampt einem bewehrten Regiment für das böse ding.
Jtzundt aber auffs neüw gebessert/ vnd mit schönen Figuren
gezieret/Dergleichen vor nie außgangen.
Gedruckt zu Franckfurt am Mayn/ M. D. XCII.

Jost Amman's fine woodcut of Adam and Eve was originally made for Feyerabend's edition of Jacob Rueff's *Hebammenbuch* (1580), but was also used to illustrate other publications from the same press, as in this edition of Albertus Magnus' 'Secrets of Women' (1592).

In the *Liber aggregationes* the author considers sixteen herbs (in this German version supplemented with the virtues of seven herbs according to the emperor Alexander), about forty-five stones and some eighteen animals, many of which are birds. The virtues ascribed to these natural objects are often indeed magical. They may allow one to become invisible, escape dangers, travel in safety, conquer the enemy, win honours, not feel pain, boil water instantly, make a rainbow appear or the sun seem blood-red, excite love between two persons, or arouse joy, sadness, overpower wild beasts, interpret any dream, etc. In brief, by the aid of the occult virtues of these natural objects one can accomplish almost anything that any other form of magic can procure.

The first herb discussed is the *Heliotrope* [Sonnenwirbel, *Cichorium*]. If plucked when the sun is in the sign of Leo in August and worn wrapped in a laurel leaf with the tooth of a wolf, it insures that the bearer of it will be addressed with none but friendly words. If a person who has been robbed sleeps with it beneath his pillow, he will see all the circumstances of the theft repeated in his dreams. If it is placed in a temple unfaithful wives will be unable to leave the premises until the herb is removed.

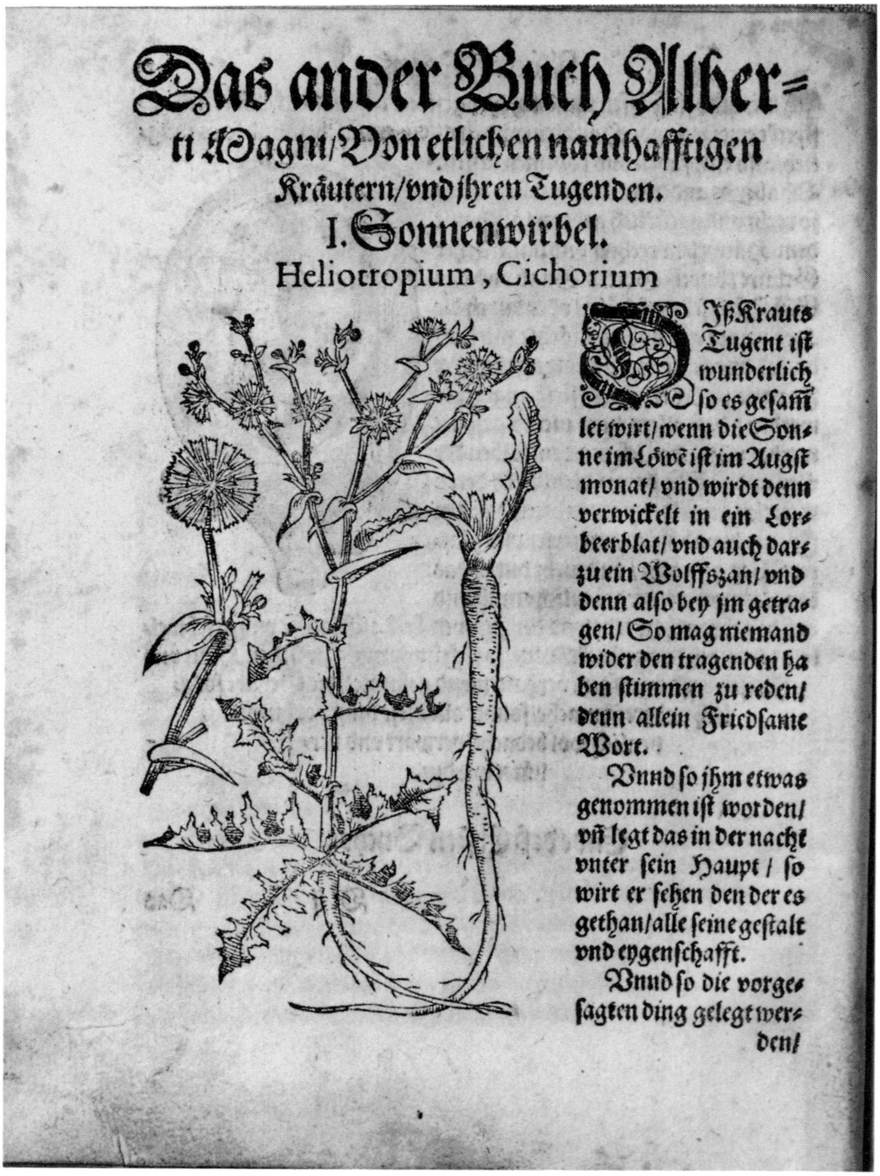

Das ander Buch Alberti Magni/Von etlichen namhafftigen Kräutern/vnd jhren Tugenden.

I. Sonnenwirbel.

Heliotropium, Cichorium

DJß Krauts Tugent iſt wunderlich ſo es geſamlet wirt/wenn die Sonne im Löwẽ iſt im Augſtmonat/ vnd wirdt denn verwickelt in ein Lorbeerblat/ vnd auch darzu ein Wolffszan/ vnd denn alſo bey jm getragen/ So mag niemand wider den tragenden haben ſtimmen zu reden/ denn allein Fridſame Wort.

Vnnd ſo jhm etwas genommen iſt worden/ vñ legt das in der nacht vnter ſein Haupt / ſo wirt er ſehen den der es gethan/alle ſeine geſtalt vnd eygenſchafft.

Vnnd ſo die vorgeſagten ding gelegt werden/

In the animal section we can read about the owl [Steinkäusslin, *Bubo*]. If the heart and right foot of an owl are placed upon a sleeper's breast, he will tell whatever he has done and answer whatever you ask him. 'And this was tested experimentally by our brothers recently'. No dog will bark at a person who carries these same parts of an owl in his armpit, and together with an owl's wing they will attract all sorts of birds to a tree from which they are suspended.

Thorndike, II, pp. 739-45; Waller 316-19 (other editions).

Alberti Magni.

Von dem Eychhörnlin.

Sciurus.

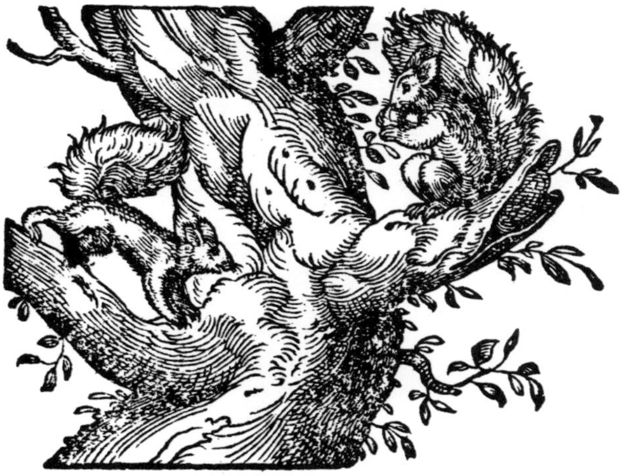

WEnn man ſeine Nägelin oder Kläwlin verbrennt vnnd befeſtiget/vnnd gibt denn das in der Speiſe/etwa einem Pferdt/ das jſſet in dreyen Tagen nichts.

The best pharmaceutical handbook of the 15th century

PRÉVOST, Nicole, latinized **Nicolaus Prepositus** (fl. 1470–80)
Dispensatorium magistri Nicolai prepositi ad aromatarios.
Lyon, Francois Fradin for Jacques Huguetan, 1505.

Quarto – *leaf*: 250 x 175 *mm*. 106 *leaves, numbered* I-CV, *the final leaf is blank. Sign.*: a-l8 m-o6 (o6 *blank*); o2 *wrongly signed* o3. *Huguetan's device on the title, colophon on* o5 *verso. Double columns, gothic types. Title leaf reinforced, wormholes throughout affecting some letters. Fine copy with wide margins. It has been removed from an old collective volume and rebound in the* 1920s *in vellum-backed boards.*

From the Ernst Matérn Collection.

An early edition of this epoch-making work in the history of pharmacy, written about 1480 by the French physician Nicole Prévost, whose name in latinized form, Nicolaus Prepositus, found in the title, has contributed to his being confused with Nicolaus Salernitanus, compiler of the *Antidotarium Nicolai*, who has been supposed to have been a principal, (*praepositus*), at the famous medical school of Salerno.

The *Antidotarium Nicolai*, attributed to a certain Nicolaus of Salerno and completed in the first part of the 13th century, is held to be the oldest formulary and became also the first published pharmacopoeia, beautifully printed by Nicolaus Jenson in Venice, 1471. Reprinted several times it must have been a very useful book, as it lists in alphabetical order formulae and preparations of 115 drugs, with indications for their medical use. The *Antidotarium Nicolai* was a trimmed-down version of the anonymous *Antidotarium magnum* or Great Antidotary, composed about 1100 by the early masters of the Salerno School with a listing of some 1200 drug formulas. Parts of these two works as well as recipes from other antidotaries written in Latin were collected and translated into Greek in the early 14th century and included in the *Dynameron* by the so-called Nicolaus Myrepsus. That extensive work of more than 2650 recipes was translated into Latin by Leonhart Fuchs in 1549 (see page 24 in this catalogue).

Towards the end of the Middle Ages there was some discord among physicians regarding their choice of authorities on writing recipes. Some prescribed after Avicenna, others after Serapion, still others upheld a recipe by Arnold of Villanova. The majority, however, used the prescriptions in the *Antidotarium Nicolai.* Though listed under the same title, one author's recipe would greatly differ from that of another in its composition. In time the text was ruined due to errors and mistakes made by the copyists, so that no two copies corresponded. Moreover there appeared numerous drugs, whose names were unfamiliar due to their Greek or Oriental origin; even medicinal plants fallen into extinction already in Ancient times were still prescribed. In the 15th century some physicians tried to bring uniformity to the pharmaceutical practice. The want of a really useful handbook for apothecaries induced Nicole Prévost to write a pharmaceutical handbook that would set all the standards necessary to practise the art of the apothecary.

The dates of Prévost's birth and death are unknown, but he studied at the University of Paris in 1472 and in 1478 became 'Magister' in Avignon before settling as physician in Tours. The first edition of his *Dispensatorium magistri Nicolai prepositi ad aromatarios* was published about 1480. Klebs lists three incunabula editions, all undated. These were followed in the 16th century by eleven more editions, the last printed at Paris in 1582. The book is divided into three parts, the first describing the *Simplicia*, the second the *Composita*, and the last third being a dictionary with translations of foreign names of drugs. This work, in most medico-historical books erroneously ascribed to the Salernian Nicolai 'Praepositus' of the 12th century, is now definitely ascribed to its real author, the French physician Nicolaus Prepositus (Nicole Prévost of Tours) thanks to the investigations made by Dr. Alfons Lutz, who has unraveled the confusion of the many 'Nicolauses' and their formularies. The book was a serious endeavour to epitomize the knowledge of the apothecary in the 15th century. With the publication of the *Dispensatorium ad aromatarios*, a work appeared, that for the first time in the history of pharmacy was so complete and concise that it for a very long time fulfilled the purpose of an indispensable aid in running a well-ordered apothecary shop.

Alfons Lutz, 'Das "Dipensatorium ad aromatarios" des Nicolaus Praepositus um 1490 und seine Bedeutung für die Geschichte der Pharmazie', in *Veröffentl. d. Intern. Gesellshaft f. Geschichte d. Pharmazie.* N.F. Band 26 (1965), pp. 87-103; Ferguson, II, pp 223-4; Wickersheimer, E. 'Nicolaus Prepositi, ein französicher Arzt ums Jahr 1500', in *Sudhoffs Archiv f. Gesch. d. Medizin,* Band V (1911/12), pp. 302-10; Castiglioni, p. 305; Waller 6859 (Lyons, 1517).

Dispensariuz magistri Nico-
lai prepositi ad aromatarios

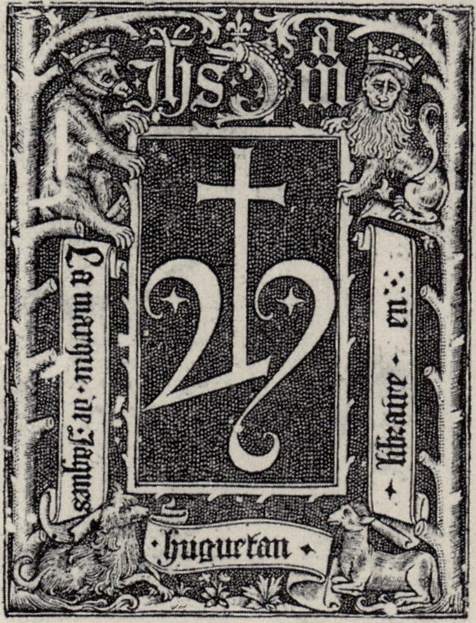

Venundantur Lugduni ab Jacobo huguetan eiusdem ciuitatis bibliopola in vico mercuriali. Et parrhisijs in vico sancti Jacobi sub diua virgine prope sanctum benedictum.

The powers and virtues of 435 plants commonly used in apothecaries' shops

[GART DER GESUNDHEIT]

Das Kreüterbuch oder Herbarius Das buch von allen kreütern, wurtzlen und anderen dingen, wie mans brauchen soll zu gesundthayt der menschen, Von newem Corrigiert und gebessert. Item wie man verstehen soll die gradus, Als wann man lisst, das kraut ist warm, kalt, trucken, oder feucht etc.

Augsburg, Heinrich Stayner, 1534.

Folio – *leaf:* 287 x 192 *mm. Incomplete copy containing* 159 (*of* 168) *leaves with* 368 (*of* 390) *woodcuts. Sign.:* a-b⁶ c⁴ A-Z⁶ Aa⁸ π⁶. *Lacks nine leaves:* B6, L2, X1-6, *and the final blank leaf. Printed in two columns. Title with a woodcut border with flowers, birds and insects, the lower part of the title page has a large woodcut showing three persons in an apothecary's shop with a door leading out to a herb garden with four persons. The title page and all the woodcuts contemporarily hand-coloured. Title leaf reinforced in inner margin, otherwise fine throughout. Modern marbled boards in grey and green, with green spine label, gilt.*

Book-plate: C.D. Carlsson.

This *Kreüterbuch oder Herbarius* is a late edition of 'the most important medieval work on natural history with illustrations' (Choulant). The *editio princeps* was published in 1485 by Peter Schöffer in Mainz, under the title of *Gart der Gesundheit*, which is indisputably the most splendid and important of the incunabula herbals. With its 435 chapters, and nearly 400 illustrations it was of outstanding importance. It was a landmark in the history of botanical illustration, one which marked perhaps the greatest single step ever made in that art. Its delineations of plants, breaking away from the traditional stylized woodcut, were not only unsurpassed, but unequalled for nearly half a century up to the appearance of Brunfels' *Herbarum Vivae Eicones* (1530), with Hans Weiditz's woodcuts of plants, all of which were drawn from nature. Textually, too, it was an original concept, giving a compendium of the whole pharmacy of that time in the vernacular. It was one of the first works on a scientific subject written in the vernacular – a Bavarian dialect.

According to the preface of the first edition the originator of the work was a wealthy amateur who received medical advice from a certain Dr. Johann von Cube, who in Chapter 76 on *Bolus Armenus* names himself : 'ist ohn zweyfel ein gewyse artzney dick mal versucht an vil endenn, von mir meyster Johann von Cube'. While the work was in progress, the compiler, discovering that many of the herbs mentioned by the Ancients did not grow in Germany, set out for the Holy Land upon a pilgrimage whose object was partly spiritual, partly botanical.

By a newly discovered manuscript, the *Codex Berleburg*, it has been proved that the editor was Bernhard von Breydenbach, author of the *Perigrinatio in Terram Sanctam* (1486), the first travel account with illustrations executed from sight. He had already in 1475 realized the importance of a German-language *materia medica* illustrated with lifelike figures of plants. He started to prepare for the work in the early 1480s, before his departure on his pilgrimage to the Holy Country. He had entrusted the compilation of the text to Wonnecke von Kaub (Johann von Cube), town physician in Frankfurt. Breydenbach left the illustrations uncompleted and engaged the Utrecht artist, Erhard Reuwish, to accompany him on his journey to the Holy Land and to draw the plants not found in Germany. Reuwich also made drawings portraying cities along the route, inhabitants of Palestine, and desert fauna, including the unicorn, which appeared in the *Perigrinatio in Terram Sanctam*. Passing through Italy and the Balkans, the travellers sailed by way of Crete, Rhodes and Cyprus to Palestine. After visiting Jerusalem, they made the customary detour to include Mount Sinai, returning through Cairo to Alexandria where they embarked for home.

'In wandering through these kingdoms and lands, I diligently sought after the herbs there, and had them depicted and drawn, with their true colour and form. And after I had, by God's grace, returned to Germany and home, the great love which I bore this work impelled me to finish it, and now, with the help of God, it is accomplished. And this book is called . . . *Gart der Gesundheit*. In this garden are to be found the power and virtues of 435 plants and other created things, which serve for the health of man, and are commonly used in apothecaries' shops for medicine.'

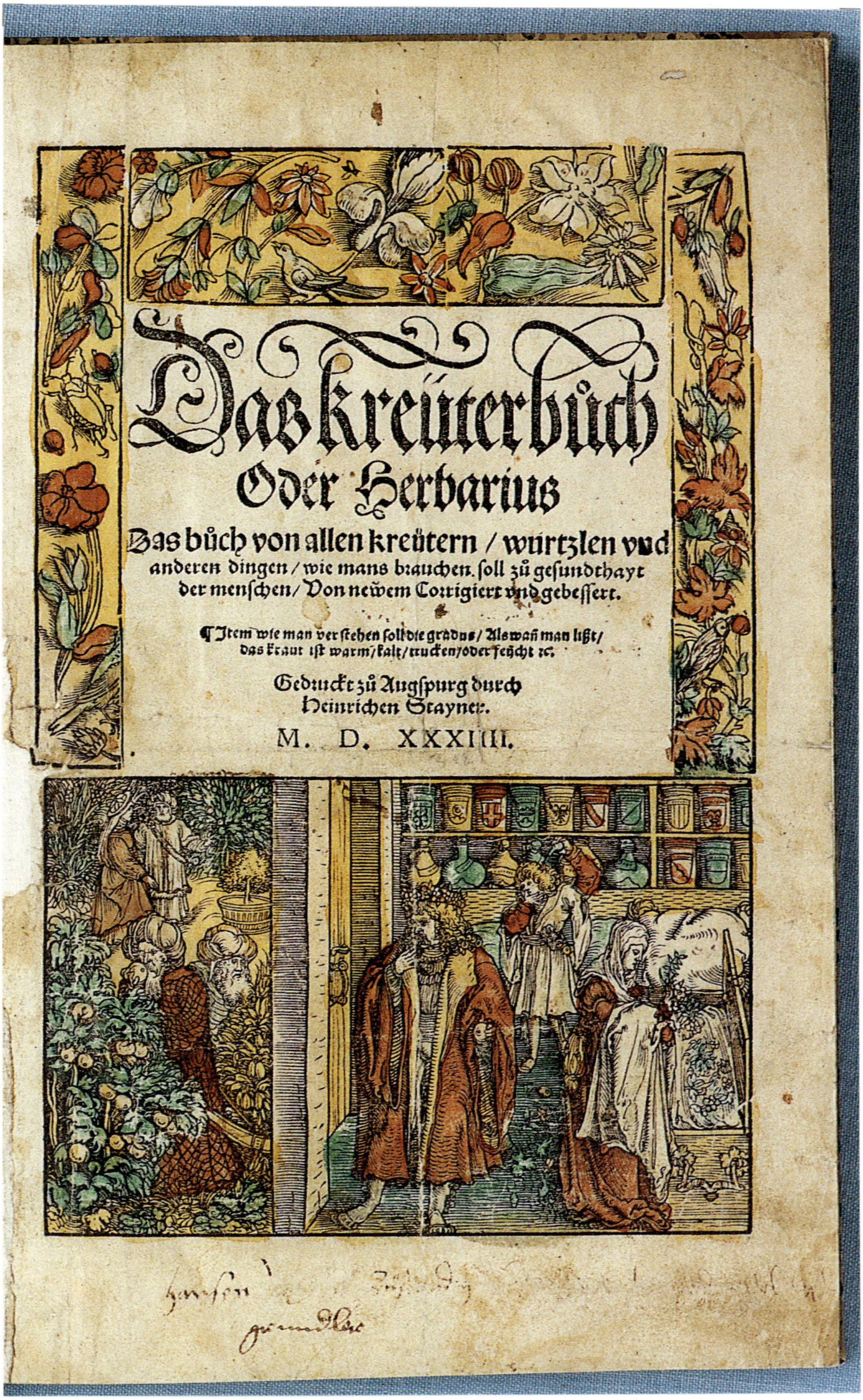
Das kreüterbůch
Oder Herbarius
Das bůch von allen kreütern / würtzlen vnd anderen dingen / wie mans brauchen. soll zů gesundthayt der menschen / Von newem Corrigiert vnd gebessert.
Item wie man verstehen soll die gradus / Als wañ man lißt / Das kraut ist warm / kalt / trucken / oder feücht rc.
Gedruckt zů Augspurg durch Heinrichen Stayner.
M. D. XXXIIII.

den kalten seych/vnd darm̃gegicht/ dise sucht mag man mit disem ö. haylen.
¶ Wider den stain ist es die allerbest artzney/ damit die lenden/ vnnd vber das gemächt geschmiert. ¶ Für das keychen vnd den alten hůsten schmier die brust außwẽdig damit. Für die gebresten der můter die do kommen von kelte / dienet diß öle fast wol/außwendig angeschmiert.
¶ Wider die auff stossung der můtter / so thů petroleum auff kolen / vnd empfahe den rauch inn die nasen / vnd bereüch dye můter von vnden auff mit laudano/so setzet sich die můter wider inn jr statt.
¶ Petroleum geschmiert auff den erkaltẽ magen/ist darzů gůt. Platearius.

Maßliebe.

Das CCCXXXIII. Capitel.

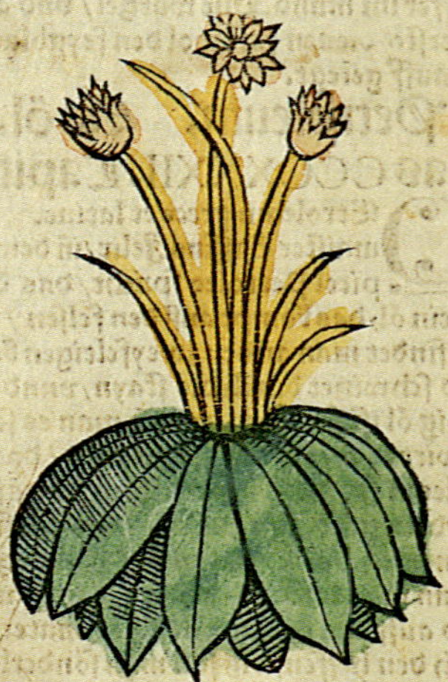

Premula veris latine. Die mayster sprechen das diß sey ein kraute das hat bletter die sind langlecht/vnd oben auß rottund/seine blůmẽ sind weyßfarb vnnd naygen sich allezeyt gegen der Sonnen. Diß kraut wechßt geren an feüchten enden/vnd brayt sich auf die erd. ¶ Paulus spricht/die wurtzel von dem kraut/sey gar nutz für die blatern an der zungen/vnd im̃ mund daruon getruncken. Diß kraut vnd wurtzel sind feüchte vnd kalt machen biß auf den andern grade. Wilhelmus spricht/das kraut soll mã samlen im̃ monat September/mit seyn blůmen vnd wurtzlen/vnd also dörren am lufft/vnd nit an der Sonnen/ das weret ein jar vnuersert an seiner krafft. ¶ Wer den krampff fast hett/ oder darzů genayget wer/der sied die inn gůtem wein/vnd trinck des so er schlaffen gehen will/er geneüßt. ¶ Für die fläcken am leyb/seüde diß kraut mit der wurtzeln inn regenwasser/vnd wäsch die fläcken damit am leib/sie vergehend. ¶ Den lamen glidern mit dem wasser gestrichen/dienet es wol.
¶ Dise wurtzel dienet wol den zerschwolnen hoden/die damit gebäwet vnden auf Auch mag man dise würtzel zerknitschen vnnd vber die geschwulst legen/es hylfft on zweyfel.

Hasenstrauch/oder hasen hauß.

Das CCCXXXIIII Capitel

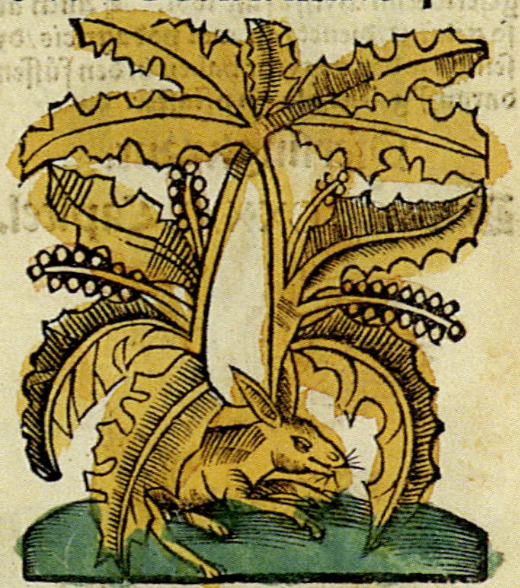

Palacium leporis latine/ Die maister sprechẽ das diß kraut sey bey nahe die disteln/allain das es lẽger bleter hat. Dises krauts wurtzel ist geleich dem stainbrech/ vnd hat kain blůmẽ vnd hat rund somen/ vnd mer rund dann staynbrech/vnd wechßt einer eln hoch in̄ die lüft/ vnd nit lenger. Dises kraut haissen etlich hasenstrauch/ vnd etlich hasen hauß/ wann so der haß darunder ist/ so förcht er sich nit/vnnd dunckt sich gantz sicher/dann diß kraut hat macht vber die melan-

The first illustrated herbal printed during the incunabula period was the *Apuleius Herbarium* (Rome, Joannes Philippus de Ligonamine, 1483), followed in 1484 by the *Herbarius Latinus* (or *Herbarius Moguntinus*), printed by Peter Schöffer in Mainz. Schöffer had served as Gutenberg's foreman and when Johann Fust acquired Gutenberg's equipment in 1455/56 he employed Schöffer to do the printing as well as cast the type for it. Later Schöffer married Fust's daughter and eventually took over the business. Like most of the early herbals his *Latin Herbarius* was a compilation from medieval writers. The *Gart der Gesundheit* must already have been in preparation for a considerable time when the *Latin Herbarius* appeared in print in 1484, and the immediate success of that book no doubt made Schöffer speed up the publication of the *German Herbarius* or *Gart der Gesundheit,* to have it ready for the 1485 Frankfurt Book Fair. The colophon is dated March 28, 1485.

Within five months a pirated edition appeared from the press of Johann (Hanns) Schönsperger in Augsburg. He had plagiarized Schöffer's *Gart* exactly, but most of the woodcuts are reversed and somewhat smaller. By 1502 Schönsperger had published no less than eight further editions, some with small woodcuts. Other printers in Strassburg, Ulm, Basel and Lübeck joined in – with the result that, in addition to Peter Schöffer's *editio princeps*, thirteen editions were published during the incunabula period – all similarly illustrated though often with small woodcuts. New editions and translations followed in the first three decades of the sixteenth century.

The present edition with small woodcuts and 'von newem Corrigiert und gebessert', was published and printed by Heinrich Stayner in Augsburg, who has adorned his title page with a fine woodcut depicting the interior of an apothecary shop and a herb garden. This woodcut had appeared earlier in Stayner's German edition of Petrarcha's *Von der Artzney bayder Glück, des guten und widerwertigen* (1532). The illustrator of that famous German Renaissance woodcut book is provisionally named the Petrarcha Master, by some identified as Hans Weiditz, who made the figures for Brunfels' herbal. Stayner's *Kreüterbuch* opens with a 26-page alphabetical listing of every disease or ailment then known, and under each such heading chapters are referred to, discussing remedies, pointing on particular paragraphs of special pertinence. The medical simples themselves are listed at the end in two indexes, with the names of the plants in German and in Latin, with reference to its chapter. There is also an additional treatise on uroscopy (Von dem Harn), a means of diagnosis used throughout the Middle Ages in which the physician examined the patient's urine by holding a flask of it to the light. Of this late Augsburg edition of *Gart der Gesundheit* (1534) we have been able to trace just two other copies, one in the British Library, and one incomplete copy sold at an auction in Austria in 1983.

Choulant, *Graphische Incunabeln*, pp. 20-61; Anderson, pp. 89-97; Arber, pp. 22-8; Blunt & Raphael, pp. 115-18; Blunt & Stearn, pp. 56-8; Gundolf Kiel, 'Gart der Gesuntheit', in *Verfasserlexikon des deutschen Mittelalters,* 2. Aufl., col. 1071-92; W.D. Müller-Jahncke, 'Das Herbar des Codex Berleburg als eine Vorlage des Gart der Gesundheit', in *Deutsche Apotheker-Zeitung*, 117 (1977), pp. 1663-71; Waller 4932 (other editions).

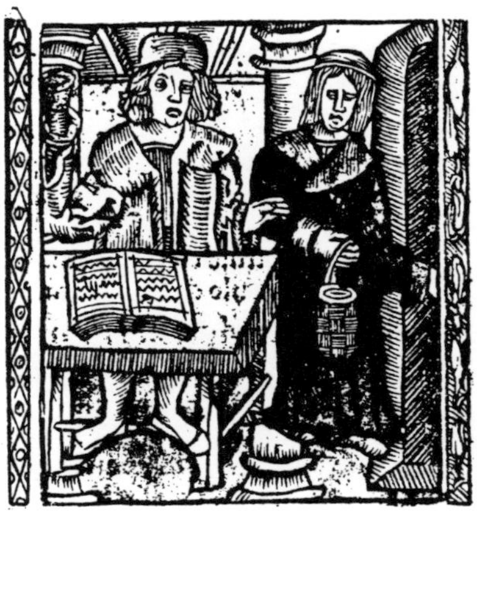

QUIRICUS DE AUGUSTIS (fl. 1450–1500)

Light shed on the art of the apothecary

Lumen apothecariorum cum nonnullis expositionibus noviter impressum.
Venice, 'per Ottinum Papiensez anno . . . domino M.CCCC.XCVII. Decimonono Kal. Septembris' [Ottoni della Luna, 1497].

Folio – *leaf*: 300 x 205 *mm*. 38 *leaves signed* a-e[6] f-g[4]. *Gothic types. Double columns, 70 lines to the page. Spaces left for initials. Title on* a1 *recto, verso blank, colophon on* g2 *verso followed by two leaves of index. Some early annotations and Ms numberings of the sections in the margins. Modern marbled boards.*

Book-plate: C.D. Carlsson

One of at least five editions printed during the incunabula period. The first edition was published at Turin in 1492 and the second one at Cremona in 1494, followed by some twenty editions published in Venice and Lyon.The book was also translated into Dutch (Brussels, 1515) followed by five more editions published at various places in the Low Countries, the last one at Rotterdam in 1623.

The author of this early textbook on pharmacology collected all that was known on this subject at the time. It became a model for later textbooks as well as an indispensable vademecum for the apothecary. Very little is known about Quiricus de Augustis de Tortona, or Ciriaco degli Augusti. According to himself, he was the son of the master N. Angelo of Tortona in Piedmont, who was a medical doctor and inventor of an ointment for the stomach. In 1480 Quiricus became the personal physician to Margareth, the daughter of Charles of Bourbon, and the wife of Philip, later Duke of Savoy. Quiricus had good knowledge of plants and pharmacy and travelled widely in Italy and France as the Duke's personal physician. When the Duke died in 1497 Quiricus established himself in Vercelli.

The *Lumen apothecariorum* deals with everything of importance for the apothecary of his day. The book is composed of 15 sections or 'distinctions', each divided into a number of descriptions, i.e. the 'prima distinctio' gives 22 aromatic confections, the second one 26 bitter electuaries, etc. There are sections on syrups, ointments, plasters, waxes, oils, pills, etc. There are well over 300 descriptions and prescriptions. Not only are the proper medicines mentioned, but there are also passages on how to make Turkish colour, dye of morellos, and the preparation of sweetmeats such as rose-sugar and marzipan, which is said to be mentioned here for the first time. Many of the descriptions bear the name of old authorities, and are taken from Mesue's *Grabadin,* Nicolaus' *Antidotarium,* from Rhazes, Galen and Avicenna, whom Quiricus calls 'the prince of medicines', and several others.

Besides giving methods of preparation Quiricus gives us information on the gathering of herbs, their preservation and the methods of keeping medicines. Theriac should be kept in a silver or leaden vessel, which should not be filled up to the brim but at least one third empty, so that the air can reach the medicine. All eye-waters should be preserved in copper vessels. The syrups made with honey can be preserved for two years, and those boiled with sugar and kept in a well-sealed vessel one year. Among the medicines are also various animal organs such as a wolf's liver, which when washed with the best wine is cleared of all impurities. Human blood, to which earthworms are added, should be taken from a healthy sanguine person.

There are six ways of preparing medicines: boiling, grinding or powdering, burning, washing, curdling and mixing. Quiricus uses fire for drying, roasting and burning. As to apparatus, he is acquainted with the water bath, boiling in a double vessel, lead-glazed earthenware vessels, stone mortars with wooden or iron pestles. He discusses weights and measures, and as there are many kinds which vary according to the nature of things, one must take good notice of these differences. He says he has often seen mistakes made with the preparation of medicines and that these are usually made by apothecaries. Quiricus is well-known for his fulmination against the apothecaries. He reproaches them for their ignorance and also warns the people against them.

The Facsimile of Quiricus de Augustis Dlicht D'Apotekers 1515, *The First Prescription Book Printed in the Low Countries,* with an Introduction by D.A. Wittop Koning. Nieuwkoop, 1967 (with list of literature).
This edition not in GW, Hain, Poynter, NLM, Osler, Cushing or Waller; Waller 23 (Cremona 1494).

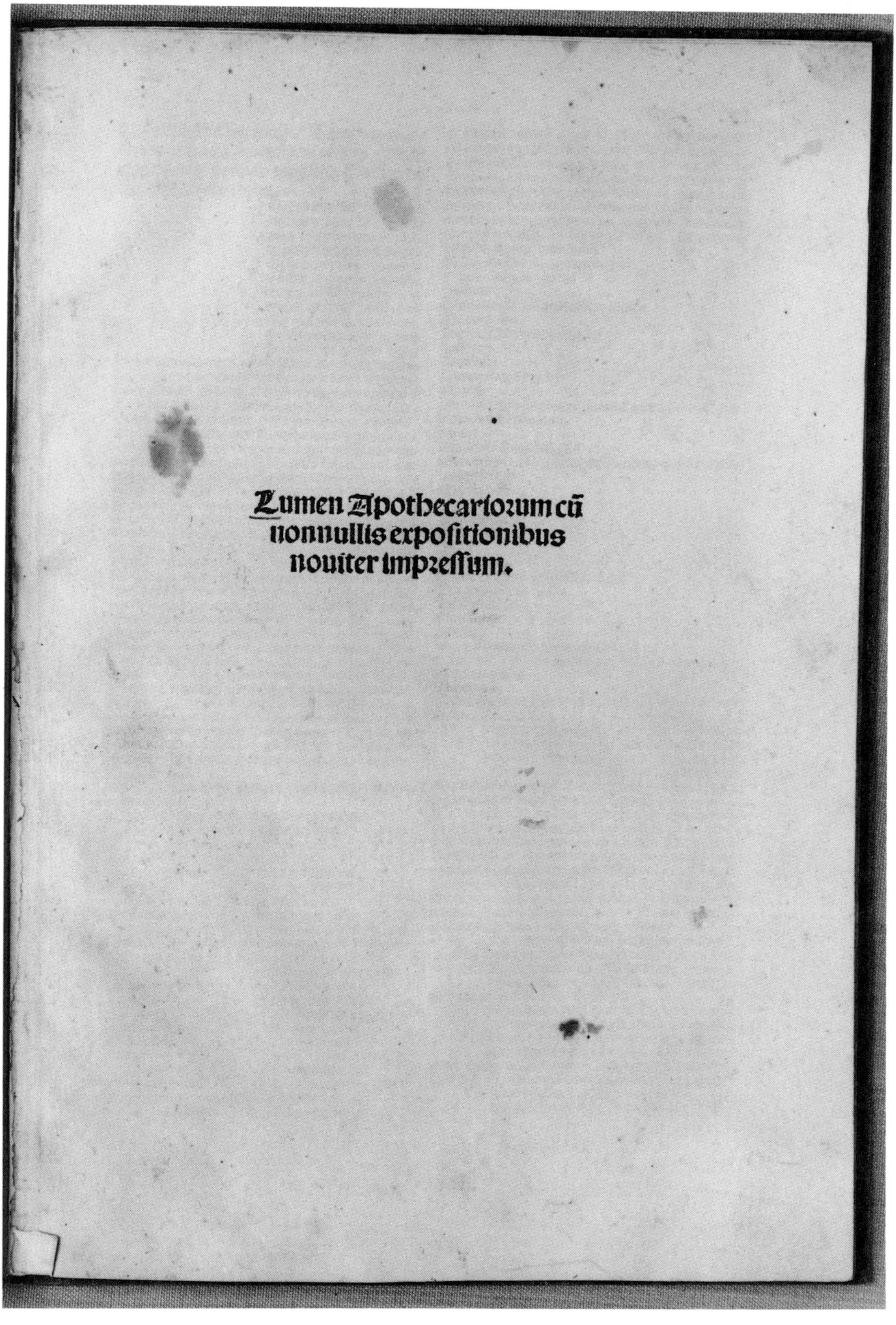

Lumen Apothecariorum cū nonnullis expoſitionibus nouiter impreſſum.

BOSSLER, Ulrich (fl.1521)

A dialogue between drugs, for and against Luther

Dialogus oder gesprech des Appostolicums Angelica und anderer Specerey der Appotecken Antreffen Doctor M. Lutterers ler und sein anhanck etc.

No place, no date; preface dated 'Prima apprilis des ein und zwentzigsten jars' [? Speyer, Johann Eckhardt, 1521].

Quarto – *leaf*: 185 *x* 140 *mm. Twelve unnumbered leaves. Sign.*: A-C4. *Title page with woodcut showing the interior of an apothecary's shop. Disbound copy preserved in modern marbled boards, black morocco label on upper cover.*

From the C.D. Carlsson Collection. *Purchased in* 1931 *from Antiquariat Max Ziegert, Frankfurt am Main, for Rm.* 110.

A rare and early Reformation pamphlet written in the form of a dialogue in an apothecary shop, where the various drugs dispute for and against the Reformation, according to their virtues. The woodcut on the title page is one of the first book illustrations to depict an early sixteenth century German apothecary shop.

This is one of two variants printed in the same year, neither of which has an imprint; the place of printing of the present one (variant A) is variously given as Speyer (Johann Eckhardt), Worms or Nuremberg. The other (variant B) was printed by Jörg Nadler in Augsburg with a quite different title page, on which the title is inscribed within an architectural border.

This type of pamphlet with title woodcuts was a popular form of pictorial propaganda for the German Reformation, often with biting satire. The present one in the form of an amusing dialogue is thought to have been composed near or at Worms during the celebrated Diet, shortly before Luther's arrival there.

In the dedication to the physician and famous astronomer Johann Fordung (i.e. Virdung, c.1465–1535) of Hassfurth, dated 'Prima apprilis des ein und zwentzigsten jars', the author states his name: Ulrich Bossler von Hassfurth. He is otherwise unknown but seems to be well aquainted with the world of the apothecary.

In the unsigned woodcut a messenger from Mainz stands in the foreground bearing a post horn, in front of an apothecary shop. On the table in the shop lies a mortar with a pestle, a spatula and a pot of ointment. On the far wall are three shelves bearing 24 apothecary jars, one shelf each for *Unguent* (ointment), *Herbe* (herbs) and *Radices* (roots). Each jar is adorned with a crest, but only the three in the middle of the shelf of herbs are identifiable: the arms of the bishoprics of Mainz, Cologne and Trier. Under the shelves is an opening from which the apprentice apothecary can be seen eavesdropping on the discussion. Indeed, Bossler says that he himself had overheard the conversation taking place between the drugs on the night of the 27th of March 1521 as he lay in his box-bed in the shop. Around midnight he suddenly heard the drugs begin to converse: the roots spoke in favour of Luther against the ointments who defended the Pope, while the herbs maintained a careful neutrality.

The dialogue form is a kind of *Dialogus Creaturarum*, [an edition of which is the earliest printed book in Sweden] except that here it is carried out between drugs rather than between animals. The main debaters are *radix Angelica* (Engelwurz, a remarkable remedy for the plague in the early sixteenth century), defending Luther, and *unguentum Apostolicum* (a brown-coloured ointment), speaking for the Curia of the Roman Catholic Church. Among the names that appear apart from Luther's are Hutten, *doctor Geckius* (Johann Eck), and *doctor Murnarr* (Thomas Murner).

Bossler may have been trying to win the educated class of physicians and apothecaries over to Luther's cause. It is an early example of one of the mass of pamphlets that appeared during the Reformation period.

München, SB, Rar 4123 [Speyer, 1521]; Herzog August Bibliothek, Wolfenbüttel [Worms, 1521]; Wolf-Dieter Müller-Jahncke, 'Die Apotheke als Schauplatz eines Reformationsdialoges: Zu Ulrich Bosslers "Dialogus oder gesprech . . ." von 1521', in *Beiträge zur Geschichte der Pharmazie* (= Geschichtsbeilage der Deutschen Apotheker-Zeitung, 27 (1975), Nr. 2, pp. 9-12; Wolfgang-Hagen Hein and Dirk Arnold Wittop Koning, *Bildkatalog* 11 *zur Geschichte der Pharmazie* (Veröffentlichungen der Internationalen Gesellschaft für Geschichte der Pharmazie e.V., Neue Folge, Band 59, 1994); Oskar Schade, *Satire und Pasquille aus der Reformationszeit,* Hannover, 1856-63, *vol.* III, *pp.* 36-58 *and* 238-43 (Kommentar); Waller 19424.

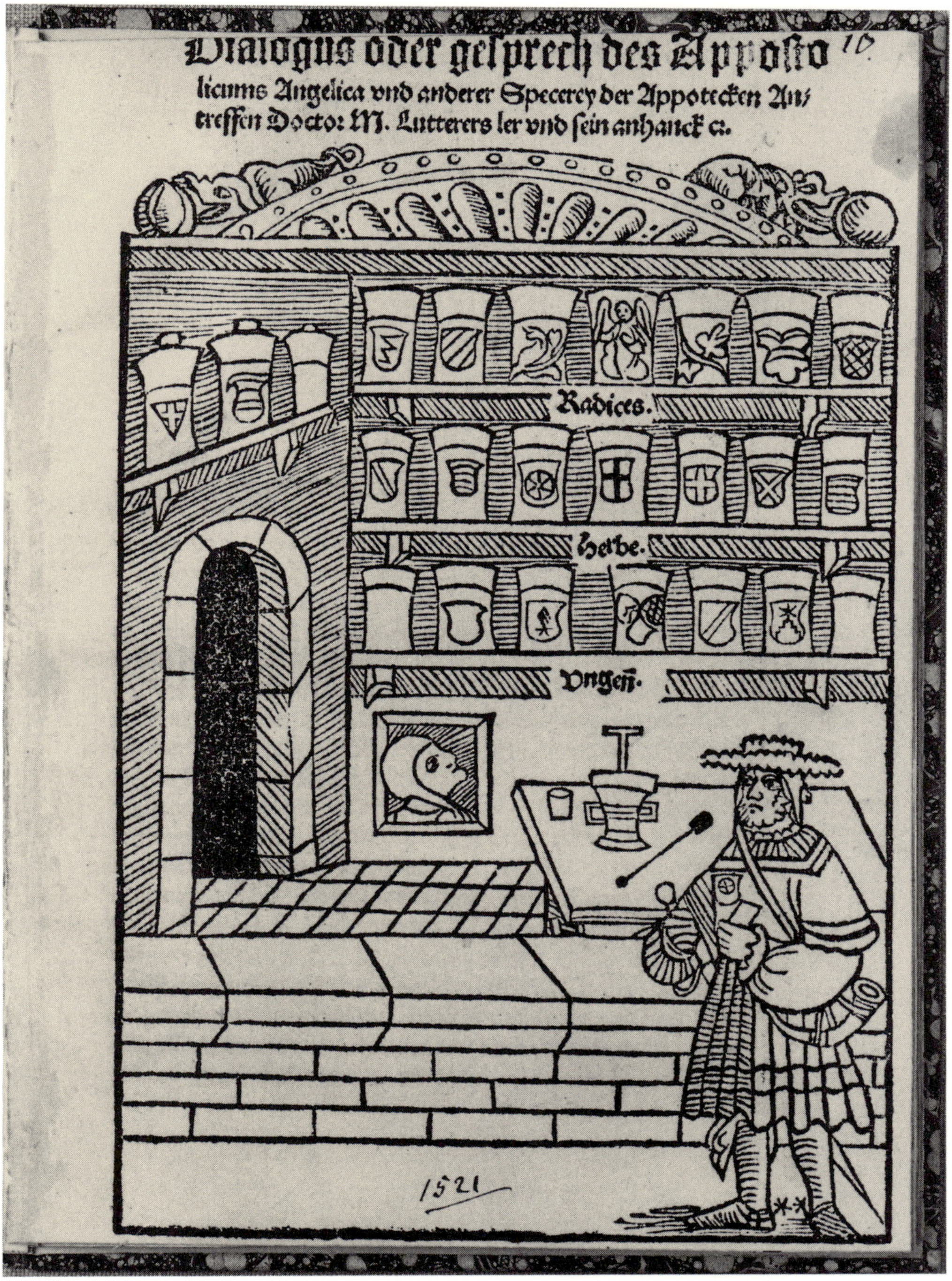
Dialogus oder gesprech des Apposto
licums Angelica vnd anderer Specerey der Appotecken An-
treffen Doctor M. Lutterers ler vnd sein anhanck &c.
10
Radices.
Herbe.
Vngeñ.
1521

An early pharmacopoeia for the poor

BRUNSCHWIG, Hieronymus (c.1450–1512)

Hauss apoteck. Zu yeden leibs gebresten, für den gemainen mann, und das arm Landt volck.

Augsburg, Heinrich Stayner, 1538.

Small quarto – *leaf*: 183 *x* 138 *mm. 76 leaves, sign.*: A-T^4. Ff. [4], I-XL (XLI *to* L *dropped*), LI-LXXXI, [1] *blank. One woodcut on the title page and three in the text. In the lower margin of the title page, beneath the woodcut, is a stamped monogram:* FG. *Modern panelled calf, gilt, red edges.*

Book-plate: C.D. Carlsson.

Early and finely illustrated edition of this popular pharmacological book, which was first published as the fifth book, or part, of Brunschwig's 1512 edition of *Liber de arte Distillandi de Compositis*, the so-called *Grosses Distillier Buch*, which impressive volume of 362 leaves covers in detail not only the techniques and technology of distillation and preparation of compound distillates but also all aspects of the pharmacological knowledge of the time. That richly illustrated book was the most popular vernacular manual of domestic pharmacology in the sixteenth century and went through numerous editions and translations. The fifth book, a home pharmacy for the poor, was independently published in various editions under the titles of *Thesaurus pauperum* or *Hauss Apoteck . . . den gemainen Mann und das arm Landtvolk*.

The present edition of the *Hauss Apoteck* is one of several printed by Heinrich Steiner in Augsburg. However, there were several more printed by other famous presses in south German towns. This Steiner edition of 1538 incorporates some very fine and famous woodcut illustrations that had been used earlier to illustrate other herbals of the period, the main purpose being to attract the reader's attention. In his *Grosse Distillier Buch* Brunschwig himself remarks on his publisher's choice of illustrations. He advices the reader not to place too much reliance on the pictures, 'for the figures are nothing more than a feast for the eyes, and for the information of those who cannot read or write'.

Very little is known about Brunschwig, or Braunschweig, other than what he tells us himself in his books. He was born c.1440-50 and was probably apprenticed to an older surgeon to learn the craft. There is no evidence that he ever studied at Bologna, Padua or Paris, as some have alleged, or that he was an army surgeon. He was an exceedingly well-read man, who possessed a far wider knowledge of medical literature than most of his colleagues. Even though we need not implicitly believe the statement that he had studied 3000 volumes, as he states in the preface to his book on distillation, his reading had certainly been vast and varied, as is clearly proved by his writings. With his decided talent for surgery and reading, he far surpassed the intellectual level of his contemporaries and became an author. His first book was *Buch der Cirurgia* (Strassburg, 1497), the first important printed surgical treatise in German. It contains the first detailed account of gunshot wounds in medical literature and is notable for its interesting woodcuts, some of the earliest medical illustrations in a printed book.

Brunschwig's *Thesaurus pauperum* is a book of popular medicine designed for self-treatment, and it became a model for later pharmacopoeias for poor people. The first chapter starts with the upper part of the body and gives a remedy for those who have lost their hair: 'make a salve of the ash of dove dung and rub the scalp with it – it helps'. With this widely read book Brunschwig became one of the most influential pharmacists of his time.

H. E. Sigerist, *Hieronymus Brunschwig and His Work*. New York, 1946; Anderson, *Herbals*, pp. 113-20; Waller 1582 (Augsburg, 1539).

Hauß apoteck. Zů yeden leibs gebresten/für den gemainen man/vnd das arm Landtuolck/Durch Hieronymum Braunschweig getrewlich zůsamenn tragen/vnnd an tag gegeben.

Der Herre hat die Ertzney vonn

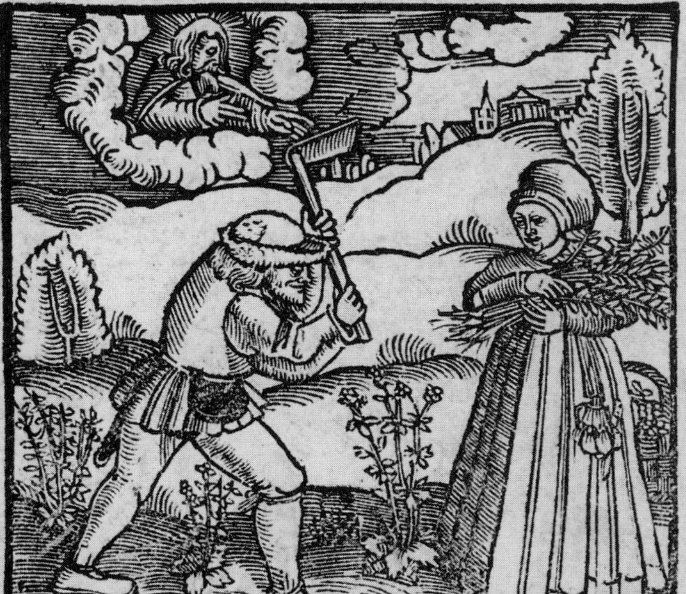

der erden erschaffen/vnnd der weyse

wirdt kain scheühen darab habenn.

Ecclesiastici. am xxxviij.

EG

The technique of distilling compounded medicines

ULSTADIUS, Philipp (early 16th century)

Coelum Philosophorum. Von heymlicheyt der Natur, das ist, wie man nit alleyn auss wein, sonder auch auss allen metallen, früchten, fleysch, ayern, wurtzlen, kreuttern, und anderen dingen mer sol distilliren Aquam Vite, zu erhaltung der gesundheyt menschliches cörpers, Eyn kurtz klares, und nützlichs Buch, durch fleiss Philippi Ulstadii von Norimberg auss Raymundo, Arnoldo de Villa Nova, und Alberto Magno, zu samen inns Latin geschriben, aber jetzunt von neuwen verteutscht, und die Capitel, welch vorhin gemangelt, hirzu gethon. Item Marsilii Vicini Regiment dess lebens, mit essen, trincken, wonungen . . . Darbei viel gütter Recept für aller handt krankheyten, dem Gemeynen Mann eyn wolfeyle unnd gar nützliche Apoteck.

Strassburg, Jacob Cammerlander, 1536.

Folio – *leaf*: 265 *x* 190 *mm. Ff.* [4], 55, [1]. *Sign.*: π^4 A-O^4. *With* 53 *woodcuts in the text. Nineteenth century red boards, yellow spine strip.*

Gift from Bertil Bjurling, 1951.

Coelum philosophorum, seu liber de secretis Naturae, per Philippum Ulstadium ex variis Autoribus accuratè selectus, variisque figuris illustratus. Nunc recens adiecimus Ioan. Anto. Campesii Directorium summae summarum Medicinae.

Lyon, Guillaume Rouille, 1557.

Sextodecimo in 8s – *leaf*: 109 *x* 77 *mm. Pp.* 431, [1], [16] *index. Sign.*: A-Z AA-EE^8 (*last blank*). *Printer's device on the title and* 65 *woodcuts in the text* (15 *full-page*), *many of which are repeated. In the first part* 24 *of the woodcuts are hand-coloured. Contemporary blindstamped pigskin over wooden boards, clasps. Seventeenth-century copper engravings with Christian motifs pasted in inside the covers.*

Owner's signature on the title: Ex. lib. Joannis Caspari Kiferix, 1608; *From the* C.D. Carlsson Collection *with his book-plate.*

This popular work on distillation, *Coelum philosophorum* [Heaven of The Philosophers] was first published in Latin around 1526 and went through some twenty editions and translations. Our library owns the Cammerlander German edition in folio and a small 'pocket edition' in Latin, the latter of which includes many of the woodcuts coloured by a contemporary hand.

Philipp Ulstad, or Ulstadius, was a physician from Nürnberg, who taught medicine at Fribourg in Switzerland. His major work is the *Coelum Philosophorum*, in which he describes the technique of distilling compounded medicines. He gives good recipes for claret, hypocras, *aqua vitae Frederici* II and other spiced wines, which were then (as now) very much in vogue. He describes the preparation of spirit of wine (*aqua vitae*) by distilling wine in an alembic with its neck packed with sponges soaked in oil, and alembics for 'circulation' (refluxing), which were thought to enrich the wine in spirit. He tested alcohol by burning it on a piece of linen where it should not leave any water after having been consumed, nor burn up the linen.

Ulstad's work was based mainly on the medieval writings attributed to Ramon Lull, Albertus Magnus, Arnold of Villanova and especially to John of Rupescissa. 'He was most clearly indebted to John of Rupescissa's doctrine of the fifth essence, namely, the substance that can be extracted from all mundane bodies by ordinary chemical methods and that is the chemically active principle of each body. Ulstad was primarily concerned with the curative and preservative properties of rectified alcohol – which he denoted variously as the fifth essence, *aqua vite, aurum potabile*, and *coelum philosophorum*. He maintained that the fifth essence, although not incorruptible, was less corruptible than the four elements and owed its medical value to its ability to regulate the bodily humours and thereby preserve the human body from decay . . . Ulstad con-

Diſer ofen iſt hie angezeigt den müſſigen künſtnern/welche wol der weil
hon/darinnen zů diſtillieren Aqua vite vnd andere ding/das da
ſenfftigklich zů ſoll ghan/Alßdañ von den Alten hochgelerten
vnnd erfarneſten Artzten zůwegen bracht/zů nutz deß men
ſchen leib in geſundtheit zůbehalten mitt Gottes hilff.

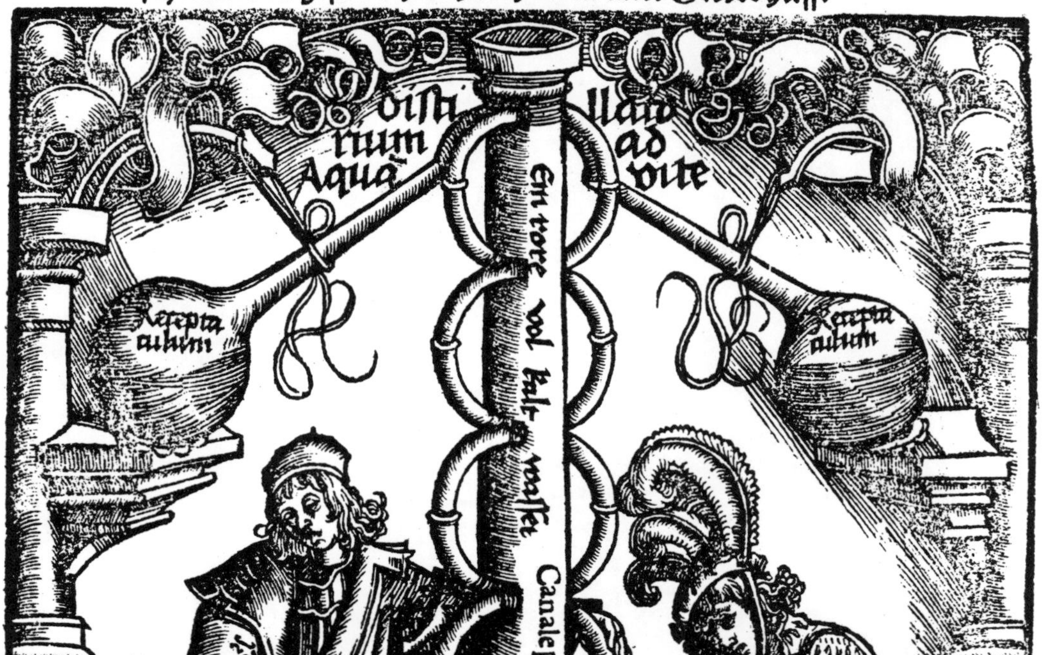

A ij Wie

The famous woodcut illustration of an early alcohol still with cooling-coil. This and most of the other woodcuts in Ulstad's *Coelum Philosophorum* had earlier been used to illustrate Brunschwig's work on distillation.

Diß ist die gestalt deß offens als hie verzeychnet.

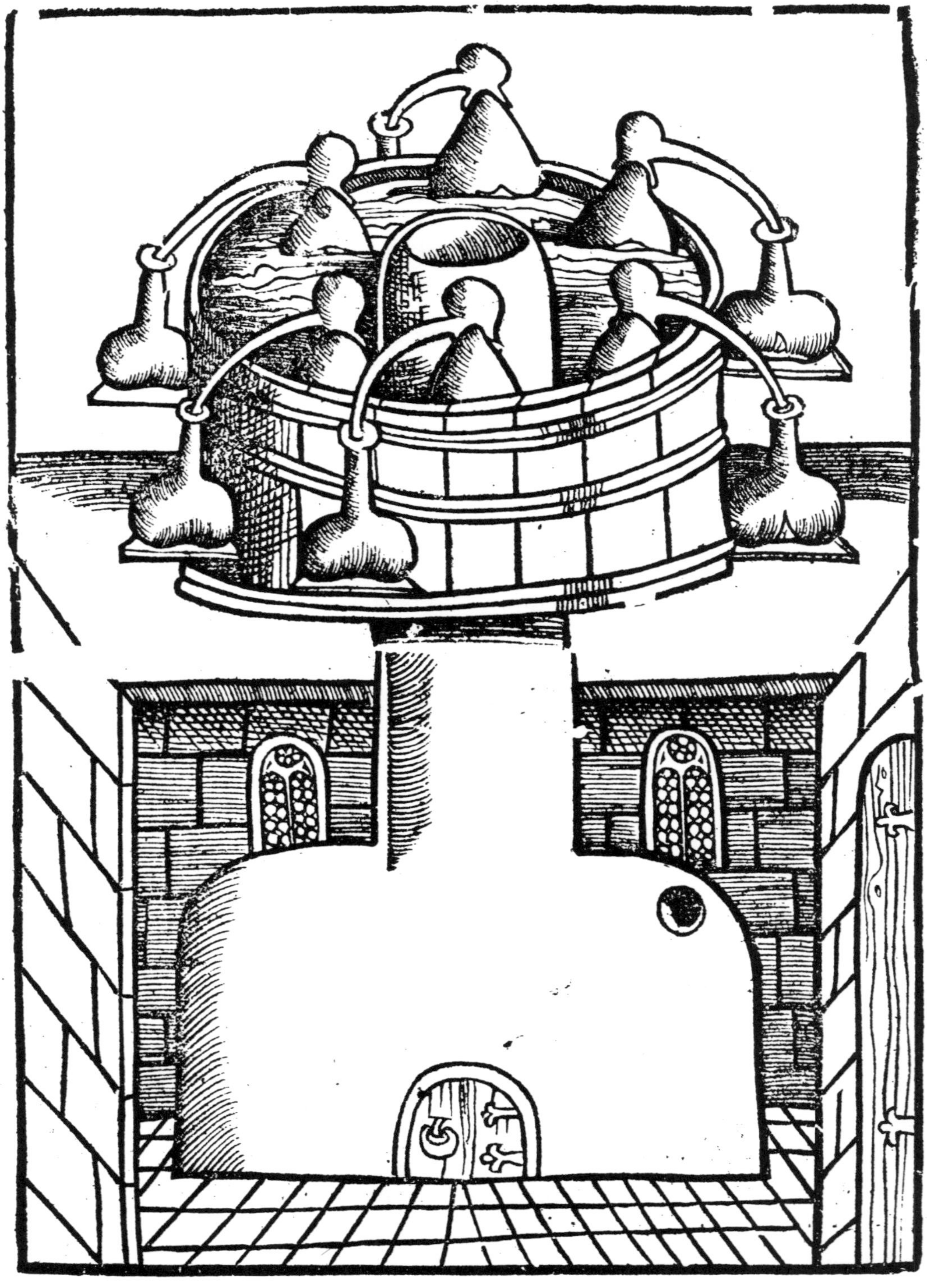

Water-bath distillation for several cucurbits, heated by a furnace, where the flue gases heat the bath through a copper dome which is emerging from the middle of the bath. This woodcut is the same as in Brunschwig's *Grosses Distillierbuch*.

tributed to the rise of iatrochemistry by demonstrating that drugs and other medicinals depend for their efficacy upon pure spirits of essences that can be extracted by the methods of chemistry.' (Martin Fichman in DSB). Distilling was a new trade and so was chemical pharmacy. Ulstad's *Coelum Philosophorum* and Brunschwig's *Grosses Distillierbuch*, with their wealth of woodcut illustrations of chemical apparatus, brought this knowledge to a wider public of apothecaries, surgeons and medical doctors, whereas hitherto the knowledge of pharmacology had been limited to a few experts, mainly in the monasteries.

Benzing, *Die Drucke Jakob Cammerlanders zu Strassburg* 1531–1548. No. 130; Partington, II, pp. 84-6; Fergusson, II pp. 482-3; Duveen, pp. 591-2; Martin Fichman in DSB, XIII, pp. 534-5; Thorndike, V, pp. 541-2; Edward R. Atkinson & Arthur H. Hughes, 'The "Coelum Philosophorum" of Philipp Ulstad', in *Journal of Chemical Education*, 16, pp. 103-07; Forbes, *Short History of the Art of Distillation* (Leiden, 1948) pp. 127-30; Waller 9742 (Cammerlander, 1536).

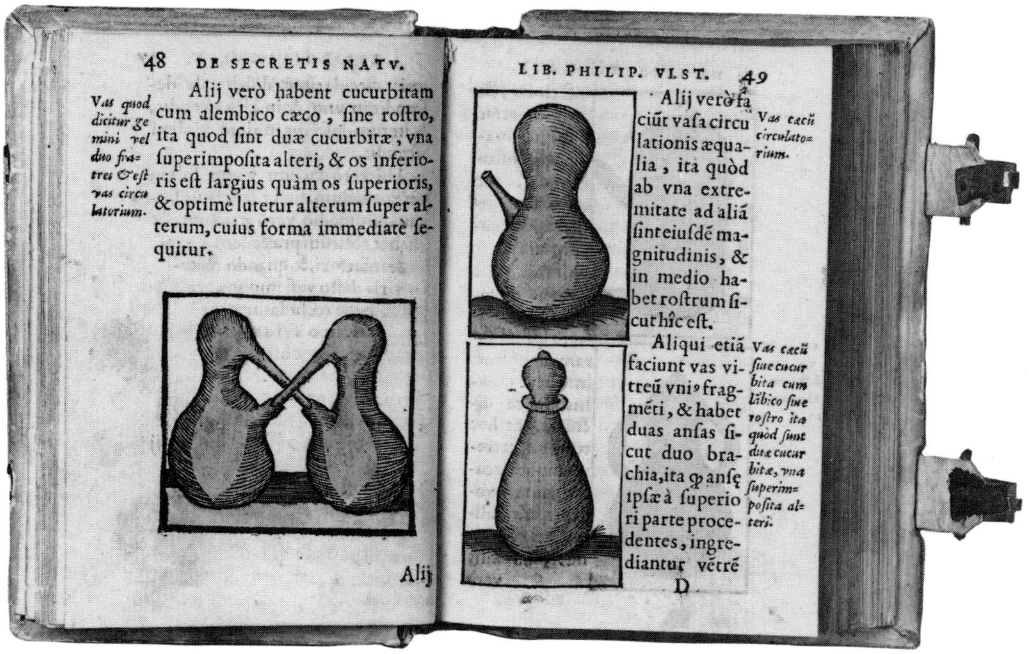

48 DE SECRETIS NATV.

Alij verò habent cucurbitam cum alembico cæco, ſine roſtro, ita quod ſint duæ cucurbitæ, vna ſuperimpoſita alteri, & os inferioris eſt largius quàm os ſuperioris, & optimè lutetur alterum ſuper alterum, cuius forma immediatè ſequitur.

Vas quod dicitur gemini vel duo fratres & eſt vas circulatorium.

Alij

LIB. PHILIP. VLST. 49

Alij verò faciũt vaſa circulationis æqualia, ita quòd ab vna extremitate ad aliã ſint eiuſdẽ magnitudinis, & in medio habet roſtrum ſicut hĩc eſt.

Vas cæcũ circulatorium.

Aliqui etiã faciunt vas vitreũ vniꝰ fragmẽti, & habet duas anſas ſicut duo brachia, ita ꝙ anſę ipſæ à ſuperiori parte procedentes, ingrediantur vẽtrẽ

Vas cæcũ ſine cucurbita cum lãbico ſiue roſtro ita quòd ſunt duæ cucurbitæ, vna ſuperimpoſita alteri.

D

Our copy of the pocket edition of Ulstad's *Coelum philosophorum* has many of the woodcuts coloured by hand. Most of them depict various types of vessels. One of these, a so-called 'double pelican' or 'twins', a medieval type of distilling vessel used for circulation, is shown above and is also reproduced in colour as a vignette on the front cover of this catalogue.

One of few surviving complete copies

EGENOLPH, Christian (1502–1555), publisher

Herbarum imagines vivae. Der kreuter lebliche Conterfeytunge. [*with*]: Imaginum herbarum, pars II. Andertheyl der Kreutter Conterfeytungenn.

Frankfurt a.M., Christian Egenolph, 1538, 1536.

Small quarto – *leaf*: 193 x 140 *mm. Part* I.: 44 *leaves, sign.* A-L4. *Ff.* 40, [4] *index. With* 226 *woodcuts of plants, five of which are repeated on the title page; Part* II.: 22 *leaves, sign.* a-e4 f2. *Ff.* 20, [2] *index. With* 65 *woodcuts of plants, three of which are repeated on the title page along with a woodcut of an idyllic landscape scene with three persons and a dog. All woodcuts are hand-coloured. Clean and almost untrimmed copy with both parts bound in one volume. Modern vellum over wooden boards.*

This very fine copy was described by Willy Heimann in *Catalogue Six* from Sandberg's Rare Book Department, item 30. The book was purchased for SEK 1200, a sum collected at the Annual Meeting of the *Apotekare Societeten* (Swedish Pharmaceutical Society) in 1951, and presented to their library. It was a pretty good investment, as a similar copy was offered for sale at the Antiquarian Book Fair in Cologne some years ago at a price one hundred times higher. A copy such as this, fully complete with the almost unobtainable second volume, and with all the woodcuts in the original handcolouring, is of extreme rarity. The experienced bookseller and scholar, Willy Heimann, found it to be practically unknown to botanical literature. He refers to Alfred Schmid, the great authority on old herbals, who in his *Ueber alte Kräuterbücher* (1939) says that the book is 'fast völlig verschwunden'. Already F.W.E. Roth (1902) said that, in spite of its being reprinted at least once, complete copies are hardly ever found, and the very few copies that have survived are worn out and incomplete.

In 1530, when the Strassburg printer Johann Schott published the first volume of Brunfels' *Herbarum Vivae Eicones* ('Living Pictures of Plants'), it was the first time that the illustrations in a herbal were based on living plants, and not copied from crudely drawn pictures of preceding centuries, as were many illustrations in the early herbals. For this purpose Schott had employed Hans Weiditz, a highly skilled artist, who is known as one of the best book illustrators of the period. In 1533, the Frankfurt publisher Christian Egenolph issued a *Kreutterbuch* in folio compiled by the town physician in Frankfurt, Eucharius Rösslin. The book was illustrated with woodcuts pirated from Brunfels' herbal but in a smaller size and reversed. Egenolph was taken to court by the Strassburg printer and was evidently legally compelled to hand over all the blocks he had plagiarized to Schott. There is no record of the actual result of the suit, but in 1534 Schott published the *Kreuterbuch contrafayt*, a German edition in quarto of Brunfels' *Herbarum*, illustrated in the main with the very cuts that had been used by Egenolph in Rösslin's *Kreutterbuch*. It was an expensive lesson, but also one that Egenolph blithely ignored, as he shortly afterwards (in 1535) issued the first volume of the above-mentioned popular edition, intended for an uneducated public, printed without text except for the names of the plants in German and Latin and with an index at the end. The second volume followed in 1536.

Egenolph was evidently a man keen on business and with a flair for picture-books to attract the public. Like many other publishers, he saw no reason to increase his expenses by engaging competent artists to depict the plants themselves, but hired block cutters to copy the illustrations in the botanical works of his competitors. In the preface to his *Historia stirpium* (1542) Fuchs refers unsparingly to the botanical mistakes in the Frankfurt books: 'Among all the herbals which exist today, there are none which have more of the crassest errors than those which Egenolph, the printer, has already published again and again'. Later on Egenolph plagiarized woodcuts from both Fuchs' and Bock's herbals. Whatever their importance in the history of botany may be, the many illustrations in the popular herbals published by Egenolph still have considerable and independent merit because of their freshness and vigor, and the unusually fluid and decorative style of the block cutters who produced them.

Pritzel, 2626 (1536, 1538); Nissen, BBI, 2344 (1535, 1538); Junk, *List* 53/37 (1538); Goldschmidt, *Cat.* 159/93, with the title page reproduced on p. 48 (first part only, dated 1535); Durling, 1350 (1536, 1538); Heimann, *Some Rare Books and Autographs,* List No. 6/30, Sandbergs Rare Book Department, 1951; Alfred Schmid, *Zwei seltene Kräuterbücher aus dem vierten Dezennium des sechzehnten Jahrhunderts.* Separatabdruck aus dem Schweizerischen Gutenbergmuseum, 1936, Nr. 3, *nebst einem bibliographischen Verzeichnis aller bekannten frühen Ausgaben der Brunfelsschen Kräuterbücher* als Anhang. Bern, 1936 (20 pp.); Schmid, *Ueber alte Kräuterbücher*, pp. 23-5, with both title pages reproduced; Arber, pp. 70-4, 209-12; Meyer, IV, p. 335 (1533!).

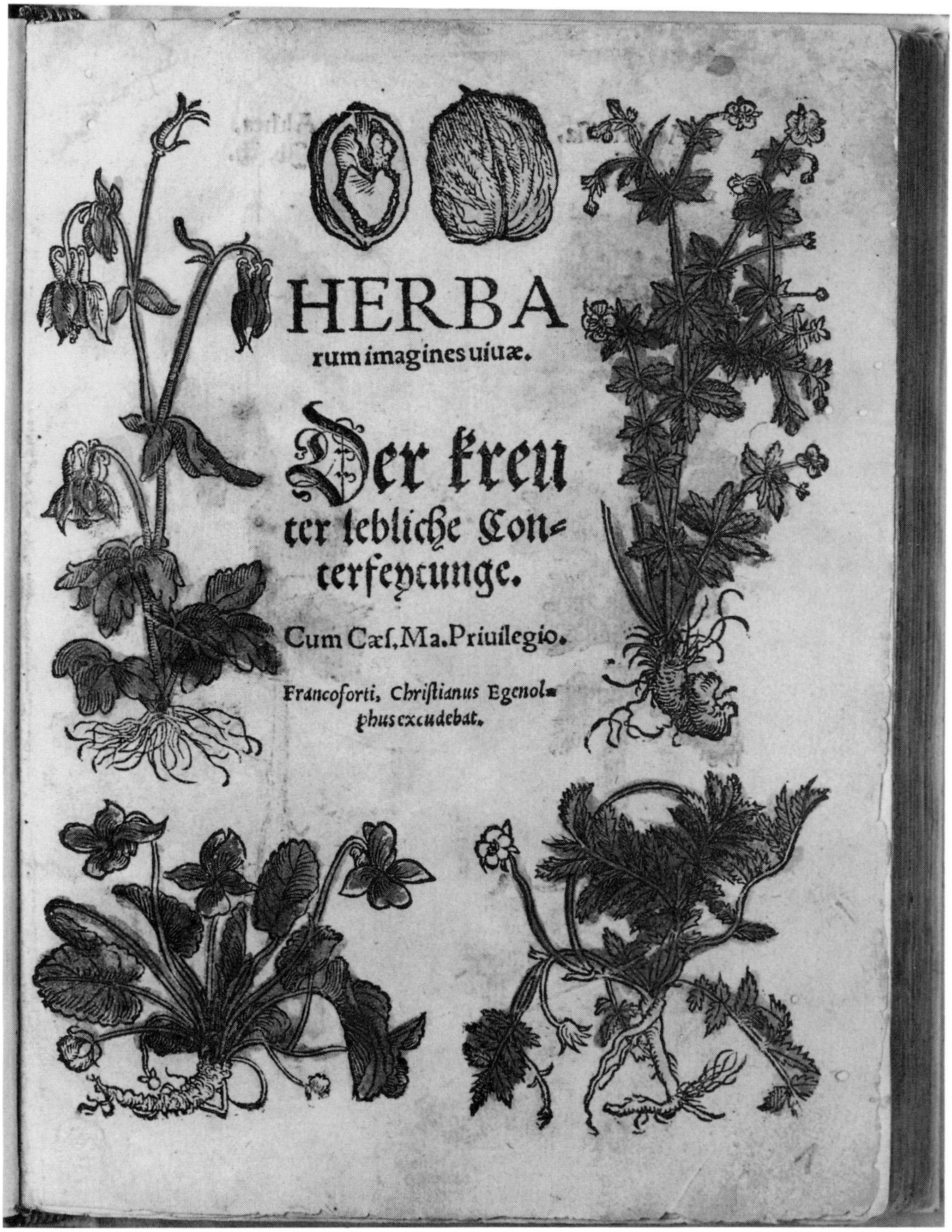

The title page to the 1538 issue of Egenolph's *Herbarum imagines vivae* is reset as compared to the 1535 issue, which has 'Contrafaytung' instead of 'Conterfeytunge' as well as typographical differences.

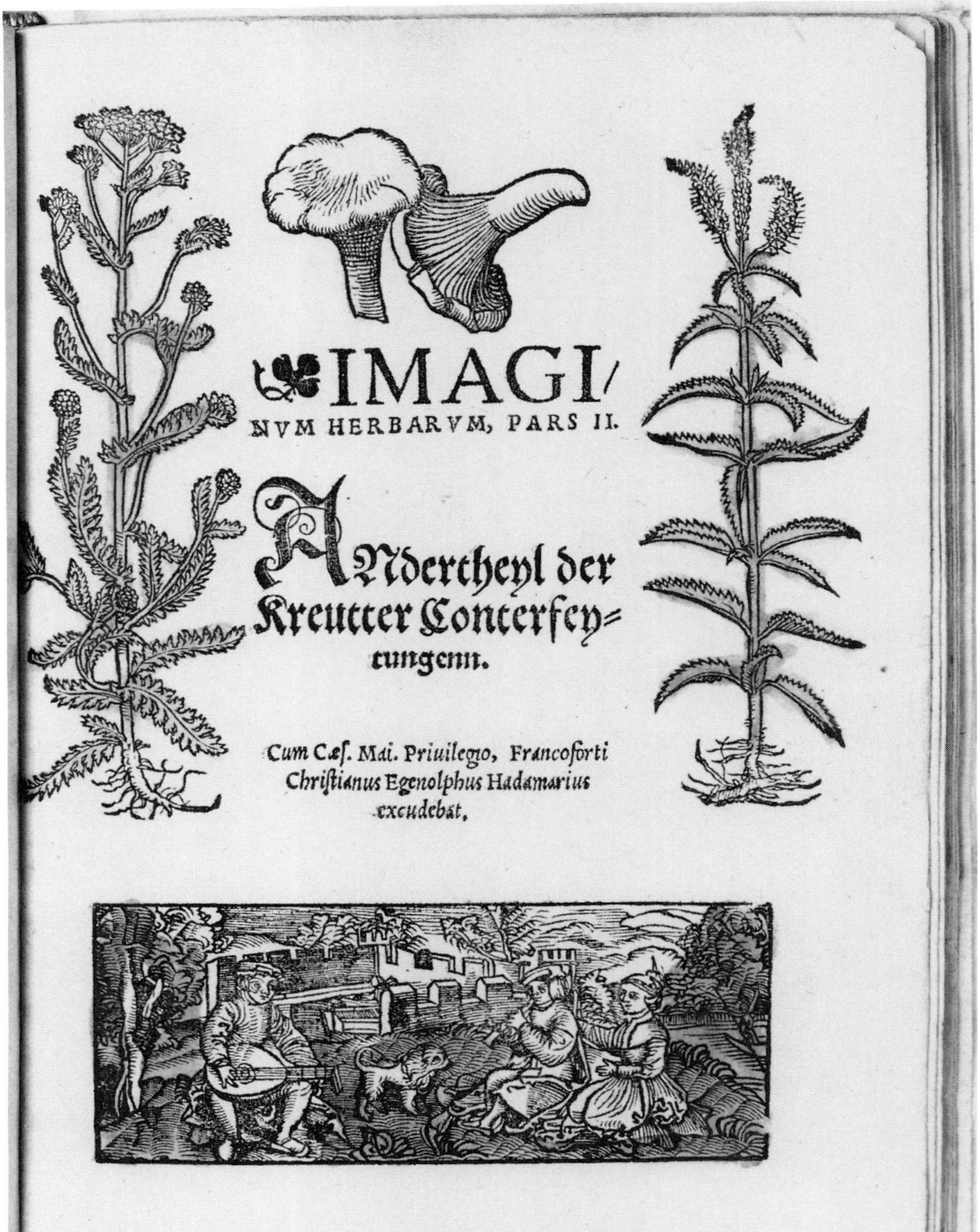
IMAGI/
NVM HERBARVM, PARS II.

Andertheyl der
Kreutter Conterfey=
tungenn.

Cum Cæs. Mai. Priuilegio, Francoforti
Christianus Egenolphus Hadamarius
excudebat.

The three botanical woodcuts on the title page to this second part of Egenolph's illustrated *Herbarum* are repeated inside the book. The vignette depicts an idyllic scenery with two musicians, one playing the lute, the other the flute; a girl and a dog are listening.

EGENOLPH, Christian (1502–1555)

Hundreds of woodcuts of plants and fabulous beasts

Herbarum, Arbarum, Fruticum ac Leguminum. Animalium præterea terrestrium, volatilium & aquatilium, . . . Kreutter, Bäume, Gesteude, unnd Früicht, Dessgleichen Gethier, zam unnd wild, im Lufft, Wasser und Erdtrich lebende. Mit sampt anderen Materialen und Simplicien, zur Artznei dienlich, recht Conterfaytet, und mit iren namen benennet.

Frankfurt am Main, Christian Egenolph, 1546.

Small quarto – *leaf:* 183 x 140 *mm. Pp.* [16], 265, [3]. *Sign.:* o^4 $*^4$ A-Z^4 a-i^4 k^6. *Lacks seven leaves:* F4, V1, a4, b4, k3, k4 *and the final blank* (k6). *Large woodcut on the title page. Illustrated throughout with c.* 800 *small woodcuts. Recased in modern vellum, new endpapers, title leaf and some other leaves restored.*

Signature in pencil, dated 1818: Carl Mangnus [Må]nson.

Book-plate: C.D. Carlsson.

Another of Egenolph's many popular picture-books, in which he made use of his large stock of woodblocks of plants and animals. Most of them were earlier used in Rösslin's *Kreuterbuch*, and later in Lonicerus *Kreuterbuch*. There are about 800 small woodcuts, of which some 660 of plants, all said to be useful in medicine.The last pages feature pictures of animals living in the air, on the earth and in the sea, including basilisk, unicorn, griffin, dragons and other fabulous beasts. In some copies the figures are coloured. There is no text other than an index in the prelims and the names of the plants and animals in German and Latin. There were many editions, all of which are rare. Few of the surviving copies are complete. The fine woodcut of a gardener on the title page is by Hans Weiditz.

Durling (NLM) 1351; Bird (Edinburgh Libraries) 785.

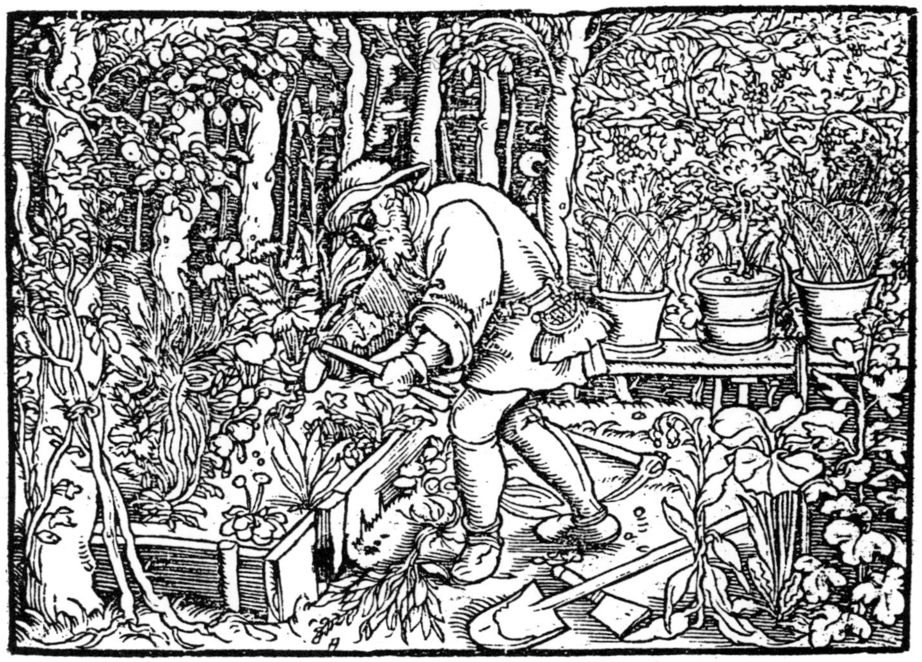

FRANCOFORTI, Apud Chr. Egenolphum.

The most complete treatise on botany since Theophrastus

RUEL, Jean (1474–1537)

De natura stirpium libris tres.
Basel, in Officina Frobeniana, 1543.

Folio – *leaf*: 325 *x* 220 *mm. Pp.* [92], 666, [2]. *Last page with Froben's device. Lacks one leaf* [*pp.* 659-60]. *Contemporary brown calf, blind fillets, inner frame with a gilt fleuron in outer corners, centrepiece with four gilt trefoils.*

Reprint of the Froben edition of 1537. The original edition which had appeared in 1536 is a typographical masterpiece and one of the finest sixteenth century French books; its superb pictorial title border depicting emblematic figures in a luxuriant garden setting, specially designed for Ruel's book, makes it the most famous book printed by Simon de Colines in Paris. Nevertheless, the present Basel edition with Froben's pigeon and serpent device on the title is also a noble folio volume.

Jean Ruel, born at Soissons in the year 1474, took his M.D. in 1508 and in the following year became physician to Francis I. Thoroughly absorbed in his own scholarly works, Ruel refused to follow the court on its frequent travels. When his wife died he entered holy orders so that he could devote himself entirely to study. The bishop of Paris obtained a canonry at the cathedral of Notre-Dame for him and Ruel was thus freed of material concerns. His first published work was his influential and excellent Latin version of Dioscorides. From the year 1516, when the first edition appeared, Latin versions of Dioscorides became numerous and for a whole century thereafter the most voluminous and most useful herbals were in the form of commentaries on the Greek pharmacist's *De materia medica*. Ruel also translated into Latin the pharmacopoeia *De medicamentorum compositione* written in about 1330 by the Byzantine physician Joannes Actuarios (1539).

Ruel is the first, next after Theophrastus – and fully seventeen centuries later – to undertake the preparation of a complete treatise on botany in general. While Hans Weiditz in Strassburg was executing the illustrations for Brunfels' herbal, Ruel in Paris was engaged in the composition of his great classic, the *De Natura stirpium*. The preparation of this thick volume confined its author during some eighteen years to a sedentary life, and may naturally account for the sudden ending of his life by cerebral haemorrhage soon after its appearance from the press in 1536. It antedates the noted books of the German Fathers of Botany except for that of Brunfels. The others: Fuchs, Bock, and Valerius Cordus, had the aid of Ruel in the identification of their plants, and Fuchs made generous acknowledgments on behalf of himself and his botanical countrymen on their obligations to the learned Parisian. Brunfels' herbal, with its life-like pictures of plants, would meet the needs of even an unlettered but intelligent peasant, as well as the apothecaries and others who wished for a book helping them easily to identify common plants – the comprehensive and unillustrated work by Ruel, however, would have no appeal to any of these, or be of much use to those unskilled in Latin and the Latin terminology of plant description.

The *De natura stirpium libri tres* is elegantly written and furnishes many vernacular plant names. The three 'Books' mainly consist of descriptions of about 600 plants. The first twenty-two chapters of Book I are of great interest since they take the form of a general treatment of botany, the first since Theophrastus, whom Ruel considered the father of botany. Instead of botanical classification, Ruel used alphabetical order, which gave the book a great practical value. In each chapter one subject only is discussed: for example, stalk, leaves, bark, flowers, germination, grafting, vegetables, cereals, and medicinal properties. He also provided information on odours and tastes of plants. The book is dedicated to Ruel's patron, Francis I, who paid for the printing.

From the preface to his *Stirpium* we learn that it must have been written during a period when this 'sedentary man' had time and strength for personal botanical exploration and that his knowledge of plants was not only acquired from books:

> 'I have walked through the vast solitudes of many different regions, traversed the pathless heights of mountains; surveyed the shores of the most inaccessible lakes, have scrutinized the cavernous places of the earth, penetrated the deepest ravines, have sometimes even imperilled my life clambering about the most dangerous precipices, all this in order that I might closely examine and well comprehend – even when still unable to identify them by their ancient names – the things about which I had the intention to write' (from Greene/Egerton, p. 600).

Greene /Egerton, II, pp. 598-657; DSB, XI, 495-6; Johnston, *Cleveland Herbals*, 51.

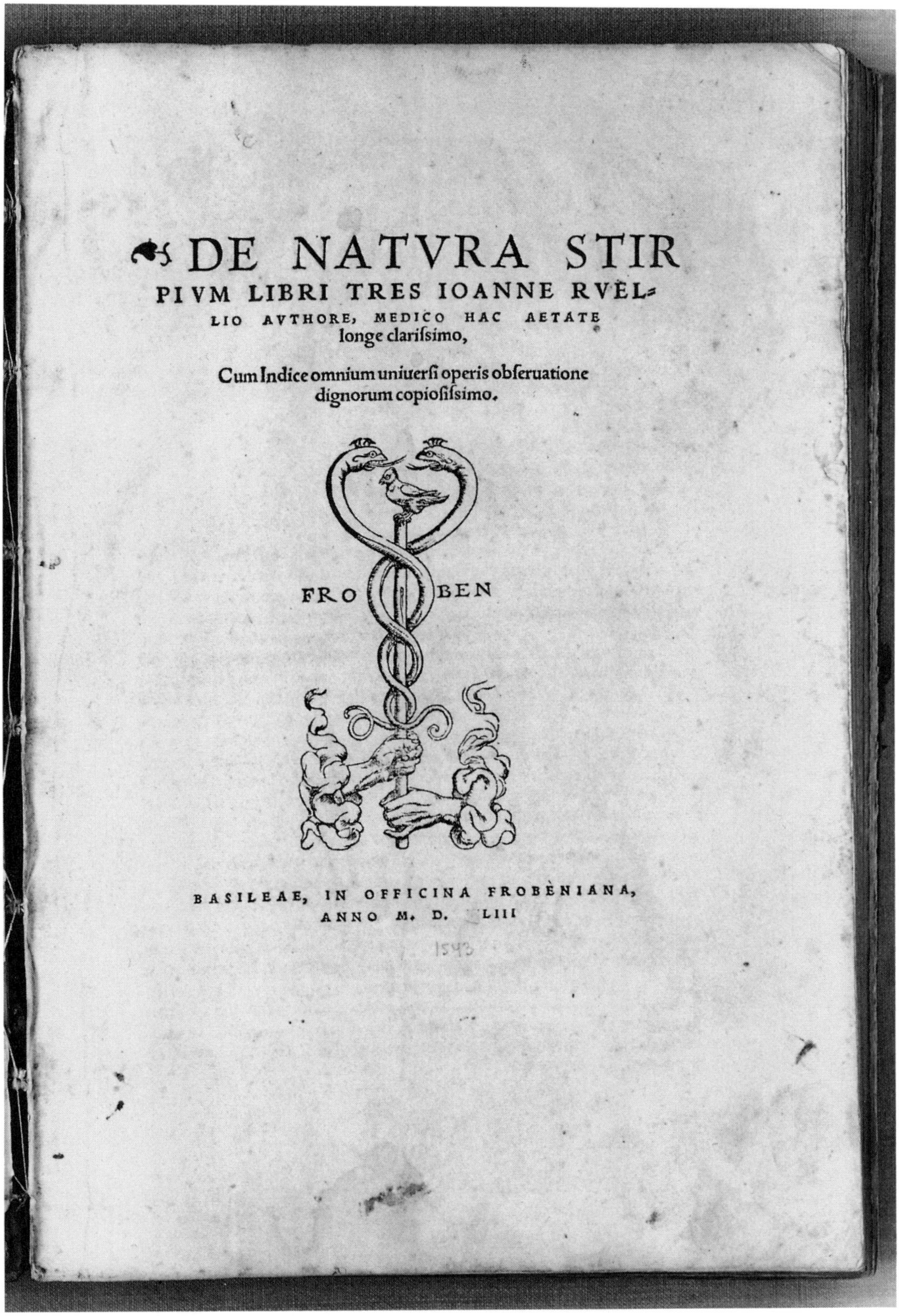

DE NATVRA STIRPIVM LIBRI TRES IOANNE RVELLIO AVTHORE, MEDICO HAC AETATE longe clarissimo,

Cum Indice omnium uniuersi operis obseruatione dignorum copiosissimo.

BASILEAE, IN OFFICINA FROBENIANA, ANNO M. D. XLIII

1543

Handbook for apothecaries

BRUNFELS, Otto (1488–1534) & **Lorenz FRIES** (c.1490–1531)
Von allerhandt Apoteckischen Confectionen, Lattwergen, Oel, Pillulen, Tränncken, Trociscen, Zucker scheiblein, Salben unnd Pflastern etc. Wie, wenn, unnd warzu man jedes brauchen soll, ein kurtzer Bericht D. Otthonis Brunnfelsii.
Gedruckt zu Franckfurdt am Mayn, durch Hermann Gülfferichen, inn der Schnurgassen zum Krug, 1552.

Small quarto – *leaf*: 183 *x* 137 *mm. 16 leaves, signed* A-D4. *Last page with full-page printer's device. Title printed in red and black with woodcut vignette of three apothecary jars. Modern grey boards.*

This rare little handbook, explaining when and for what ailments each remedy is to be used, is another compilation of the notorious plagiarist and compiler Walter Hermann Ryff, who in the preface to the reader uses the pseudonym Q[uintus] Appolinaris. The text is compiled from works of Otto Brunfels and Lorenz Fries. Ryff admits here that 'ist diss Büchlein auch nicht mein, sondern zum theyl Laurentii Friesenn, unnd Otthonis Braunfelsii, beid erfarne Doctores . . . auss den alten Artzten durch ihren fleiss zusamen geschrieben . . .'

It was first printed by Jacob Cammerlander in Strassburg about 1540, which edition, besides two woodcut figures in the text, also has two large woodcuts on the title page, one depicting three persons collecting herbs, the other an apothecary in his shop crushing herbs in a mortar, not found in the above edition.

Benzing, *Ryff*, No.3; Benzing, *Cammerlander*, No. 104; The title page of the Cammerlander edition is reproduced in Joachim Telle (ed.), *Pharmazie und der gemeine Mann* (Herzog August Bibliothek, Wolffenbüttel), 2nd ed., 1988, p. 54; Waller 1563.

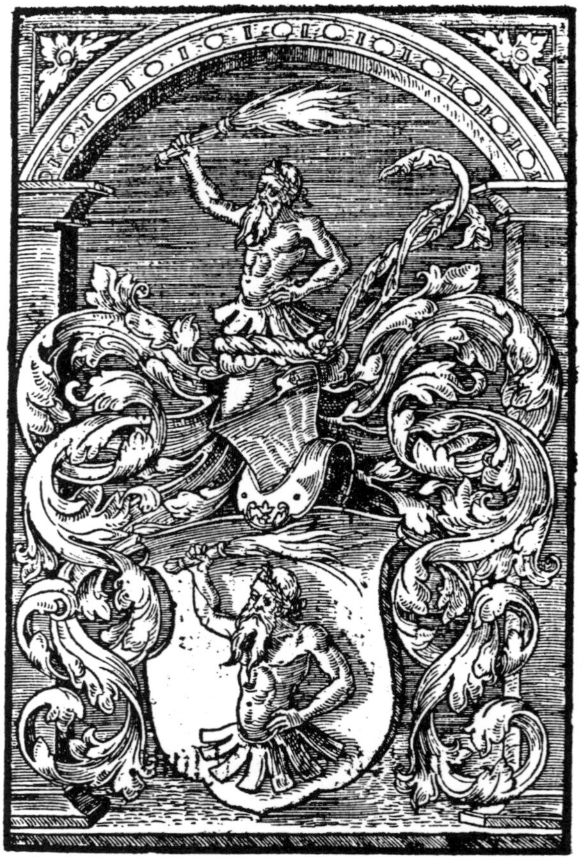

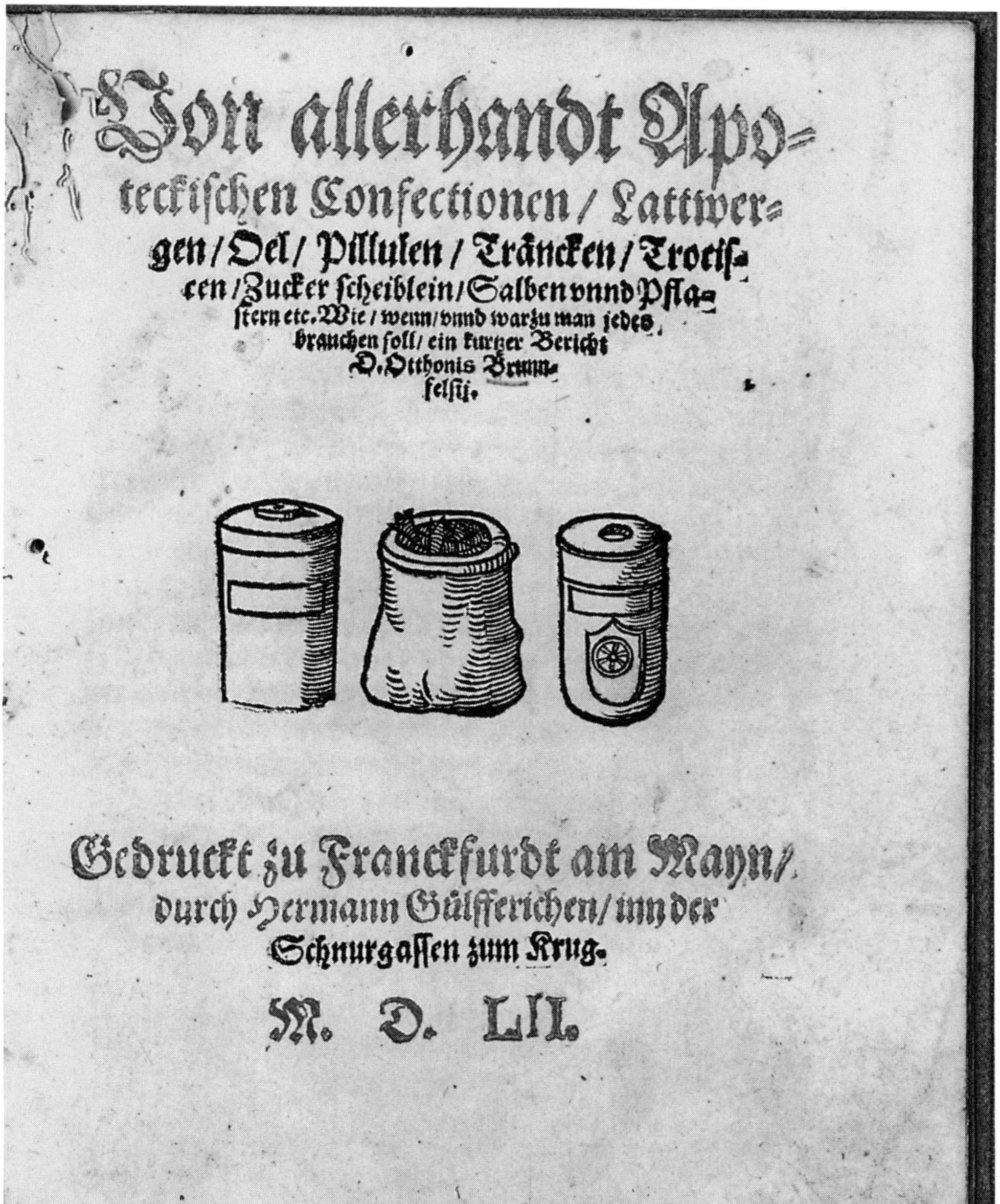

Von allerhandt Apo-
teckischen Confectionen / Lattwer-
gen / Oel / Pillulen / Träncken / Trocis-
cen / Zucker scheiblein / Salben vnnd Pfla-
stern etc. Wie / wenn / vnnd warzu man jedes
brauchen soll / ein kurtzer Bericht
D. Otthonis Brunn-
felsii.

Gedruckt zu Franckfurdt am Mayn /
durch Hermann Gülfferichen / inn der
Schnurgassen zum Krug.

M. D. LII.

RYFF, Walther Hermann (c. 1495–1548)

Rechter und nutzlicher gebrauch, ordenliche vermischung und zubereyttung aller Laxativen, purgierender oder treibender artzney, eynfacher, gemeyner unvermischter stuck, auch vermischter und zusamen gesetzter, treibender artzney, mancherley Compositzen von Latwergen, täflin, getränck, pulver, Clyster, stulzäplin, Pillen unnd dergleichen vermischung, den leib zureinigen und purgieren, wie solche diese zeyt bey den erfarnesten ärtzten im brauch, unnd in allen rechtgeschaffnen Apotecken bereyttet werden, Sampt nutzlicher unnd notwendiger erklärung ir natur, eygenschafft, krafft und würckung, auch wie solche auff das best erwölet, warhefftig erkennet, rechtgeschaffen bereyttet und zugericht werden sollen, Für mancherley kranckheyt, fäl und gebrechen menschlichs leibs. Zu neüwer Reformation der Apoteckerey, vast nutzlich, und hoch von nöten.

Colophon: Strassburg, Balthasar Beck, 1541.

Quarto – *leaf*: 193 *x* 152 *mm. Ff.* [4], 163, [5]. *Sign.*: A-Z4 a-v4 (*last leaf blank*). *Contemporary white pigskin, three double bands, richly blindstamped in panels. Remains of leather ties. A very fine copy.*

Book-plate: C.D. Carlsson.

This is the first edition of what in the following year came to form the third part of Ryff's *Der kleynen Teütschen Apoteck oder Confectbüchlein* (Strassburg, the heirs of Balthasar Beck, 1542).

Walter [Gualtherus] Hermann Ryff, a native of Strassburg, was one of the most prolific and voluminous writers of his generation within the domain of medicine, pharmacy and allied sciences. He was the editor of Dioscorides, Pliny, Albertus Magnus and the alchemist Raymond Lull, and also an industrious compiler. His literary talents were exploited by several business-minded German publishers, who in Ryff found a golden goose for the compilation of medical books in the vernacular, that had a market not only for medical practitioners but for the general public. People who suffered from any ailment whatsoever could with the help of these books treat themselves instead of consulting a doctor, which of course promoted the widespread quackery of the day. In composing his numerous publications on medicine, pharmacy, surgery, obstetrics, distillation, etc., Ryff had no scruples in appropriating material wherever he could find it. Ryff is known as one of the most notorious plagiarists who robbed the works of others, and therefore brought on himself the wrath of his contemporaries, who showed no mercy for his shortcomings, either as a man or as an author.

Conrad Gesner in his *Bibliotheca universalis* (1545) pilloried Ryff as an absolutely unpardonable ignoramus and plagiarist who published a steady stream of books, especially in medicine, anatomy, pharmacy and surgery, fields in which he knew nothing, with commentaries that were worthless except for what was copied from others, particularly from the works of Leonhart Fuchs, Hieronymus Bock, Andreas Vesalius and Gesner himself. The *Nürnbergische Gelehrten-Lexicon* (1757) states that Ryff came to Nürnberg and became municipal physician. However, its editor, Georg Andreas Will, also calls Ryff a shameless plagiarist, who did nothing but invent splendid titles and translate the works of Fuchs, Gesner, and other famous physicians into German, passing them as his own compositions.

Ryff not only copied the most famous obstetrical textbook, Roesslin's *Rosengarten,* but even more unfortunately added antiquated theories and prescriptions which he found in earlier medical works. Vesalius writes in a letter to his printer, Johann Oporinus, that 'the fellow in Strassburg played a scurvy trick on scholars in that he so shamefully cramped the engravings [from Vesalius' *Fabrica*] and issued them as his own, wretchedly reproduced, and reduced in size out of all reason'. Fuchs called Ryff the most brazen of mortals and was involved in a serious polemic with Ryff's publisher in Frankfurt, Christian Egenolph.

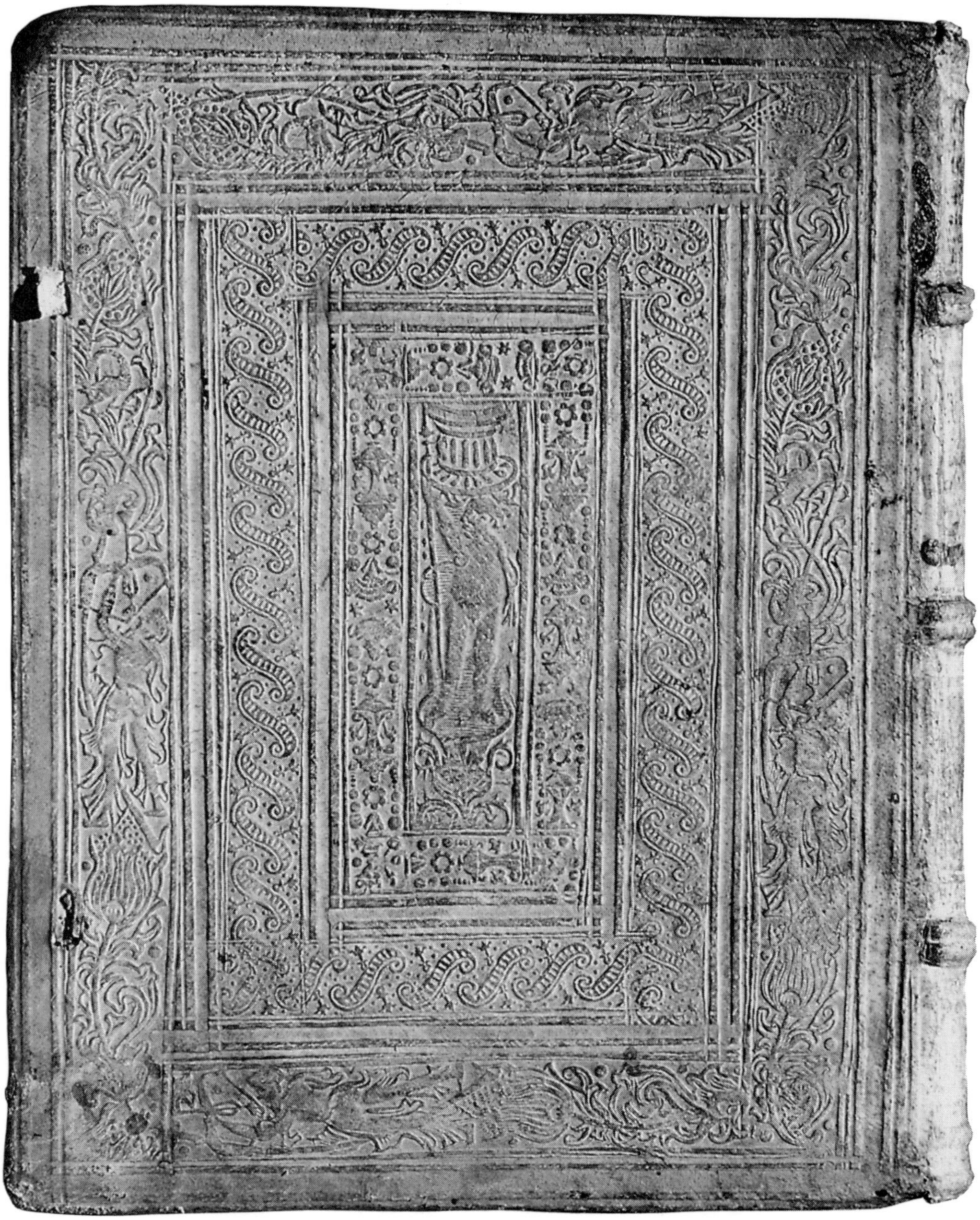

The greater part of sixteenth century medical literature was formed of speculating enterprises rather than serious medical publishing. That the publishing of these often beautifully printed and excellently illustrated popular books was a lucrative business is proved by the many editions the books went through. Benzing in his bibliography of Ryff lists no less than 194 items, which proves that Ryff was successful as the author of many best sellers. The often thick volumes with long and wordy titles were usually richly illustrated with splendid woodcuts, most of which were also copied from the works of others.

Benzing, 100.

How to prepare sweetmeats

RYFF, Walther Hermann (c.1495–1548)

Confect Büchlin, und Hauss Apoteck. Kunstlich zu Bereyten, Einmachen, und recht gebrauchen, mancherhandt nutzbare Confect, Latwergen, Conserva oder Conditen, Sirop, Julep, und andere künstliche getränck, zum lust und noturfft, Sampt notwendigen stücken ausserhalb leibs zebrauchen, als Öl, Pflaster, Salben, Bäder, Behungen, etc. Item was zu güttem Geruch und lieblichem Geräuch dienet, als Pom Ambre, Bisam säcklin, wolriechende pulver, unnd Seyffen küglin. Aqua vitae, unnd ander bewerte Krafft wasser. Alles so diser gestalt dem gemeynen man zu täglicher noturfft dienlich unnd nütz, gnügsame und treuliche underrichtung. Dabei kurtze Erklerung ieder Mass, Zal, Gewicht, und aller einfachen stück, vonn Kreuttern, Wurtzeln, Blümen, Samen, Frücht, Gethier, unnd Gesteyn, zu Artzney dienlich unnd zebrauchen.

Frankfurt am Main, Christian Egenolff, 1544.

Quarto – *leaf*: 190 *x* 140 *mm. Ff.* [32], 159, [1] *blank. Sign.*: x4 a-g4 A-Z4, a-r4. *Title printed in red and black with two small woodcuts. Illustrated with* 55 *woodcuts of plants and pharmaceutical equipment. Bound together with Ryff's* New Kochbuch *in contemporary richly blindstamped pigskin over wooden boards, three double bands, brass clasps.*

Book-plate: C.D. Carlsson.

First edition of Ryff's *Confect Büchlein*, one of the most popular cookery books in Germany, which went through a dozen editions. It is probably the best book of the period on how to prepare sweetmeats and drinks for the household with a large collection of recipes for various healthy mixtures.

The book opens with costly medicaments as *Teriaca Andromachi* and *Aurea Alexandrina* as well as drugs called *Narcotica* or *Opiate*. The second part describes a multitude of various sweetmeats from flowers, fruits, herbs, etc., prepared with honey and sugar. It is followed by a great variety of drinks, syrups, oils, salves and even various aromatic substances burnt for their fragrance. There is also a recipe for *Aqua vitae*, a distilled strong drink. All is illustrated with small woodcuts in the text.

Benzing, 135.

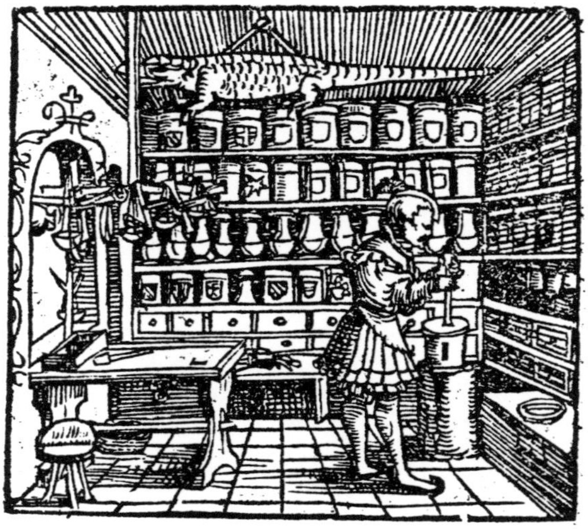

Confect Büchlin/

vnd Hauß Apoteck.

Kunstlich zu Bereyten/ Einmachen/ vnd recht gebrauchen/ mancherhandt nutzbare Confect/ Latwergen/ Conserua oder Conditen/ Sirop/ Julep/ vnd andre künstliche geträncк/ zum lust vñ notturfft/ Sampt notwendigen stücken ausserhalb leibs zebrauchen/ als Öl/ pflaster/ Salben/ Bäder/ Behungen ꝛc. Item was zu güttem Geruch vnd lieblichem Geräuch dienet/ als Pom Ambre/ Bisam säcklin/ wolriechende puluer/ vnnd Seyffen küglin. Aqua uitæ, vnnd ander bewerte Krafft wasser. Alles so diser gestalt dem gemeynen man zu täglicher notturfft dienlich vnnd nütz/ gnügsame vnd treuliche vnderrichtung.

Dabei kurtze Erklerung ieder Maß/ Zal/ Gewicht/ vnd aller einfachen stück/ vonn Kreuttern/ Wurtzeln/ Blůmen/ Samen/ Frücht/ Gethier/ vnnd Gesteyn/ zu der Artzney dienlich vnnd zebrauchen. New ann tag geben/ Durch

Gualtherum H. Ryff, Argent. Medicum.

Mit Keyserlichen Gnaden vnd Priuilegio.

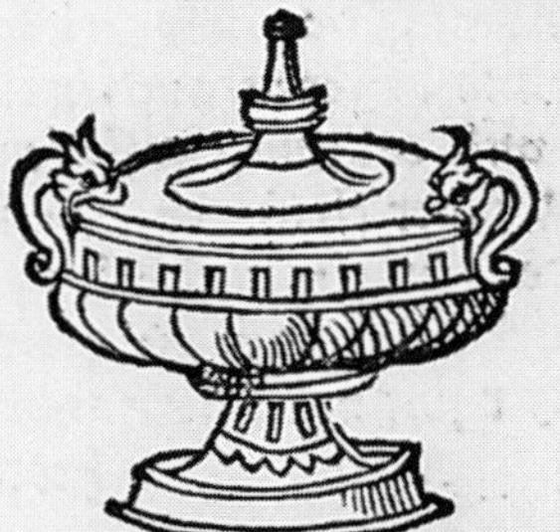

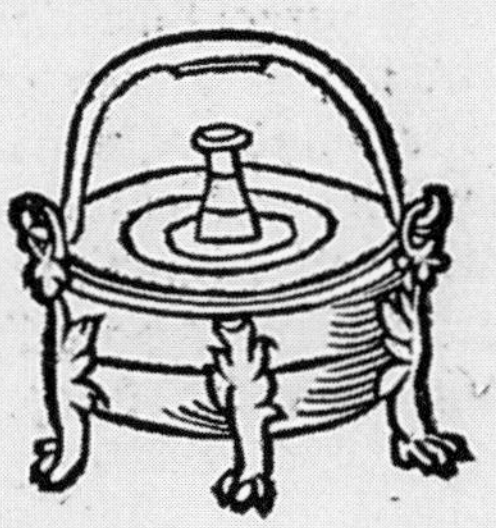

Zu Franckfort/ Bei Christian Egenolff.

RYFF, Walther Hermann (c. 1495–1548)

Cook-book for the sick

New Kochbuch, Für die Krancken. Wie mann krancker Personen, In mancherley Fehl und Gebrechen des leibs pflegen, Mit zurichtung unnd Kochung viler nützlicher gesunder Speiss, Getränck, und allen eusserlichen dingen warten sol. Den Kranckenwartern, unnd sunst iederman in der noturfft zu underweisung gestelt, . . .

Frankfurt am Main, Christian Egenolff, 1545.

Quarto – *leaf*: 190 *x* 140 *mm. Ff.* [4], 152. *Sign.:* π4 A-Z4 a-p4. *Title with a woodcut depicting an interior of a kitchen and a sickroom, printed in red and black. A few woodcuts in the text. Bound together with Ryff's* Confect Büchlein *in contemporary richly blindstamped pigskin over wooden boards, three double bands, brass clasps.*

Book-plate: C.D. Carlsson.

First edition of one of Ryff's own works dealing with dietetics and cooking for the sick. At the beginning of the text is a woodcut of a sick-room.

It seems that the pharmacological works of Ryff are the only that show some independence. Ryff had evidently started his career to learn the apothecary's trade, which he practised in Güstrow in Mecklenburg. Here he also got married to Anna from Rostock. He later lived in Strassburg and may have served there as town physician, thus being a successor of Hieronymus Brunschwig. He names himself *Medici* or *Chirurgi* on the title pages of his books from this period. Here he also started his literary career writing under the pseudonym of Q. Appolinaris. His first works were printed by the famous publisher of popular books, Jacob Cammerlander. Later on he became the house-author of Balthasar Beck until he early in 1544 was engaged by Christian Egenolph in Frankfurt am Main, who was the leading publisher of popular medical books in Germany. After a productive period at Egenolph's, Ryff moved to Nuremberg where he translated Vitruvius into German and published his perhaps greatest work, this time on architecture and perspective, the so-called Ryff's *Architectur*, one of the most richly illustrated Nuremberg imprints of the post-Dürer period, a book that is often called the Bible of the German Post-Renaissance. It went through three editions, the last printed by Sebastian Henricpetri in Basel, 1582. Eventually Ryff settled in Würzburg where he died on 29 September, 1548.

Benzing, 160; Waller 8356.

Von vnmessigen bauchfluß/
oder durchbruch des leibs.

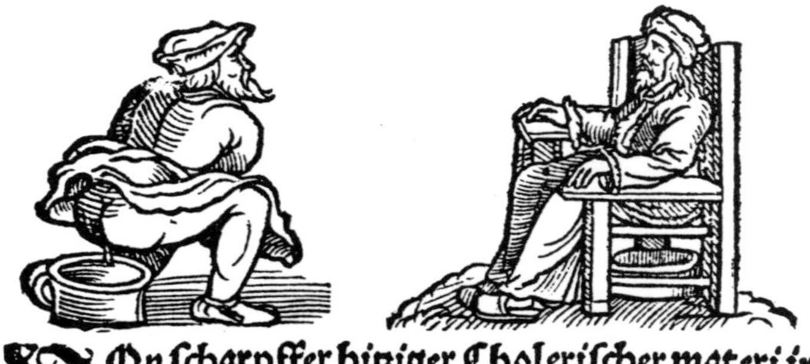

VOn scharpffer hitziger Cholerischer materi in scharpffen hitzigen febern vnnd gebrechen/ erhebt sich auch vnderweilen ein hefftiger vnmessiger durchbruch des leibs/vnd durchlauffen/Wo dann solcher fehl nit beschicht zu einem endzeychenn der kranckheyt/sol er gestopfft werden. Vnd magst in solchem fall dem Patienten vnderweilen nützlichen geben des sirops/oder safft Latwergen von Mir-

B

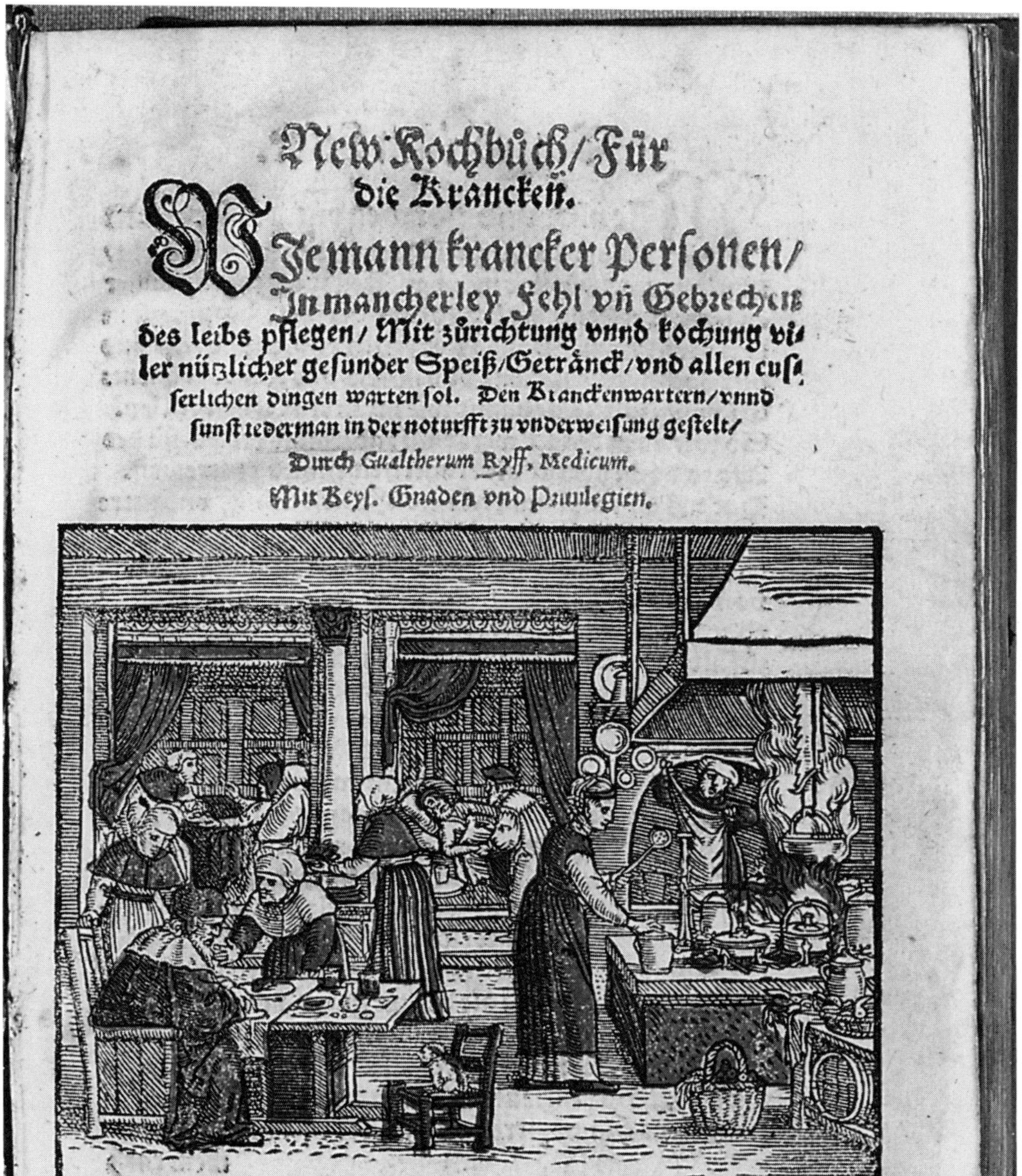

New Kochbůch/ Für
die Krancken.
W Je mann krancker Personen/
In mancherley Fehl vñ Gebrechen
des leibs pflegen/ Mit zůrichtung vnnd kochung vi-
ler nützlicher gesunder Speiß/Getränck/vnd allen eus-
serlichen dingen warten sol. Den Kranckenwartern/vnnd
sunst iederman in der notturfft zu vnderweisung gestelt/
Durch *Gualtherum* Ryff, *Medicum*.
Mit Keys. Gnaden vnd Priuilegien.

Illustrated with 166 hand-coloured woodcuts

RYFF, Walther Hermann (c. 1495–1548)

Reformierte Deütsche Apoteck Darinnen Eigentliche Contrafactur der Fürnembsten und Gebreüchlichsten Kreüter, sampt ihrer Underscheidung, Art, Natur, Krafft, Vermögen unnd Würckung. Auch was von den selbigen von APOTECKISCHEN stucken, unnd dergleichen vilfaltigen Vermischungen, der Speis und Artznei dienstlich, bereidt werden mögen, als Syrup, Lattwergen, Confect, Einbeitzung oder Einlegung und Conserven. Safft, auss gebrandte Wasser, gekreüttert Wein, Essig, öly, Salsen, und Condimenten, zu der Speis, Pflaster, Salben, unnd dergleichen vil andere mehr vast gebreüchliche Stuck, so dem Menschen nit allein in mancherlei Kranckheit, sonder auch den selben in Leiblicher Gesundtheit zu fristen und erhalten, vast nutzlich und uber die mass gebreuchlich unnd hoch von nöten. Item Beschreibung der Eltisten Lattwergen oder Confecten, des gerechten Tiriacks unnd Mithridats, sampt vilen andern alten, gebreüchlichen zusamen gesetzten und vermischten stucken, Auch Pomambre, Bisam säcklin, wolriechende Pulver, wie solliche alle Recht kunstlich gemacht unnd gebraucht werden sollen. Dergleichen von Recht nutzlichem gebrauch, auch Ordenlicher Vermischung und Zubereitung aller Laxativen, Purgierender oder Dreibender Artzney, Einfacher gemeiner unvermischter auch vermischter stuck, mancherley Compositzen, den Leib zu Reinigen und Purgieren. Sampt einem Nutzlichen Regiment, wie man sich inn Sterbens leüffen und Pestilentzischen Fiebern bewahren und verhalten soll. Alles durch den Wolgelehrten D. Gualtherum H. Ryff, Argent. Medicum beschriben, und zuvor im Truck nie aussgangen.

Strassburg, Josia Rihel, 1573.

Folio – *leaf*: 326 *x* 208 *mm. Ff.* [10], 262, [16] *last blank,* 128, [6]. *Title printed in red and black. With 166 hand-coloured woodcuts. Four leaves with Ms index inserted before the text* (*fol.*1). *Title leaf mounted. Rebound in early nineteenth century half calf, marbled boards, red edges, new endpapers.*

C.D. Carlsson Collection (*no book-plate*). *Two early owners' signatures on the title, both partly worn out and unidentified. One* 'Peter W . . .' [Wilde *?*], *dated* 1674, *the other dated* 1696. *One of them may have written the Latin and Swedish names found throughout the book beside the plant figures.*

This is the first edition of the herbal published under the title of the *Reformierte Deutsche Apoteck*. It is a collection of Ryff's previous publications on the subject, which the publisher, Rihel in Strassburg, here has gathered together and produced on his own in one folio volume published after Ryff's death. The statement at the end of the title that the book was 'zuvor im Truck nie aussgangen' is true with some reservation, as the long and wordy title of no less than 33 lines, given in full above, incorporates almost in verbatim many of Ryff's previous titles, which all had gone through numerous editions from the Egenolph press in Frankfurt. Rihel was the printer and publisher of the illustrated edition of Hieronymus Bock's *Kreuterbuch,* and the present book has the same charming woodcuts by David Kandel that were used to illustrate Bock's herbal. The woodcut of the *Carnation* on fol. 153 is signed and dated 'DK 1545' on the flowerpot.

The book is divided into three parts, with no subtitles for the *Ander* or *Dritte Theil*. All the woodcuts are in the *Erster Theil* only and all are coloured by hand. Besides plants there are a few of apparatus, presses, etc. and a bee-keeping scene on A^1 recto.

Hunt 1, 114; Benzing, *Ryff*, 106; Nissen, BBI, 1707; Waller 8363.s

Weiß Seeblůmen.

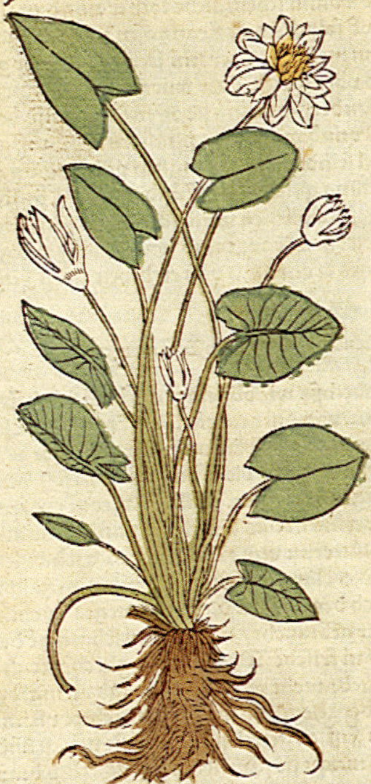

Gäl Seeblůmen.

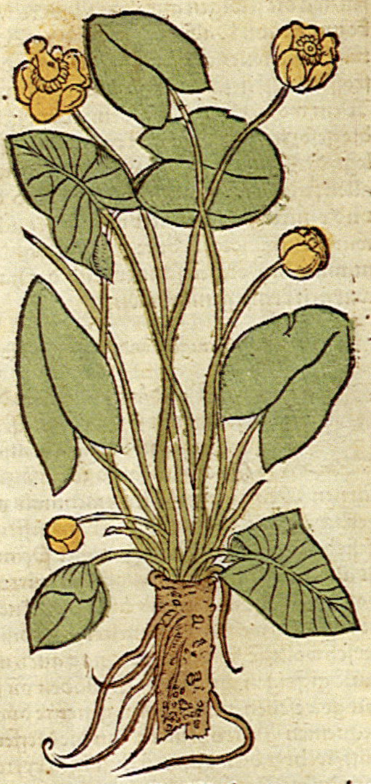

tzel setzet sich ein mit vilen neben zaseren inn das můr der tieffen Weiher/ wogen/ vnd
seen/ auff welchen die runden breitten bletter oben schwimmen/ fast dick vnd steiff wie
ein Leder / auff einem glatten/langen/holen/rundē Bintzen stengel wachsend/ je eins
auff einē stengel allein/auff solchem Bintzen stengel thůn sich auch gegen dem Meyen
vnnd Brachmonat schöne braun grüne/langlechte knöpff herfür / die sich naher eröff
nen/dann erscheinen die schönen weissen Seeblůmen/anzůsehen/wie ein schöne gefül
te weisse Lilgen / aber mit vil mehr blettlin/ dann solche weisse Seeblůmen/etwann
auff xxi. oder xxviij. blettlin haben/ inn mitte ein schöne gälbe Sonne/ mit vilen gel
ben zaseren. Nach dem die weissen vnd eüssersten grünen blettlin hinweg fallē/ nimpt
das knöpflin zů darauff die gelb Soñe steht / würt groß vnnd langlecht/rund wie ein
langs spitzigs Mon heüptlin oder Magsamen klüpfflin anzůsehē/ in solchem Heüpt
lin würt ein schwartz breittes sämlin gefunden. Die wurtzel ist etwann arms dick/ ligt
nach der zwerch auff der Erden/mit vil neben zaseren angehenckt / dise wurtzel hatt
vil knöpff/darauß sie järlichen newe frische bletter vnd stengel stosset/ꝛc.
Die ander gelb Seeblům ist der weissen in allen dingen änlich/mit blettern/wur
tzel vnd stengel/allein das die knöpff der blůmen schön rund seind/vnd die blům schön
gelb würt/So würt auch das Heüptlin so den samen dregt nicht wie der weissen lang
lecht rund / sonder gantz scheüblecht rund/ꝛc.

Wachsung oder pflantzung der Seeblůmen.

GElb vnd weiß Seeblůmen mögen nicht gepflantzet werden/dann sie können on
wasser nicht sein / dann wa sie gleich von jhnen selbst inn dieffen Weyhern ge
nůgsamlichen eingewurtzlet haben / vnd jhn aber das Wasser entgeht oder ent
zogen

From the Adam Horn library

PARACELSUS. Theophrastus Philipus Aureolus Bombastus von Hohenheim (1493–1541)

OPERA. Bücher und Schrifften, so viel deren zur Hand gebracht: und vor wenig Jahren, mit und auss ihren glaubwürdigen eigener hangeschriebenen [*sic*] Originalien collacioniert, vergliechen, verbessert: und durch Ioannem Huserum . . . in zehen unterschiedliche Theil, in Truck gegeben. Jetzt von newem mit vleiss ubersehen, auch mit etlichen bisshero unbekandten Tractaten gemehrt, und umb mehrer Bequemligkeit willen, in zwey unterschiedliche Tomos und Theil gebracht, . . . [*&*] Ander Theyl. Darinnen die Magischen und Astrologischen Bücher, sampt ihren Anhängen und Stücken, auch von dem Philosophischen Stein handlene Tractatus, begriffen, . . .

Strassburg, Lazarus Zetzner, 1603.

Folio – *leaf*: 317 *x* 200 *mm.* Volume I: *Pp.* [12], 1127, [53]. *Title page in red and black within an elaborate woodcut border incorporating the author's portrait.* Volume II: *pp.* [8], 691, [13]. *Title and last leaf mounted. With c.*150 *woodcuts in the text. Two leaves in the index* (Nn2 *and* Nn3) *wrongly bound. Lacks two leaves: pp.* 261-2 *and* 593-4. Volume I *in contemporary vellum with green ties.* Volume II *in modern vellum.*

This is the Strassburger folio edition in two volumes. This set was purchased from Björck *&* Börjesson, *Catalogue* 250/1614 (1930). Its first volume has two early signatures on the title: Martin *&* Henr. Möinichen. It has later belonged to Adam Horn (1717–1778), and bears his signature and his red seal on the title page (cf. Carlander II: 495-9, *Fogelviks Bibliotek*). His fine library of several thousand volumes was dispersed, but the main part, rich in alchemy and the hermetic arts, was acquired by the Royal Library in the late 1860s at the bargain price of SEK 1200 (Carlander). This folio edition was based on Johann Huser's quarto edition in ten volumes, which was the first definitive edition of Paracelsus' collected works (Basel, 1589–1590). Our library is also proud to have the sixth volume of the Huser edition, which is of particular pharmaceutical interest as it contains the 'Archidoxa' (*Die Neun Bücher der Archidoxen Alles zum fleissigsten Corrigiert auss Theophrasti eignem Handschrifften).* This handbook was considered by Paracelsus' disciples as a key to his therapeutical teaching and jealously guarded as a 'secret' in manuscript copies:

Sechster Theil Der Bücher und Schrifften . . . In disem Tomo feind begriffen solche Bücher, in welchen des mehrer theils von Spagyrischer Bereitung Natürlicher dingen, die Artzney betreffend, gehandelt wird. Item, ettliche Alchimistische Büchlin, so allein von der Transmutation der Metallen tractiren.

Basel, Conrad Waldkirch, 1590.

Quarto – *leaf:* 240 x 160 *mm. Pp.* [8], 440, [24]. *Full-page woodcut portrait of Paracelsus on fol.* a2 *and at the end. Title in red and black.*

From the C.D. Carlsson collection.

This copy of the sixth volume of the Huser quarto edition is bound in limp vellum on which the originally gilt stamps and lettering has faded [transmuted?] with time. The upper cover bears the date 1632 and the arms and initials of Gabriel Bengtsson Oxenstierna (1586–1656): H[*err*] G[*abriel*] O[*xenstierna*] B[*engts*] S[*on*] F[*riherre*] T[*ill*] M[*örby*] O[*ch*] L[*indholmen*]; the lower cover bears the arms and initials of F[*ru*] A[*nna*] B[*anér*] G[*ustafs*] D[*otter*].

A complete set of the valuable Huser edition, a copy bearing the book-plate of Emil Starkenstein, Professor of Pharmacology in Prague, is described and reproduced in colour in Hagelin: *Rare and Important Medical Books in the Library of the Swedish Society of Medicine*. Starkenstein was, after a visit to Dr. Erik Waller at Lidköping, the first to pay attention to Waller's great medical library (*Philobiblon*, 10, 1938). He seems himself to have had a fine collection, from which books have recently turned up in Oregon, U.S.A. (Phillip J. Pirages, *Catalogue*, 1993).

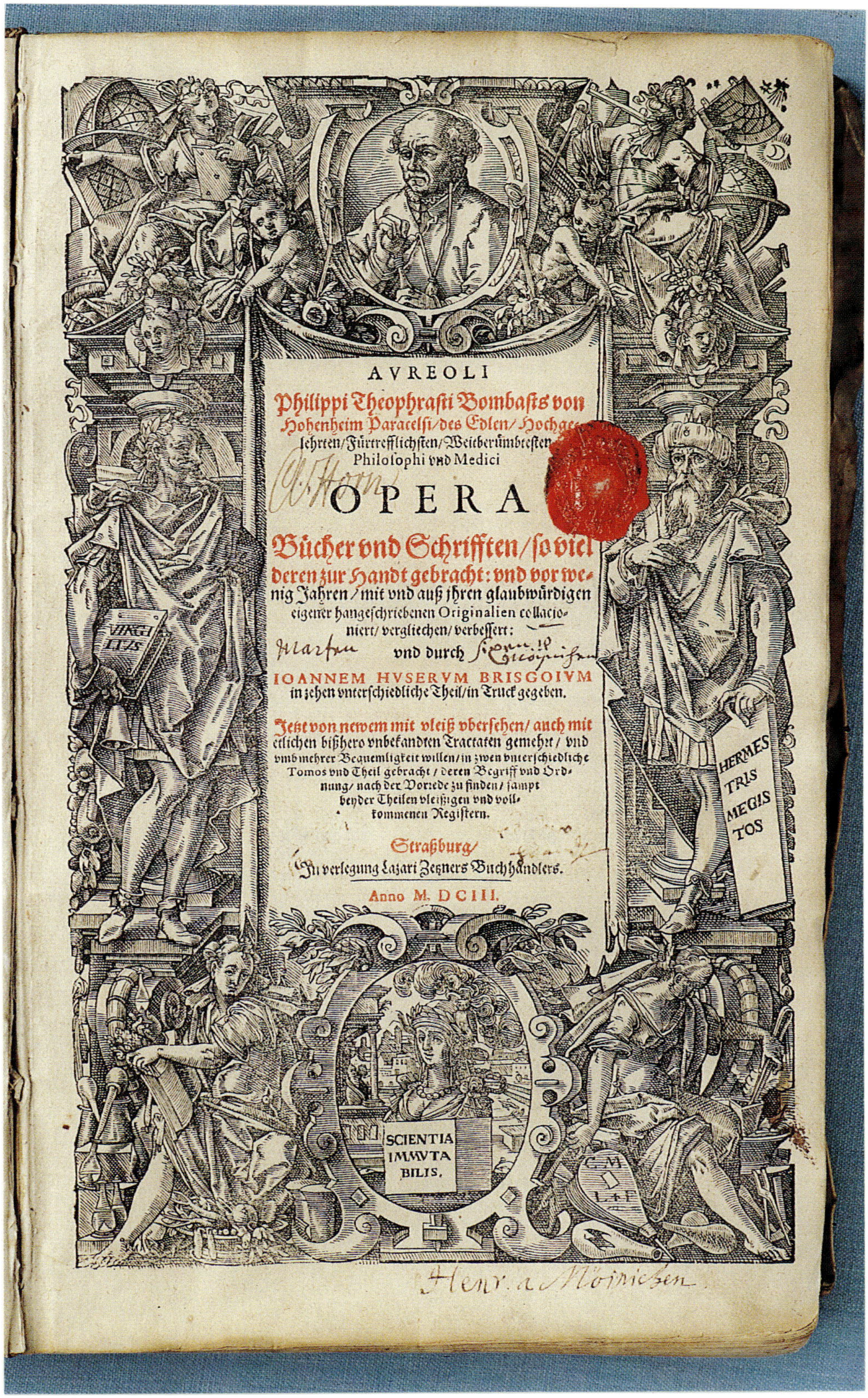

AVREOLI

Philippi Theophrasti Bombasts von Hohenheim Paracelsi/des Edlen/Hochgelehrten/Fürtrefflichsten/Weitberümbtesten Philosophi vnd Medici

OPERA

Bücher vnd Schrifften/so viel deren zur Handt gebracht: vnd vor wenig Jahren/mit vnd auß jhren glaubwürdigen eigener hangeschriebenen Originalien collacioniert/vergliechen/verbessert:

vnd durch

IOANNEM HVSERVM BRISGOIVM

in zehen vnterschiedliche Theil/in Truck gegeben.

Jetzt von newem mit vleiß vbersehen/auch mit etlichen bißhero vnbekandten Tractaten gemehrt/vnd vmb mehrer Bequemligkeit willen/in zwen vnterschiedliche Tomos vnd Theil gebracht/deren Begriff vnd Ordnung/nach der Vorrede zu finden/sampt beyder Theilen vleißigen vnd vollkommenen Registern.

Straßburg/

In verlegung Lazari Zetzners Buchhändlers.

Anno M. DCIII.

Theophrastus Bombastus von Hohenheim, known as Paracelsus, was one of the most controversial and remarkable characters of the sixteenth century – an eccentric who was destined to exert an epochal influence on medicine and chemistry. Of the c.364 works attributed to him – some of doubtful authenticity – only a very few were published during his lifetime. But he left a mass of manuscripts, which were passed on by his factotum, Johannes Oporinus, to Bodenstein and Michael Toxites, both of whom published some of them in the decades following Paracelsus' death. Their publication reached a peak in about 1570 with the *Archidoxa*, which went through many editions after the first, issued at Cracow in 1569.

All the printed and manuscript material was assembled by Johann Huser, who published at Basel in 1589–1590 the first collected edition of Paracelsus' works in ten quarto volumes and an appendix, which is still considered the best edition. The above folio edition in two volumes (Strassburg, 1603), is a reprint of the Huser edition, but according to Sudhoff, not without faults. An appendix to this folio edition, the *Chirurgische Bücher*, prepared after Huser's manuscript notes, followed in 1605, but that volume is missing in our set. In 1922–1933, Karl Sudhoff, the eminent German medical historian, who spent fifty years critically studying Paracelsus' writings, published a collection of Paracelsus' medical works in fourteen volumes (reprinted 1954), which is also available in our library.

Theophrastus was born in Einsiedeln in Switzerland. His father was a physician, who gave his son his first education including instruction in medicine and surgery. When Theophrastus was nine years old the family moved to Villach, in Carinthia, a mining district, where he probably attended the School of Mines founded by the Fuggers of Augsburg. In 1510 he went to the University of Basel and later to Würzburg to study with the abbot Trithemius, the renowned alchemist. He then started his *Wanderjahre* lasting from 1517 to 1527 during which time he travelled all over Europe as a physician, serving also as military surgeon in different armies. While serving in the Danish army under Christian II he may have witnessed the bloody Stockholm Massacre of 1518. During his travels he collected information from every source, and by his acquaintances with barbers, executioners, bathkeepers, gypsies, midwives, and fortune-tellers, he learned a great deal about medical practice, and incidentally acquired an unusual knowledge of folk-medicine and a permanent taste for low company. Paracelsus thought and spoke in the language of the people, was 'popular' as no other physician before him. He returned to German territories at the age of about 32, his experience qualifying him to make a lasting impression as a practising physician.

Paracelsus' successful treatment of the Basel printer Frobenius (who died soon after!) made a strong impression on Erasmus and Oecolampadius. On the latter's recommendation, Paracelsus was appointed city physician of Basel in March, 1572, and he was also allowed to lecture at the university. Here his violent opposition to the accepted authorities and his aggressive temper soon brought him into conflict with the medical faculty. His lectures, which he held in German, not Latin, were very unconventional and greatly offended the physicians at Basel, whom he is said to have invited to a lecture on the greatest secret in medicine; he began by uncovering a pan of excrement, whereupon his audience fled in anger, Paracelsus shouting after them: 'If you will not hear the mysteries of putrefactive fermentation, you are unworthy of the name of physicians'. Another story goes that he publicly burnt the works of Galen and Avicenna (two large and expensive books) in a brass pan with sulphur and nitre. After losing a case in February 1528 in which he had sued the canon of Basel, he hurriedly left the city never to frequent academic halls again; he left his properties in the care of Oporinus, his amanuensis, who later became the printer of Vesalius' *Fabrica* (1543). According to Oporinus, Paracelsus often spent the night drinking in taverns with peasants. After such nights, he would sleep on the tavern floor, visiting patients the following day. He seldom undressed and was intoxicated when dictating his books. Although fond of drinking, Paracelsus is said by another pupil never to have been more than reasonably merry ('gemeiniglich lustig'). Gesner (1545) claimed that Paracelsus was an imposter and frequently resorted to narcotics containing opium in his practice.

For the next thirteen years Paracelsus led a wandering life, unkempt, commonly drunk, passing from one town to another, practising, writing, quarrelling, defending his views, and attacking his opponents. Finally he arrived at Strassburg, broken in health and old beyond his 48 years, and died there in 1541. His enemies asserted that he died in a low tavern (at the sign of the *White Horse*) in consequence of a drunken

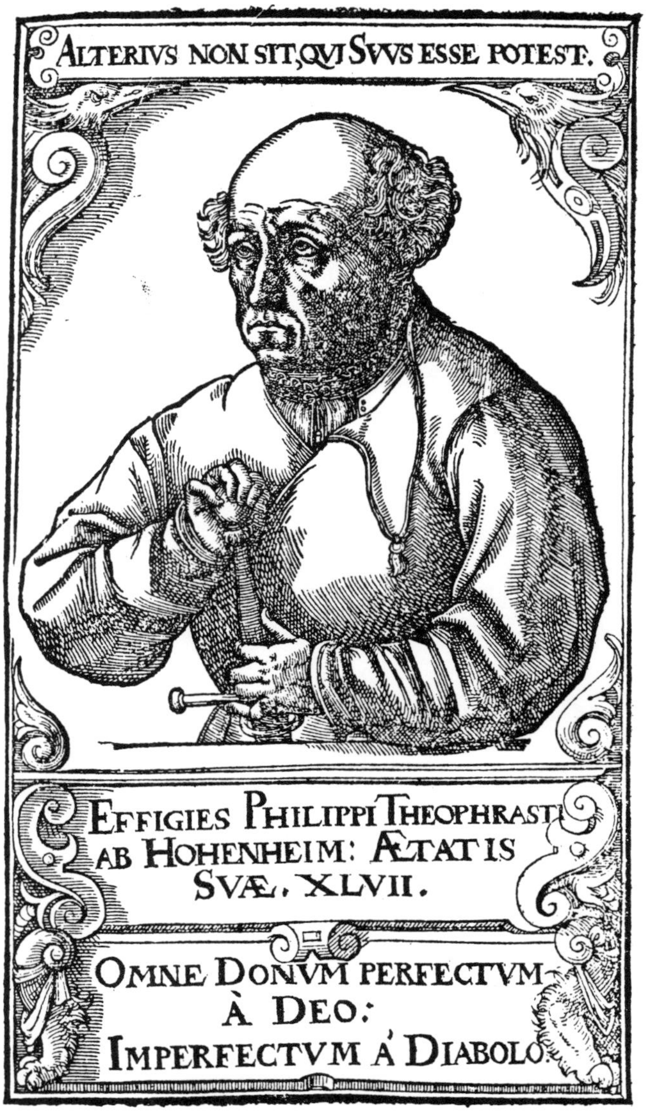

debauch of some day's duration. Others maintain that he was thrown to his death by some hired thugs either of the physicians or of the apothecaries, both of whom were grieviously harassed by Paracelsus during his lifetime. The latter legend was disproved in 1891 by C. Aberle, who showed that the injuries to the skull were caused during the exhumation.

Paracelsus' importance to pharmacy lies in his studies of drugs and their effects leading to the introduction of metals into internal therapy and the dawn of pharmaceutical chemistry. He was the first to propose that disease is a disturbance of the body chemistry, a theory of highest pharmaceutical importance. Such a disturbance, according to his argument, could be cured by the use of proper chemicals. He not only introduced chemicals for internal use into the *materia medica*, but also tried to find new and efficient methods for the preparations of tinctures and of liquid extracts containing the essential virtues of the extracted drug, his so-called 'quintessences'. Paracelsus is sometimes called the father of the pharmaceutical revolution that questioned Galenic ideas and emphasized chemical remedies.

Sudhoff, *Bibliographia Paracelsica*, 256, 257; 221; Walter Pagel in DSB, x, pp. 304-13; Partington, II, pp. 115-51; Major, *History*, pp. 383-93; Encycl. Britt. 11th ed., vol. xx, pp. 749-50; Stillman, *The Story of Alchemy*, pp. 308-28; Garrison, pp. 204-07; *Printing and the Mind of Man*, 110; Kremers & Urdang, pp. 37-8; Cowen & Helfand, pp. 59-60; These editions not in Waller.

The German edition of the most splendid herbal of the Renaissance

FUCHS, Leonhard (1501–1566)

New Kreüterbuch, in welchem nit allein die gantz histori, das ist, namen, gestalt, statt und zeit der wachsung, natur, krafft und würckung, des meysten theyls der Kreüter so in Teütschen unnd andern Landen wachsen, mit dem besten vleiss beschriben, sonder auch aller derselben wurtzel, stengel, bletter, blumen, samen, frücht, und in summa die gantze gestalt, allso artlich und kunstlich abgebildet und contrafayt ist, das dessgleichen vormals nie gesehen, noch an tag kommen. . . Mit dreyen nützlichen Registern, . . . auch deren sich die Apotecker gebrauchen begreiffen . . .

Basel, Michael Isengrin, 1543.

Folio – *leaf*: 375 *x* 240 *mm*. 444 *unnumbered leaves: ff.* [16] *title, preface, index,* [428]. *Sign.:* [π^6 $\pi\pi^6$ $\pi\pi\pi^4$] a-z A-Z Aa-Zz^6 AA^6 BB^8. *With* 517 *full-page woodcuts of plants. Full-length portrait of the author on verso of the title leaf, three half-length portraits of the illustrators and the engraver on verso of the penultimate leaf. Title and last leaf with the publisher's device (an olive tree enclosing a printer's platen, a symbol of peace, while the Latin edition of* 1542 *uses a holly tree, a symbol of the Reformation), recto blank. The first* 150 *woodcuts are coloured by hand at a later date. Contemporary blindstamped pigskin over thick wooden boards, five double bands, two brass clasps.*

Early signature on the title page: Ludwig Edlibach; *Book-plate:* C. D. Carlsson.

This is the first edition of the German translation of the *De historia stirpium,* the most famous herbal of the sixteenth century and one of the most beautiful ever to be published. It is the first edition written in the vernacular and featuring six more woodcuts than the previous Latin edition together with revisions in the text.

Leonhard Fuchs was born at Wemding, Bavaria, where his father and grandfather were *Burgermeister*. When Leonhard was four years old his father died, and his grandfather assumed responsibility for the family. He took his grandson on walks in the countryside and taught him the names of plants. At a very early age Fuchs entered the University of Erfurt, where he passed the examination after only three semesters, before he had reached his fourteenth year. After that he opened a private school in his native town. In 1519 he entered the University of Ingolstadt, where he devoted himself chiefly to classical studies and became a Master of Arts. He then turned his attention to medicine and took his M.D. in 1524 and practised as physician for two years in Munich, where he also met and married Anna, with whom he had four sons and six daughters. In 1526 he was back again in Ingolstadt as professor of medicine.

Two years later he resigned from the university for a more honourable post as court physician to Margrave George of Brandenburg in Anspach, where he in 1529 gained wide respect for his treatment of a very fatal epidemic, which one reads of as the plague [identified with sweating sickness], when he received calls from the University of Pisa and from the King of Denmark. It was during this period that his career as an author began. In 1531 he published his *Compendiaria,* a work intended to help students to appreciate the works of Hippocrates and Galen properly. Revised and greatly enlarged, this work went through some ten editions under the new titles of first *Methodus*, and later on *Institutiones Medicinae,* with additional chapters on the theory and practice of *Materia Medica*. Upon another outbreak of the plague in Anspach Fuchs with his wife and children fled the place. In 1535 he became professor of medicine in the newly established Protestant University of Tübingen, where he remained for the rest of his life, that is for thirty-one years.

Fuchs is however best known for his pharmaceutical herbal, *De historia stirpium* (1542), followed in the succeeding year by his German translation, called the *New Kreuterbuch*. He is the third of the three men referred to as the 'German Fathers of Botany', the other two being Otto Brunfels and Hieronymus Bock, both authors of celebrated herbals. Fuchs was far better educated than his predecessors and was the first after Brunfels to illustrate from nature (the first edition of Bock's herbal was unillustrated). The illustrations were based on plants growing in Fuchs' garden at Tübingen, largely those that were in common medical use. To create the impressive illustrations, which so substantially came to contribute to the book's fame and beauty,

D. Leonhart Fuchs/seins alters im XLII. Jar.

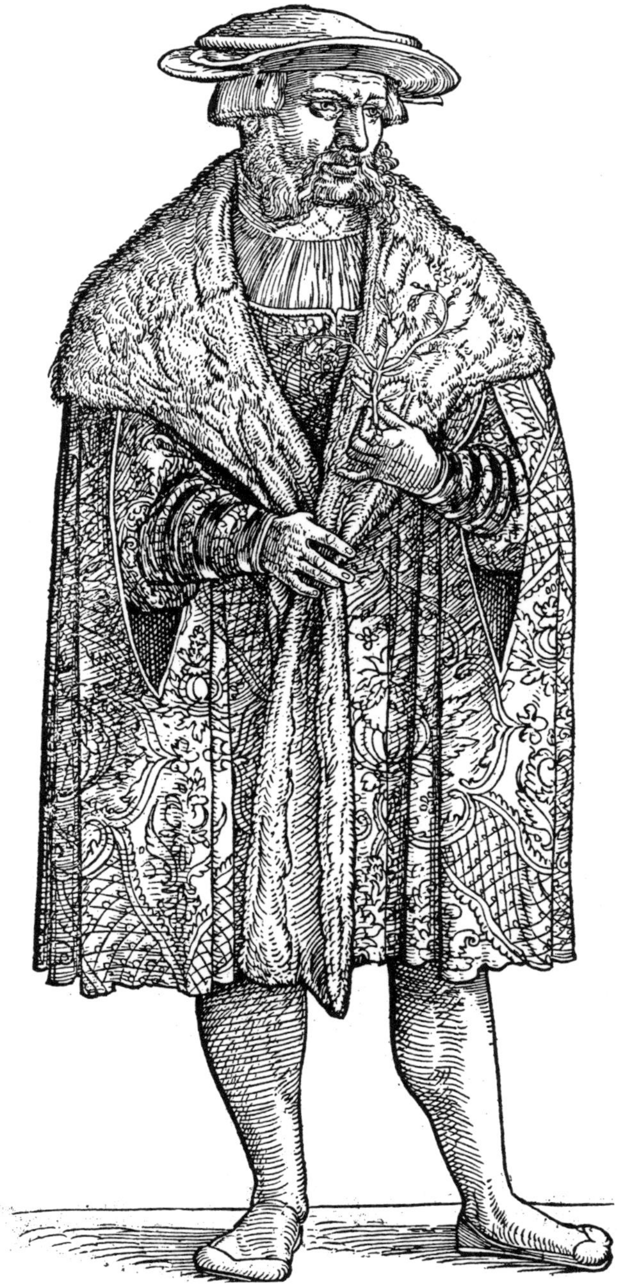

Fuchs employed the best artists then available in Basel: Albrecht Meyer, who, under Fuchs' supervision drew the plants, in life-size when possible, Heinrich Fuellmaurer, who transferred the drawings to the wood blocks, and Veit Rudolf Speckle, the best wood engraver in Strassburg, who did the woodcutting. All three of Fuchs' skilful collaborators are commemorated with portraits at the end of the book, and it is the first time that book illustrators themselves are portrayed and named in a printed book. In the beginning of the book is a full-length portrait of Leonhard Fuchs himself as he appeared in 1542, when he was full professor at the University of Tübingen. He is holding the medicinal plant *Veronica officinalis* in his left hand.

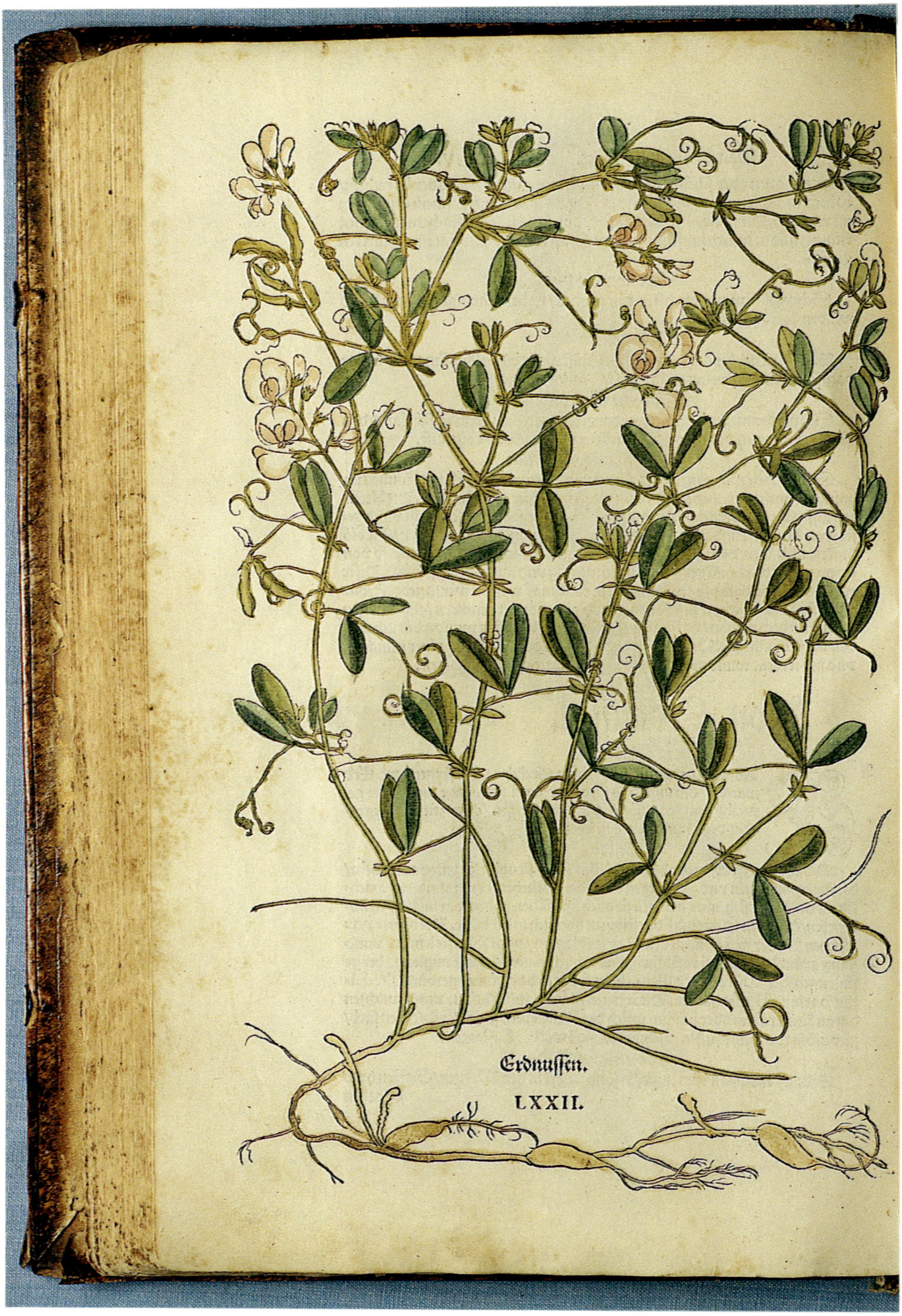

APIOS, **Erdnussen** (*Lathyrus tuberosus* L., Earth-nut-pea). This is one of the figures that was on so large a scale that the plant had to be curved in order to fit onto the page. It creates a decorative spirit that fills the rectangular space almost in the manner of an all-over wallpaper pattern, that may have inspired William Morris, who owned a copy of the first edition of Fuchs' herbal and often sang the praise of its artists.

Maler.

Heinrich Füllmaurer. Albrecht Meyer.

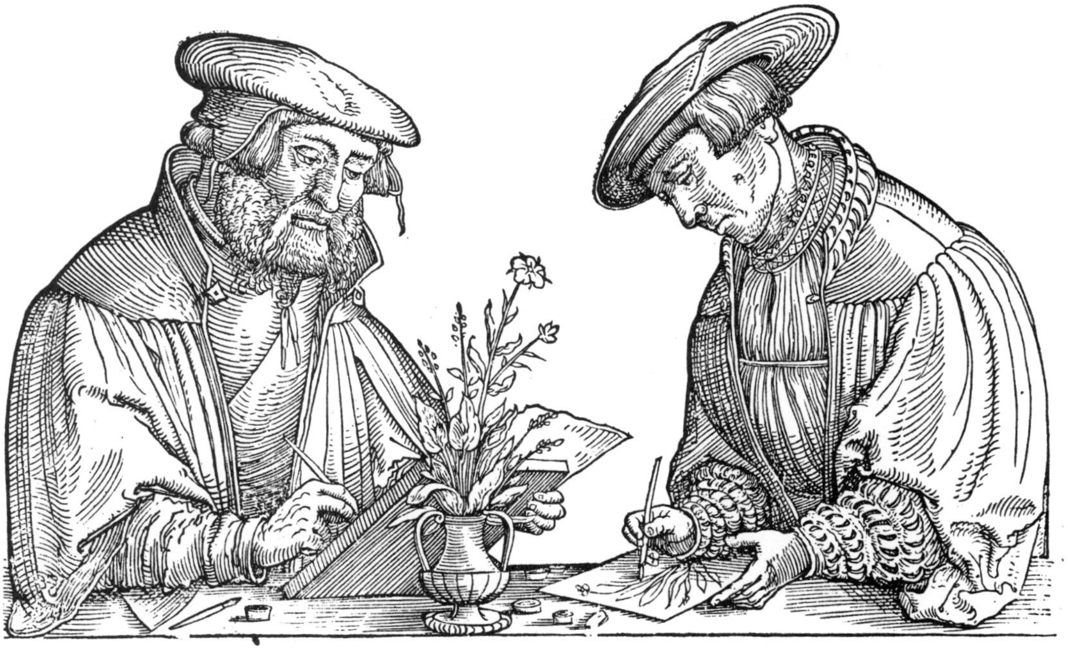

Veyt Rüdolff Speckle formschneider.

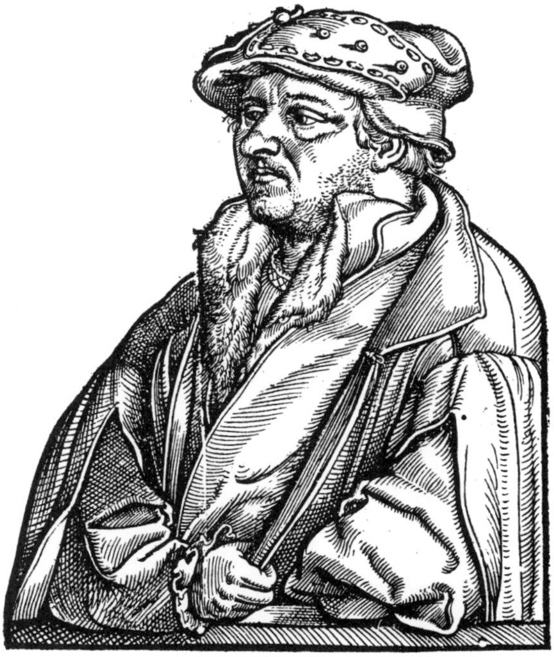

The portraits of the artists who so substantially contributed to the fame and beauty of Fuchs' herbal: Albrecht Meyer, who drew the plants from nature, Heinrich Fuellmaurer, who transferred the drawings to the wood blocks, and Veit Rudolph Speckle, who cut the blocks. It is the first time that the illustrators are portrayed in a book, besides the author.

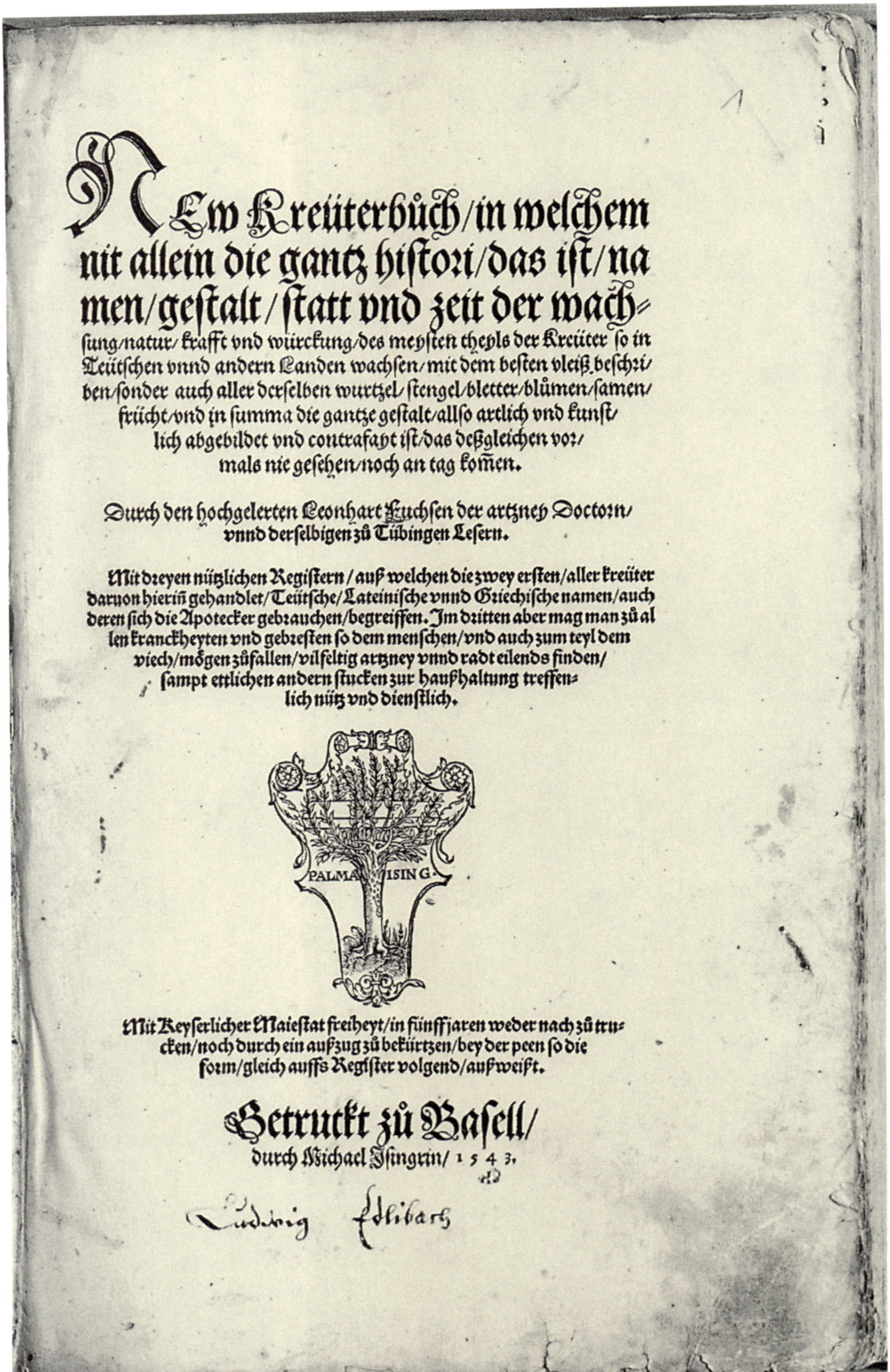
New Kreüterbůch/in welchem
nit allein die gantz histori/das ist/na
men/gestalt/statt vnd zeit der wach=
sung/natur/krafft vnd würckung/des meysten theyls der Kreüter so in
Teütschen vnnd andern Landen wachsen/mit dem besten vleiß beschri/
ben/sonder auch aller derselben wurtzel/stengel/bletter/blůmen/samen/
frücht/vnd in summa die gantze gestalt/allso artlich vnd kunst/
lich abgebildet vnd contrafayt ist/das deßgleichen vor/
mals nie gesehen/noch an tag komen.

Durch den hochgelerten Leonhart Fuchsen der artzney Doctorn/
vnnd derselbigen zů Tübingen Lesern.

Mit dreyen nützlichen Registern/auß welchen die zwey ersten/aller kreüter
daruon hierin gehandlet/Teütsche/Lateinische vnnd Griechische namen/auch
deren sich die Apotecker gebrauchen/begreiffen. Im dritten aber mag man zů al
len kranckheyten vnd gebresten so dem menschen/vnd auch zum teyl dem
viech/mögen zůfallen/vilfeltig artzney vnnd radt eilends finden/
sampt etlichen andern stucken zur haußhaltung treffen=
lich nütz vnd dienstlich.

PALMA ISING.

Mit Keyserlicher Maiestat freiheyt/in fünff jaren weder nach zů tru=
cken/noch durch ein außzug zů bekürtzen/bey der peen so die
form/gleich auffs Register volgend/außweißt.

Getruckt zů Basell/
durch Michael Isingrin/1543.

The title page to the German edition (1543) of Fuch's herbal. It bears Isengrin's device with an olive tree enclosing a printer's platen, a symbol of piece, while the Latin edition of 1542 uses a holly tree, a symbol of the Reformation.

The illustrations in Fuchs' herbal 'represent the high-water mark of that type of botanical drawing which seeks to express the individual character and habit of each species, . . .' (Arber). Fuchs states in the preface that 'we have devoted the greatest diligence to secure that every plant should be depicted with its roots, stalks, leaves, flowers, seeds, and fruits . . . We have purposely and deliberately avoided the obliteration of the natural form of the plants by shadows, and other less necessary things, by which the delineators sometimes try to win artistic glory'. Many of the figures were on so large a scale that the plants frequently had to be curved in order to fit even on the folio pages. Sometimes a peculiarly decorative spirit is shown in the form of a pattern that fills the rectangular space of the page and may well have inspired William Morris for his design of wallpapers. Both Morris and John Ruskin owned a copy of the first edition, purchased from Bernard Quaritch, and Morris often and loudly sang the praise of the artists. The book was ready for the press around 1538 but was not published until 1542. It is a folio of breathtaking splendour and its success seems to have been speedily assured. To a generation that had been accustomed to such books as the *Hortus Sanitatis*, filled with the most wretched caricatures of plants, Meyer's true representation of over 500 plants (compared to Weiditz's 135 for Brunfels' herbal) was really wonderful.

Fuchs' herbal depicts many species never before figured, e.g. the Foxglove (*Digitalis purpurea*) and several plants from the New World, among which were the first representations of the pumpkin and of maize, the familiar corn, which Fuchs, mistaking its country of origin, called Turkish Corn [turkey = the American bird]. From comments in the catalogues of rare book dealers, such as: 'In the original fresh state, absolutely free of any colour', it is evident that plain, uncoloured copies have always been preferred by collectors. But there were also original coloured copies made for the publisher Isengrin, who presumably made use of the artist's original drawings. The colouring of the first 150 plates in the present copy is, however, of a later date.

The woodcuts in Fuchs' herbal were to have far-reaching influence on botanical illustrations for many years to come. In the preface to a later edition Fuchs complained bitterly of the way in which his plates had been pirated. The blocks were copied and used in many later herbals all over Europe and designs based on the plates have been used in countless of botanical books well up to the present time. In 1774, a certain Salomon Schinz, who had somehow obtained the original woodblocks, used them to illustrate his book called *Anleiting zu der Pflanzenkentniss*. He had the woodcuts coloured by the children of an orphanage – an economic method of producing *editions de luxe*.

A collection of some 1525 drawings made for the first edition of *De historia Stirpium* and for two further volumes, which Fuchs was never able to publish, turned up in 1954. They are contained in nine volumes and were acquired by the Austrian National Library, Vienna.

In 1703 the French botanical explorer Charles Plumier honoured the great herbalist giving the name *Fuchsia* to a superb South American genus, which, however, Leonhard Fuchs had never seen. Scholars today consider Fuchs' herbal to be one of the significant landmarks of pre-Linnaean botanical literature.

It is remarkable that Fuchs' *Stirpium*, Vesalius' *Fabrica* and Copernicus' *De Revolutionibus*, were all published within the span of one year. The authority of Dioscorides, Galen and Ptolemy, names held sacrosanct for 1500 years, were in one year conclusively and irrevocably shattered. Botany, anatomy and astronomy were to enter new eras beginning in 1542.

Norman, *One Hundred Books Famous in Medicine,* 17; PMM 69; Garrison &Morton 1808; Stillwell 640; *Tax. Lit.* 1910; Arber, pp. 64-70, 212-21; DSB, xv, Suppl. 1, pp. 160-2; Blunt/Stearn, pp. 64-71; Blunt/Raphael, pp. 123-9; Greene, *Landmarks*, 1, pp. 271-303; Anderson, pp. 137-47; Johnston, *Cleveland Herbal*, 62; Nissen, *Kräuterbücher*, p. 63; Albert E. Lownes, *Renaissance Books of Science*, 6; Wightman, *Science and the Renaissance*, 1, pp. 213-17; Stübler, E. *Leonhart Fuchs, Leben und Werk* (1928); Sprague & Nelmes in *Journ. Linn. Soc. Bot.*, 48 (1931), pp. 545-642; Facsimile edition of the *New Kräuterbuch* (Leipzig, 1938; Munich, 1964); Waller 11512 (Latin ed. of 1542 only).

The first illustrated pocket flora

FUCHS, Leonhard (1501–1566)

De historia stirpium commentarii imagines.
Lyons, Balthazar Arnoullet, 1551.

Octavo – *leaf:* 154 x 100 *mm. Pp.* [32, *the last two blank*], 852, [12]. *Printer's device on the title, woodcut portrait of Fuchs on verso of the title leaf, and* 519 *woodcuts of plants, most of which are coloured by hand at a later date. Contemporary vellum.*

Early owner's signature on the title: Arnoldi Gillenii, *dated Basel,* 1608. *The title page also bears the signature of* Dr J.S. Neomeyzonio, bavarico-castrenis emerito, *dated* 2 *July,* 1879. *In a most minute and fine humanistic hand he has written botanical and bibliographical annotations on the fly-leaves and in the margins throughout the book and has also added the German names for most of the depicted plants, which nearly all are coloured by hand, possibly by himself.*
Book-plate: C. D. Carlsson.

The folio editions of Fuchs' herbal were costly volumes too expensive for the ordinary student and far too heavy for the field botanist to take along into the countryside. Soon, therefore, convenient pocket editions were issued by various publishers in Basel, Paris and Lyon, illustrated with woodcuts in reduced size, with or without text other than the names of the plants in Latin and German. Some were octavos with four figures to a page, others were miniature duodecimos with a single figure to each page.

The present edition by Arnoullet in Lyon is a re-issue of his 1549 edition with a new title leaf. The woodcuts of the plants were commissioned from Clémont Boussy by Arnoullet in 1547 and first used in the 1549 edition. Both the portrait of Fuchs and the illustrations of plants were based on the full-page woodcuts in the first folio edition printed by Isengrin in Basel, 1542.

It may be of some interest that the printer, whose beautiful device (a sea horse with sword and scales) adorns the title page, was soon after the printing of the above book involved in the barbaric heresy trial of Servetus, 'one of the sorriest episodes in history' (Fulton). It was in Arnoullet's Vienna atelier that the printing of Servetus' *Christianismo restitutio* was undertaken in the greatest secrecy during the autumn of 1552. Arnoullet was imprisoned and all the c. 1000 copies of the book, of which only three have escaped, were burnt on order of the Inquisition.

Hunt, 1, 61 (1549 ed.); Mortimer, *French*, 240 (1549 ed.); Nissen BBI, 667; Fairfax Murray, *Early French Books*, 1, 181 (1549 ed.); Blunt/Raphael, p. 128.

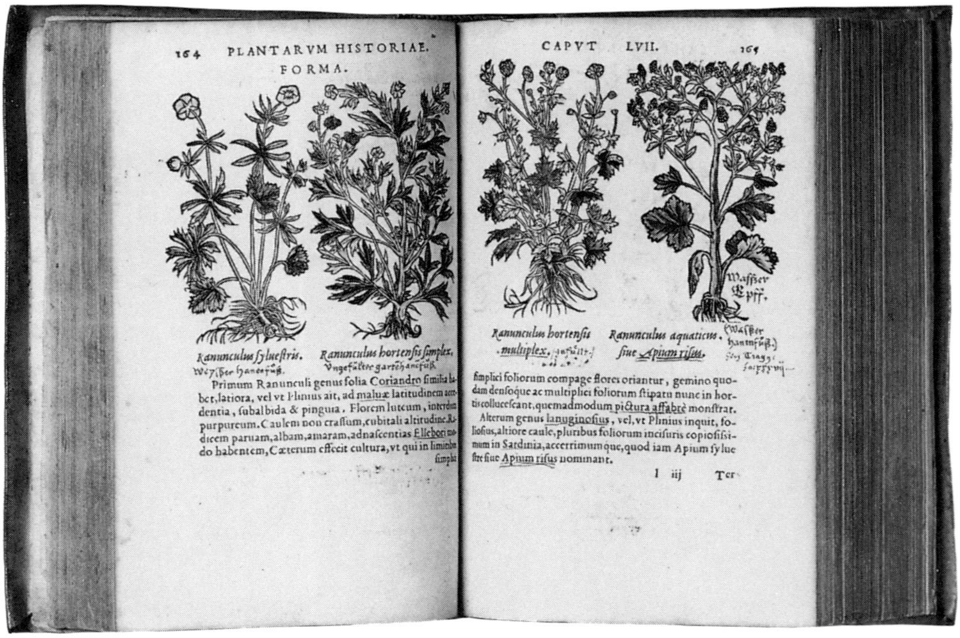

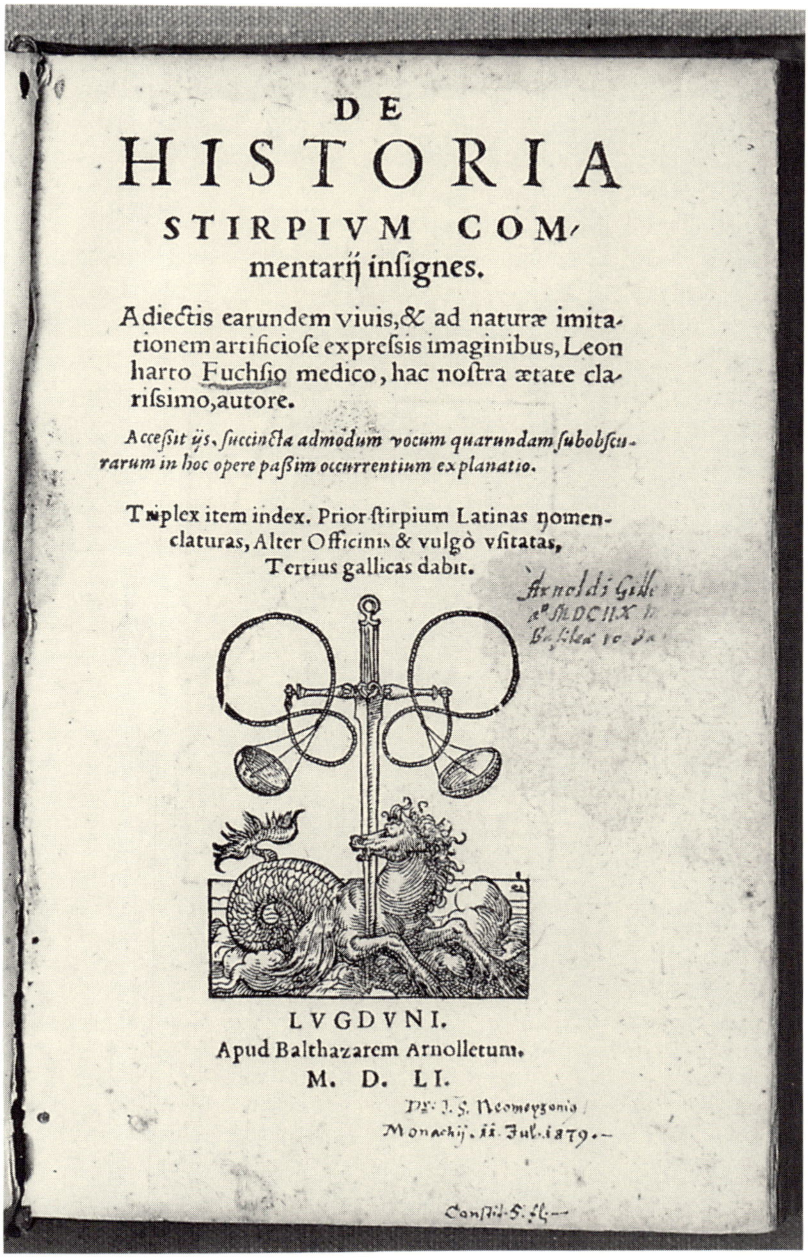

DE
HISTORIA
STIRPIVM COM-
mentarij insignes.

Adiectis earundem viuis, & ad naturæ imita-
tionem artificiose expresſis imaginibus, Leon
harto Fuchſio medico, hac noſtra ætate cla-
riſsimo, autore.

*Acceſsit ijs, ſuccincta admodum vocum quarundam ſubobſcu-
rarum in hoc opere paſsim occurrentium explanatio.*

Triplex item index. Prior ſtirpium Latinas nomen-
claturas, Alter Officinis & vulgò vſitatas,
Tertius gallicas dabit.

LVGDVNI.
Apud Balthazarem Arnolletum.
M. D. LI.

A forerunner of Linnaeus

BOCK, Hieronymus (1498–1554)

Kreütterbuch, darin underscheidt, Namen und Würckung der Kreütter, Staüden, Hecken unnd Beumen, sampt ihren Früchten, so inn Teutschen Landen wachsen, auch der selben eigentlicher unnd wolgegründter Gebrauch inn der Artzney, fleissig dargeben, Leibs gesundtheit zu fürdern und zu behalten, sehr nützlich und tröstlich, bevorab dem Gemeinen und Einfaltigen Mann. Item von den vier Elementen, zamen und wilden Thieren, auch Vöglen und Fischen, Milch, Käss, Butter, Honig, Wachss, Zucker, Saltz, Brot, Wein, Essig, Oely, Eyer, Blut, Schmaltz, Unschlit, allerhand Kochkreütter, Specerei und Gewurtz. Auch wie alle Speiss und Dranck, Gesunden und Krancken, dargereicht werden sollen. Alles durch H. Hieronymum Bock, auss langwiriger und geweisser erfahrung, beschriben. Jetztund auffs new mit allem fleiss ubersehen, unnd mit vilen nützlichen Experimenten gebessert und gemehret. Auch wie man die Kreütter zu rechter Zeit samlen und Distillieren soll. Durch den Hochgelehrten MELCHIOREM SEBIZIUM . . .

Strassburg, Josia Rihel, 1580.

Folio – *leaf*: 335 *x* 218 *mm. Ff.* [30], 450, [24]. *Lacks fol.* 432 *(supplied in photo copy) and also the final blank leaf* (H6). *Title printed in red and black with hand-coloured device, portrait of Bock* (a6 *recto) and the arms of Count Philip of Nassau on verso. With* 550 *woodcuts of plants, four of furnaces and one of an oilpress; the appendix,* 'Speisskammer', *has* 19 *woodcuts with genre scenes. All woodcuts are in the original colouring. Contemporary blindstamped pigskin over wooden boards, five double bands, red edges. Remnants of clasps. The inner panel on the upper cover has the portrait of Emperor Charles* V, *and the one on the back cover the portrait of Johann Friedrich* I *of Saxony, each with a legend below.*

Provenance: Bibliotheca Collegii S. Maria Coronaea Papie *in manuscript on the title page and a stamp in lower margin:* B. Coll. S.M. Can. no. PP. *The beautiful title page is reproduced as frontispiece in this catalogue. From the* C. D. Carlsson collection.

This is a reprint of the 1577 edition, which was the first published under the editorship of Melchior Sebitzius (1539–1625) with a fourth book (or part), the '*Teutsche Speisskammer*', added at the end. It is a neatly hand-coloured copy in its original binding.

Hieronymus Bock (latinized Tragus) was born at Heidersbach. Little is known about his early life other than that he was intended for a monastic life by his parents. Hieronymus himself preferred medicine and may have studied at the University of Heidelberg. In 1523, when he was twenty-five years old, we find him settled as a schoolteacher in Zweibrücken under the appointment of Count Palatine Ludwig V. There he married Eva; out of the ten children born to him, eight died young and Bock also survived their mother. He was also superintendent of the gardens of the Count Palatine, and no doubt his highly practical botanical knowledge was gained there. Following the death of his patron nine years later Bock became pastor of a Lutheran church in the nearby Hornbach, where he also practised medicine and devoted his leisure time to botanical excursions in the wild surroundings, disguised as a peasant.

For a period of two years Bock was driven away from Hornbach due to the effects of the Counter-Reformation, and was invited to stay in the castle of Landgraf Philip II of Nassau in Saarbrücken, whom Bock had earlier cured of a serious illness. He acted as the Landgraf's personal physician and gardener until 1551 when he returned to his beloved Hornbach, where he died in 1554.

Bock was a pioneer of descriptive botany (phytography). It is Bock, rather than Brunfels, who with his *Neu Kreutter Buch* (1539) introduced a new era in botany. Traditionally the main purpose of writers of medico-botanical works was to trace the plants back to Dioscorides and inform about their medicinal properties by quoting Arabic physicians and earlier authorities – a task performed by studying old books rather than through first-hand observations in the field.

Von der Krafft vnd Würckung.

DIE Nüßlein seind etwas warmer Natur/den Sewen/Meusen vnnd Kramat vögeln/zů Winters zeitten/ein angeneme Speiß/werdẽ selten inn der Artzney genützt.

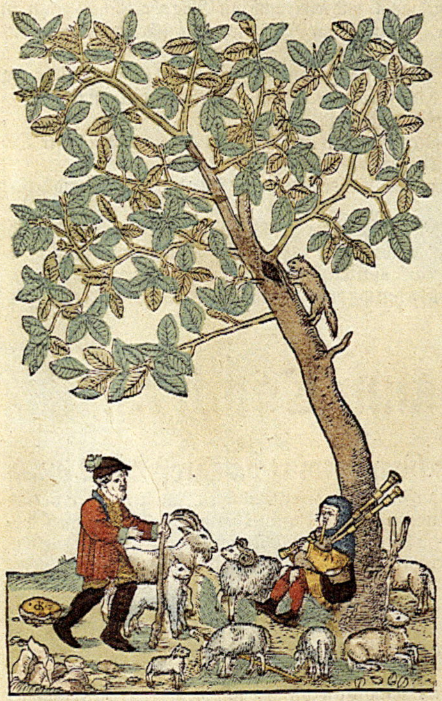

Eusserlich.

Geschwulst.

DAS grün Büchenlaub zerstossen/ vnnd vbergelegt/ zertheilet alle hitzige geschwulst.

Vsus ligni.

Auß dem Holtz machet man vil Werckgezeug/ als Laden / Arcken / Truhen/ Gefäß / ist wärhafftig inn Wasserbewen/darinn würt es desto steiffer.

Weidäschen.

Auß den faulen Büchbeumen brennet man Weid äschen zů ferben.

Grind vnd Raud.

Das Wasser/so inn den holen Büchbeumen funden würt/ ist ein köstliche Artzney für allerhand Rauden/ Grind vnnd Flechten/ darmit gewäschen. Das hab ich erfahren an Menschen vnd dem Rind Vihe.

Lib.2. cap.85.

Joannes Ruellius sagt/ man vertreibe die gifftige Ottern/ zů Latein Vipera / mit einem Büchbeumen reißlein. Ein wunderbarliche Natur des Büchbaums.

Stein.

So man Büchecker/zů äschen gebrendt / die selbig äschen mit Häner oder schweinem Schmaltz mischet/ vnd auff die Lenden warm legt/ helffen sie wider den Stein.

Hanbůchen. Cap. lxxiij.

Forma.
Vsus.
Verg. Eclog. 6. Quibus ille solebat Cantando rigidas deducere montibus ornos.
Columel. lib. 5. cap. 6.

VNder allem Holtz / so in vnsern Wäldẽ wächßt/ ist kaum eins so hart/als der Hanbüchen / von farben weiß vnnd satt/ wie Buxbaum/reißt vngern/würt derhalben zů Spindel/ zů Schrauben/ vñ zů den Kampffredern inn den Mülen erwehlet/gibt auch gůte Fackeln vñ Spän/die trüben Wein lauter zů machen.

Das laub am Hagenbüchen ist aller ding dem Rüstholtz ähnlich/ zů rings vmbher ein wenig zerkerfft. An disem baum wachsen die Vogelszungen / die vergleichen sich schier der Linden blůet / doch die zünglein am Hagenbüchen sein gantz hart/ vnd solches ist der samen/den pfleget man inn der Artzney zůbrauchen.

Von

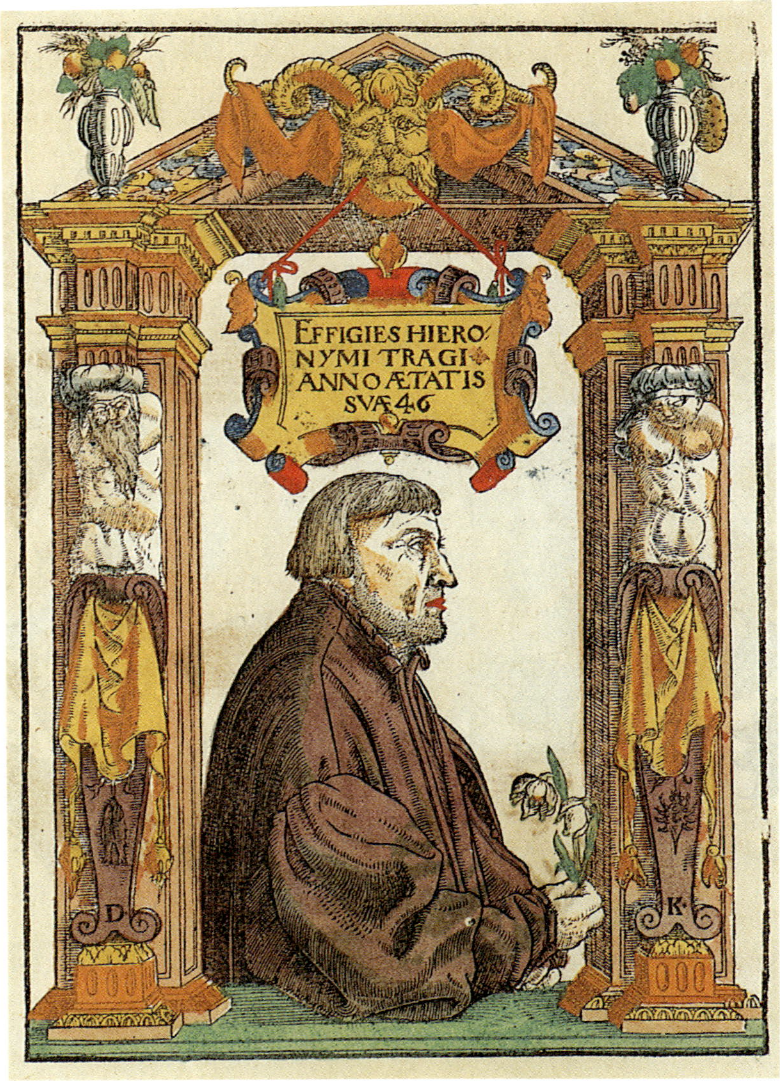

Bock fundamentally differs from his predecessors in that he only describes the local plants he himself had examined, and he mistrusted superstition and folklore until he had personally checked them. As he was probably unable to persuade his publisher to pay for artists and woodcutters, the first edition of his *Neu Kreutter Buch* (1539) had no illustrations, but Bock's detailed written descriptions of the plants served as well as Weiditz's naturalistic pictures in Brunfels' herbal. Bock writes in a simple and vivid German intelligible to the layman, whose botanical knowledge would be limited to local plants and their vernacular names.

Bock gives a detailed description of the plant's structure and nature, its size, roots, stem and foliage, flowers, fruit, colour, scent, time of flowering, locality, economic and medicinal use, etc. He was one of the first to consider the stamen and pistil as essential parts of the flower even if he was innocent of the sexuality of plants and could thus not attribute to them their proper reproductive functions. Rather than use a confusing alphabetical order he groups the plants according to a certain system. Like Theophrastus two thousand years earlier he divides them into three groups: herbs, bushes and trees, and within these main groups into sub-categories according to appearance, nature, and other common features. In this Bock is sometimes referred to as 'the first forerunner of Linnaeus'.

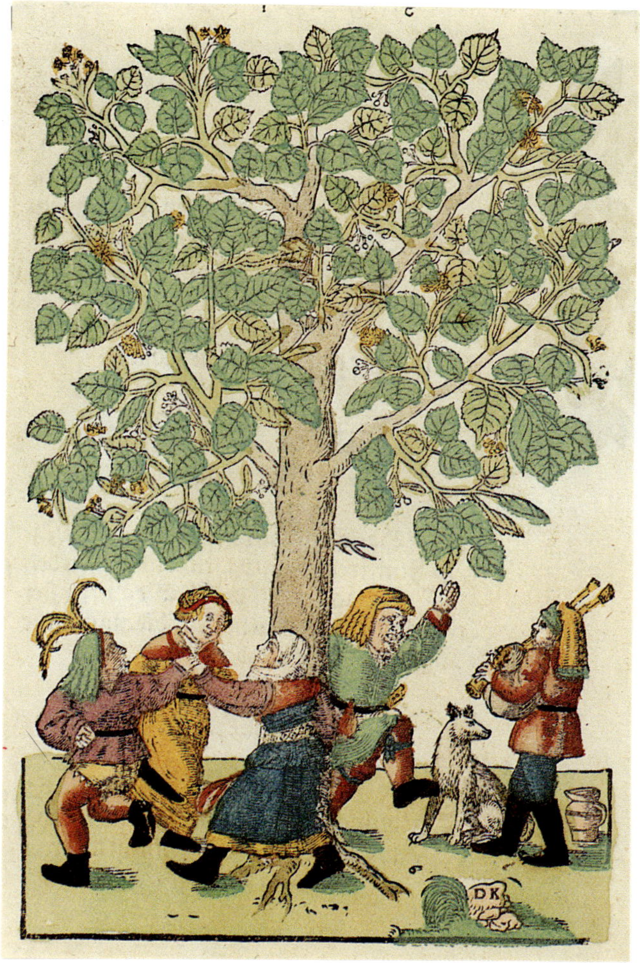

The first unillustrated edition was no great success, but in 1546 Wendel Rihel published a new edition, this time illustrated with 550 woodcuts by David Kandel, a self-taught artist from Strassburg, whose initials 'DK' can be seen on some of the blocks. Most of the pictures were adapted from the herbals of Brunfels and Fuchs but Kandel's own illustrations are at once charming, intelligent, and informative, especially in the third part where the depictions of trees are enlivened by the introduction of genre scenes with animals and people, whose activities allude to the particular uses and character of the trees. Especially famous is his picture of the fig-tree, under which a boy with his trousers down drastically illustrates the purgative effects of figs.

Bock's illustrated herbal was a great success and went through some fifteen editions. From 1577 on it was edited by Melchior Sebitzius and enlarged with a fourth book (or part), the *Teutsche Speisskammer*, illustrated with charming woodcuts attributed to Tobias Stimmer and Christoph Maurer. When Bock's publisher wished to issue a Latin edition for a wider international public he engaged a young scholar named David Kyber to translate Bock's Bavarian dialect, a task he accomplished in 1552, just one year before succumbing to the plague at the age of twenty-eight. In the botanical world Bock is known under the latinized form of his name, Tragus. He is commemorated by Charles Plumier (1703), who named the genus Tragia (*Euphorbiacede*) in his honour. This name was also used by Linnaeus (1753) who owned a copy of the 1552 Latin edition.

Greene/Egerton, I pp. 304-59; Arber, pp. 59-61, 151-3; Nissen, BBI, 182; Jerry Stannard in DSB, II, pp. 218-20; Johnston, *Cleveland Herbals* (other editions); *Tax. Lit.* 575; Anderson, pp. 130-6; Albert E. Lownes, *Renaissance Books of Science*, 7; Blunt/Raphael, pp. 129-32; Hoppe, *Das Kräuterbuch des Hieronymus Bock*, Stuttgart, 1969 (412 pp.); Waller 11463 (Latin ed., Strassburg, 1552).

RICETTARIO FIORENTINO

The first European pharmacopoeia

El Ricettario del l'Arte, et Universita de Medici, et Spetiali della citta di Firenze.
Florence, Lorenzo Torrentino, September, 1550.

Folio – *leaf*: 330 *x* 225 *mm. Pp.* 186, [2] *blank,* [20]. *With the ducal Medici arms on the title page and on the verso of the last leaf. On the second last leaf is a woodcut of the Virgin with the Child, the sign of the Florentine Guild of Physicians. Sign.*: a-p^6 q^4 r^6 s^4. *Very fine copy printed on thick paper with wide outer margin* (70 *mm*). *Modern binding by Fr. Ljunggren, Göteborg, in mottled calf with five raised bands, gilt. Preserved in a slipcase.*

From the Ernst Matérn Collection.

Second edition of of the Florentine pharmacopoeia. Our library is proud to possess not only this extremely rare edition but a further seven editions of this milestone in pharmaceutical literature: the third edition of 1567, the editions of 1574, 1597 and 1696 (the last edition with the engraved frontispiece), all being in folio; a duodecimo edition (Venice, Valgrisi, 1556), and the *Antidotarium* by Charles de L'Ecluse (Clusius) being his Latin translation of the above 1550 edition of the Florentine Ricettario. Clusius' *Antidotarium* is present both in the octavo edition printed by Christopher Plantin in Antwerp, 1561, and in the duodecimo edition printed in Lyon in the same year, both of which Hunger in his *Clusius Catalogus* (1926) regards as the rarest of all of Clusius' works. All of these treasures were recieved in the Ernst Matérn donation to our library, except the 1597 edition, which is from the C.D. Carlsson donation.

A *Pharmacopoeia* may be defined as a collection of formulae for medicinal preparations issued under the authority of some publicly recognized body. It embodies a list of approved drugs and describes the various methods of preparing them for administration or use, together with the proper weights and measures to be employed for accurate compounding. One of the chief objects of such an official publication was to ensure uniformity in the composition of the preparations and the purity of the substances used. It was in fact the apothecary's 'Bible', to which he was enjoined to conform in preparing the medicines prescribed by the physician. The name has also been applied to similar compendiums under various names such as *Antidotary, Dispensatory, Receptario*, etc., issued by private individuals or medical societies without legal government sanction.

The first edition of the Florentine pharmacopoeia, the *Nuovo Receptario,* is an extremely rare incunabula known to exist in only three copies, two in the Biblioteca Nazionale in Florence and one in the British Library. There are two variants, dated 10 resp. 21 Jan. 1498, the former containing the name of the author: Girolamo dal Pozzo Toscanelli, physician in Florence. It has often been called the first European pharmacopoeia, but it emanated from the Guild of Physicians and Pharmacists of Florence. It lacked government sanction, and therefore cannot be considered an official pharmacopoeia but a formulary for internal use of the Florentine guild. It took about half a century until the example of Florence was followed by official pharmacopoeias in the German Imperial Free Cities of Nuremberg (Valerius Cordus, 1546), Augsburg (1564) and Cologne (1565).

A pharmacopoeia of one's own gradually became a matter of national ambition, a part and a proof of national sovereignity and unity. In his article 'Pharmacopoeias as Witnesses of World History', the historian of pharmacy, Georg Urdang, makes the interesting observation that the various editions of the Florentine pharmacopoeia mirror, through their title pages and frontispieces, the political evolution in Florence in the sixteenth century, with particular reference to the rise to power of the Medici family.

The first edition of 1498 contains none of the dedicatory prefaces or phrases so common in those times of autocratic government and no coat of arms or marks save for two simple woodcuts beneath the colophon on the last page: the seal of the Guild of Apothecaries in Florence, the Virgin with the Child, and the printer's mark. The reason for this is that in early 1498 there was nobody in the city of Florence to whom such a dedication could properly be directed: the Medici family had by then been driven from the republic and the power of Savonarola was rapidly fading. The religious reformer was in fact condemned to death and perished at the stake in the very year of publication of the *Receptario.*

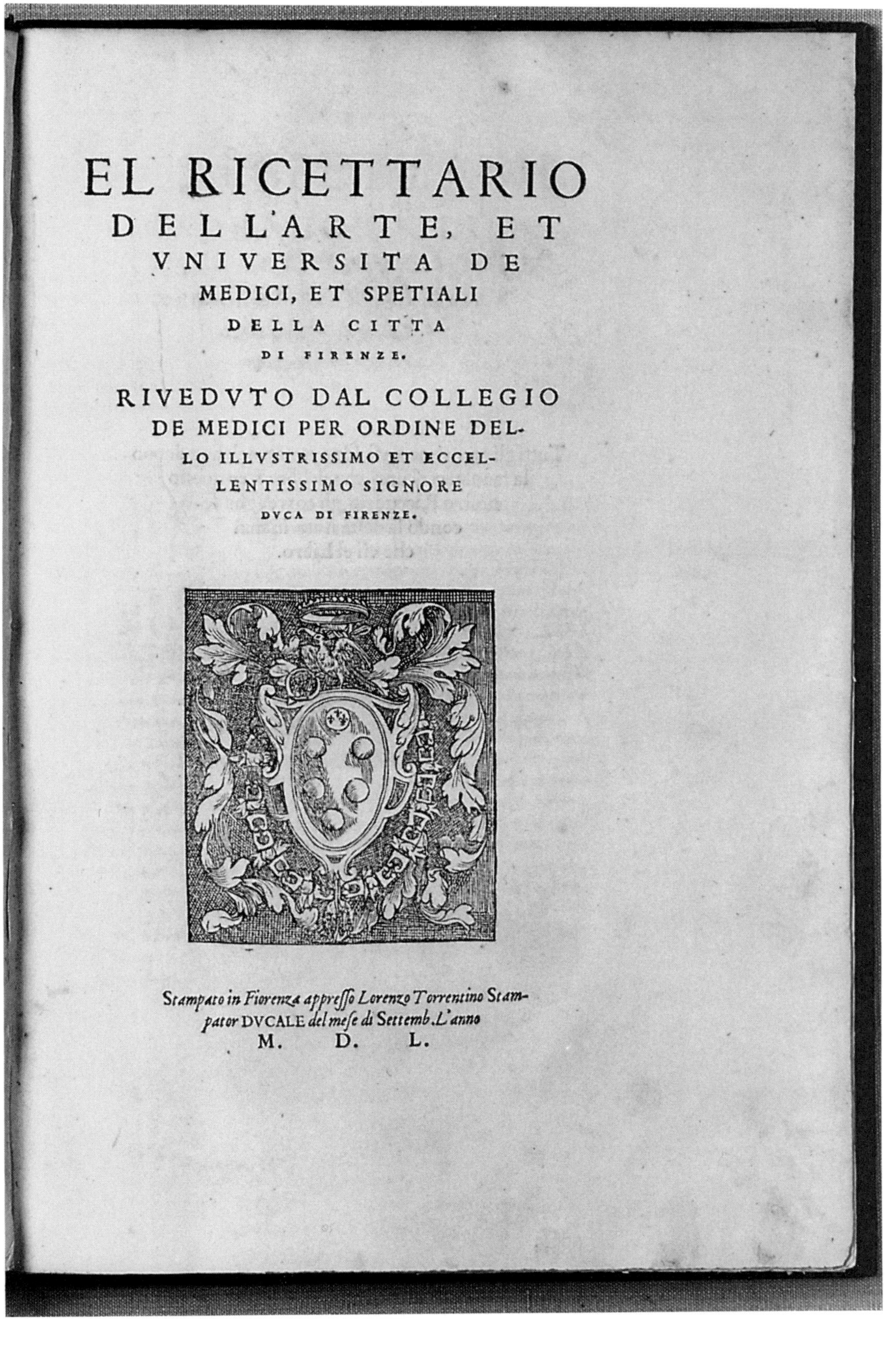
EL RICETTARIO
DELL'ARTE, ET
VNIVERSITA DE
MEDICI, ET SPETIALI
DELLA CITTA
DI FIRENZE.

RIVEDVTO DAL COLLEGIO
DE MEDICI PER ORDINE DEL-
LO ILLVSTRISSIMO ET ECCEL-
LENTISSIMO SIGNORE
DVCA DI FIRENZE.

Stampato in Fiorenza appresso Lorenzo Torrentino Stampator DVCALE *del mese di Settemb. L'anno*
M. D. L.

By 1550 the Medici had returned and ducal rule been installed, so the second edition of the pharmacopoeia, from now on entitled *Ricettario*, was prepared by order of the Duke of Florence, Cosimo I. Now to be found on the title page are the arms of the Medici family, evolved, however, from the original six simple balls set against a shield into something far more elaborate. Here a coronet surmounts the blazon and the royal lilies of France have been added, referring to Catherine de Medici's 1533 marriage to the French Dauphin, later King Henri II of France. Also present are the chain of the Imperial Order of the Golden Fleece, bestowed on Cosimo by the Emperor Charles V, and the dove symbolizing the peaceful intentions of the Duke.

The 1567 edition further illustrates political change: by now the Guild was more dependent on the Duke, a fact that is made evident by the almost sycophantic dedication to Cosimo, who is now referred to as *Duca et Principi de Fiorenza et Siena,* as he had now annexed Sienna to his territory. The coat of arms on the magnificient Renaissance frontispiece, which appears in this edition for the first time, is adapted to the new order. The peaceful dove, no doubt considered inappropriate after a period of conquest, has been replaced by a Florentine lily and the Imperial Order of Charles V has been omitted – the Medici had by now become too powerful to associate themselves with another ruler. The coronet is even more ornate, a fact that would be further accentuated in the next edition. This edition was also issued with the sanction of Pope Pius V, which suggests the intention of having this pharmacopoeia used on a broader national scale in the whole of Italy. In the 1573 edition (a reprint of the 1567 edition) Cosimo is called Grand Duke and Prince of Tuscany, a title conferred to him by Pius V in 1569. In that edition the Medici blazon is more splendid than ever, having been carefully described in the papal bull that created Cosimo's rank.

The last edition to include the famous frontispiece appeared in 1696. The next official Florentine pharmacopoeia was published in 1789, by which time the Medici had become extinct, which is why this frontispiece, tailored for the Florentine family, was never used again.

Alfons Lutz, 'Studien über die pharmazeutische Inkunabel "Nuovo Receptario" von Florenz', in *Veröff. d. Intern. Gesellsch. f. Geschichte der Pharmazie*, N.F. Band 13 (1957) pp. 113-28; Georg Urdang, 'Pharmacopoeias as Witnesses of World History', in *Journal of the History of Medicine & Allied Sciences* (1946), pp. 46-52; Cowen & Helfand, p. 68; Waller 7941 (1567 ed. only).

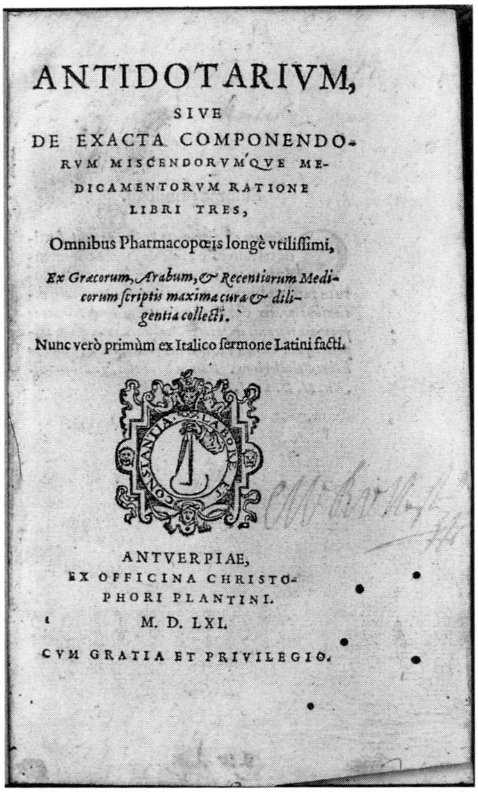

ANTIDOTARIVM,
SIVE
DE EXACTA COMPONENDORVM MISCENDORVMQVE MEDICAMENTORVM RATIONE
LIBRI TRES,
Omnibus Pharmacopœis longè vtilißimi,
Ex Græcorum, Arabum, & Recentiorum Medicorum scriptis maxima cura & diligentia collecti.
Nunc verò primùm ex Italico sermone Latini facti.

ANTVERPIAE,
EX OFFICINA CHRISTOPHORI PLANTINI.
M. D. LXI.
CVM GRATIA ET PRIVILEGIO.

The title page of Clusius' *Antidotarium* (Antwerp, 1561), being his revised Latin version of the second edition of the *Ricettario Fiorentino* (1550). It became one of the main sources for the *Dispensarium Coloniense* of 1565 (see p. 100. For Clusius, p. 120).

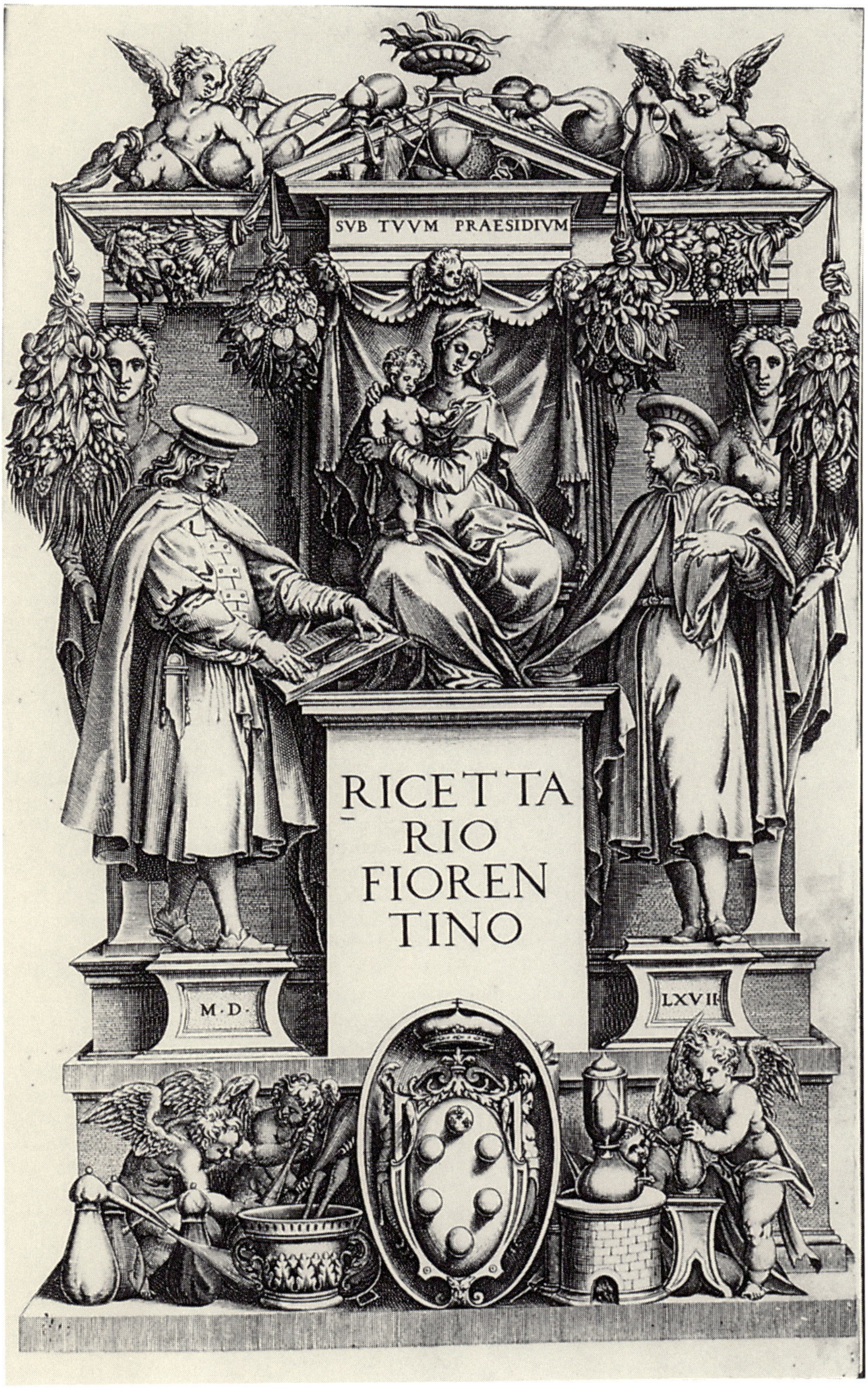

The magnificent engraved frontispiece, here in its 1567 version, represents the Virgin with the Child, the sign of the Florentine Guild of Apothecaries, seated on a pedestal and flanked by two figures. The one on the right bears the attributes of the apothecary, a spatula and ointment box, while the figure on the left represents a physician perusing an open herbal. In the four corners are putti busying themselves with alchemists' and pharmacists' equipment.

CORDUS, Valerius (1515–1544)

The first official pharmacopoeia

Pharmacorum conficiendorum ratio. Vulgo vocant Dispensatorium. Nuremberg, Johannes Daubman, 1551.

Octavo – *leaf*: 153 x 98 *mm. Pp.* [32], 1-64, 67-98, 97-508. *Sign.*: 2A-B8 A-Z8 a-h8 i6 *(lacking the two final blank leaves). Contemporary blindstamped pigskin over wooden boards with three raised bands. Inner panel surrounded by a roll-produced floral border. Upper panel with four pineapples flanked by crescents. Below is the date* 1554. *Early Ms notes inside the covers and in the text. Brass clasps intact.*

From the Ernst Matérn Collection.

A very rare early edition of the first official pharmacopoeia ever to be published, that of the city of Nuremberg. The undated first edition had appeared after the author's death (c.1546) and was quickly followed by the likewise undated second edition (c.1547). The first edition is an extremely rare book of which a facsimile appeared in 1934, with an introduction by Ludwig Winkler. The present (pirated?) edition, an incorrect copy of the first two editions, was probably published without the permission of the Nuremberg council. It was printed in 1551, by Johannes Daubmann, in Nuremberg, who had been landed several times in the town dungeon for similar escapades. In 1554 he became the first printer in Königsberg.

Valerius Cordus was the son of Euricius Cordus, who was professor of medicine at the then newly founded (1527) University of Marburg. He is famous as a gifted humanist, poet and botanist; he laid out a botanical garden and was the first German professor to organize excursions for studying plants. Valerius was thus brought up in a scholarly, stimulating atmosphere and became somewhat of a prodigy. He obtained his bachelor's degree at the University of Marburg at the early age of 16. His father instructed him in botany and the preparation of medicines. Valerius completed his training in the apothecary shop of his uncle, Johannes Ralla, at Leipzig, where he moved in 1533 and enrolled at the university. In the year 1539 he is lecturing at the University of Wittenberg on pharmacy and the *materia medica* of Dioscorides.

In Wittenberg Cordus developed close ties to a local apothecary shop and here completed his *Dispensatorium*, a collection of medical recipes, chiefly selected from earlier writings. This work was considered so valuable that, after it had been examined and tested by the local physicians, it was published in 1546 under the auspices of the Nuremberg town council. For the first time order was brought to the unsystematic corpus of medicaments and Cordus' pharmacopoeia soon became the obligatory standard work for all Germany. With its selection of formulas and its brief but clear annotations, it met the needs of the practising pharmacists to such an extent, especially in the version edited by the Antwerp apothecary, Peter Coudenberg, in 1568, that is was copied and reprinted again and again until the end of the seventeenth century in about forty editions in various European cities. A very fine copy of the Coudenberg edition (Antwerp, Plantin, 1568) is also in our Ernst Matérn collection. In addition to describing approximately 225 medicinal plants and minerals, Cordus refers, with careful commentary, to the origin and adulteration of drugs. Cordus traveled widely in Germany in search of plants, but as he had always longed to see the plants of which the ancients had written under their native skies, he came to spend two years in Italy visiting Padua, Bologna, Florence, Sienna, and other cities. In the late summer of 1544 in the company of two friends he reached Rome, where he contracted a severe fever (malaria), which was reputedly aggravated after he was kicked by a horse, causing his death at the early age of 29. Since he was regarded a heretic his corpse would have been thrown into the Tiber had it not been rescued by his two countrymen. The body found its resting place in the Church of Santa Maria dell' Anima. The grave is long since destroyed as a result of one of several church restorations.

All of Valerius Cordus' published works are posthumous, compiled partly from finished manuscripts and partly from notes taken by his students. He is generally called the discoverer of ether (c.1540) after a recipe found in his annotations on Dioscorides, published by Conrad Gesner in 1561. He was a brilliant botanist of unusual capacity, who, but for his early death, might have become one of the most renowned herbalists of the sixteenth century. To the three German Fathers of Botany, Brunfels, Bock and Fuchs, a fourth name should be added, that of Valerius Cordus.

Garrison-Morton, 1810 (first ed.); Rudolf Schmitz in DSB, III, pp. 413-15; Greene /Egerton 1, pp. 368-72; Arber, *Herbals*, pp. 74-6; Waller 2128-30 (later editions).

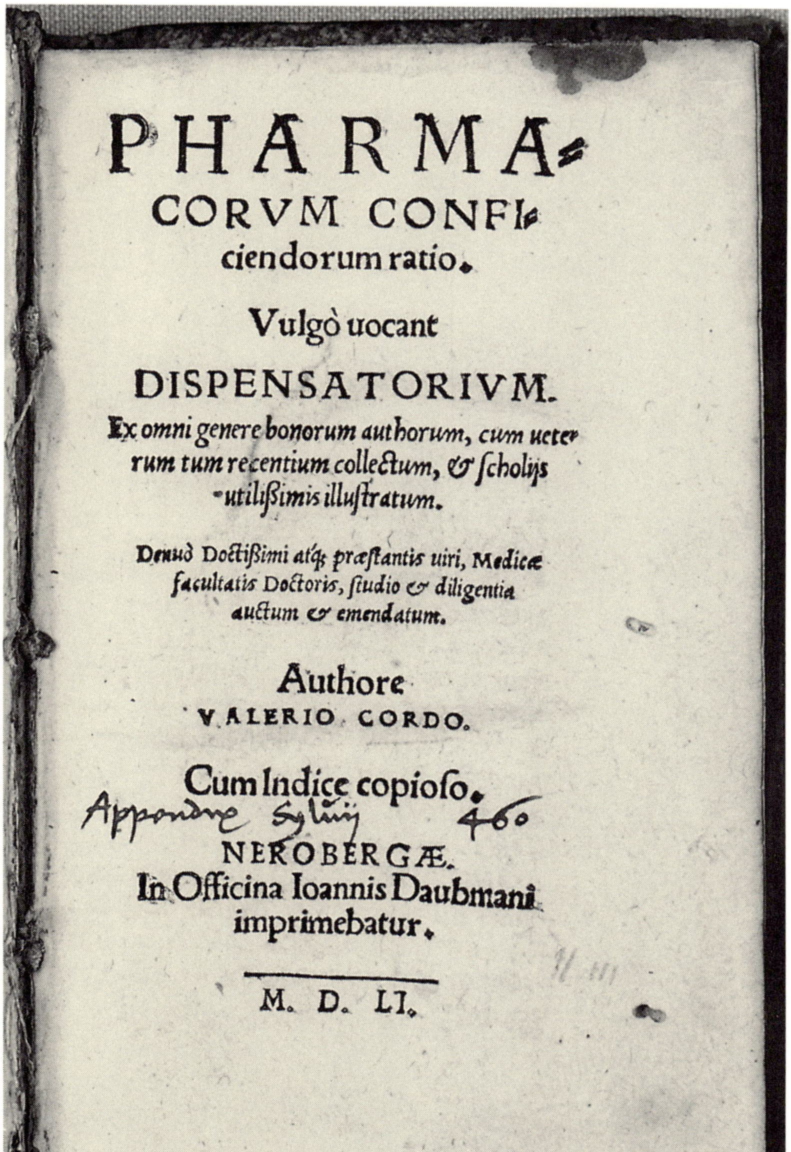
PHARMA-
CORVM CONFI-
ciendorum ratio.

Vulgò uocant

DISPENSATORIVM.

Ex omni genere bonorum authorum, cum ueterum tum recentium collectum, & scholijs utilißimis illustratum.

Denuò Doctißimi atq; præstantis uiri, Medicæ facultatis Doctoris, studio & diligentia auctum & emendatum.

Authore
VALERIO CORDO.

Cum Indice copioso.

NEROBERGÆ.
In Officina Ioannis Daubmani imprimebatur.

M. D. LI.

The most widespread of all herbals

MATTIOLI, Pietro Andrea (1500–1577)

Commentarii in sex libros Pedacii Dioscoridis Anazerbi de Medicina materia . . . Adiectis plantarum, & animalium Iconibus, supra prioris editiones longe pluribus, ad vivum delineatis, . . .
Venice, Valgrisi, 1570.

Folio – *leaf*: 327 *x* 215 *mm. Pp.* [168], 956, [12]. *Title and last page with Valgrisi's snake device. With* 1023 *smaller woodcuts in the text of which* 88 *are of animals and the rest of plants. The appendix of* 12 *pages,* De ratione distillandi aquas, *has* 6 *full-page woodcuts of furnaces and distilling apparatus. Contemporary blindstamped pigskin over thick wooden boards, five bands, brass corners, two brass clasps.*

Provenance: G.A. Bernardi, *with his signature and Ms monogram (initials) in red ink on the title page, repeated on the last woodcut of a furnace;* Christoph Wenzel Graf von Nostitz (1643–1712), *with his signature on the title.*

Mattioli's Commentary on Dioscorides' *De materia medica* was one of the most popular herbals of the sixteenth century. Dioscorides' descriptions of some 600 medicinal plants, written in the first century A.D., was the largest collection of drugs described in classical antiquity. It was copied throughout the Middle Ages and provided, along with Pliny and Galen, the principal sources for the description of plants and their medicinal uses. Before 1544, when the first edition of Mattioli's commentaries was published, there had appeared some 35 editions, translations and commentaries. These early editions of Dioscorides were of more appeal to the scholar and philologist than to the physician. Mattioli's purpose was to provide doctors and apothecaries with a practical treatise in Italian with a commentary that would enable them to identify the medicinal plants mentioned by Dioscorides.

Pietro Andrea [Pierandrea] Mattioli was born in Siena. He was the son of a physician and his early life was spent in Venice, where his father practised. Pierandrea was destined for the law but chose to follow in his father's footsteps. After studies in Padua he set up a practice in Siena and in 1520 in Rome, where he remained until the barbarous sack of that city in 1527. Mattioli was fortunate to survive and spent the next fourteen years in Valle Anania, near Trento, where he became very popular. After that he moved to Gorizia, where he worked as town physician for a further fourteen years.

The first edition of the work that was to make Mattioli famous was published in Venice in 1544 by Nicolo de Bascarini. It was an annotated Italian version of Dioscorides' *De materia medica*, a modest, unillustrated book, which, judging from its rarity, may have had a small print run. It is possible that Mattioli was dissatisfied with his publisher, as the next edition of his Italian translation was published in 1548 by the prestigious Valgrisi press in Venice, the publishers or co-publishers of the majority of Mattioli's books. It was soon followed by two more Italian editions in 1550 and 1552 with rewritten commentaries.

In 1554 Valgrisi published the first Latin edition, which took the book to the rest of Europe. It was a publishing success. The addition of synonyms drawn from various languages was a decided advantage to the physician, the apothecary, and the professional herb collector, all of whom benefitted by this additional information. What most of all contributed to its success was the inclusion of 562 small illustrations of uniform size, more than five hundred of which were of plants. These woodcuts were the joint work of Giorgio Liberale of Undine and of a German named Wolfgang Meyerpeck. This imposing production of an important work made Mattioli known throughout Europe and it aroused special interest in Prague, since in the same year Mattioli was invited there by the Holy Roman Emperor, Ferdinand I, to treat his son, the Archduke Maximillian. Mattioli remained in the imperial service for more than twenty years, and there appeared in 1562 a Bohemian edition translated into Czech published by Georg Melantrich, who collaborated with Valgrisi in Venice. That edition and the 1563 German translation by Georg Handsch, also printed in Prague, were the first to be illustrated with large full-page woodcuts. These large blocks were also produced by Liberale and Meyerpeck and are far more accomplished and impressive, with details executed with great skill. The whole series of just over 900 of plants and almost 100 of animals were incorporated into Valgrisi's Latin edition of 1565, which brought the book back to Venice. This fourth Latin edition is the first to be augmented by Mattioli's fuller notes and has always been the most valued due to its completeness.

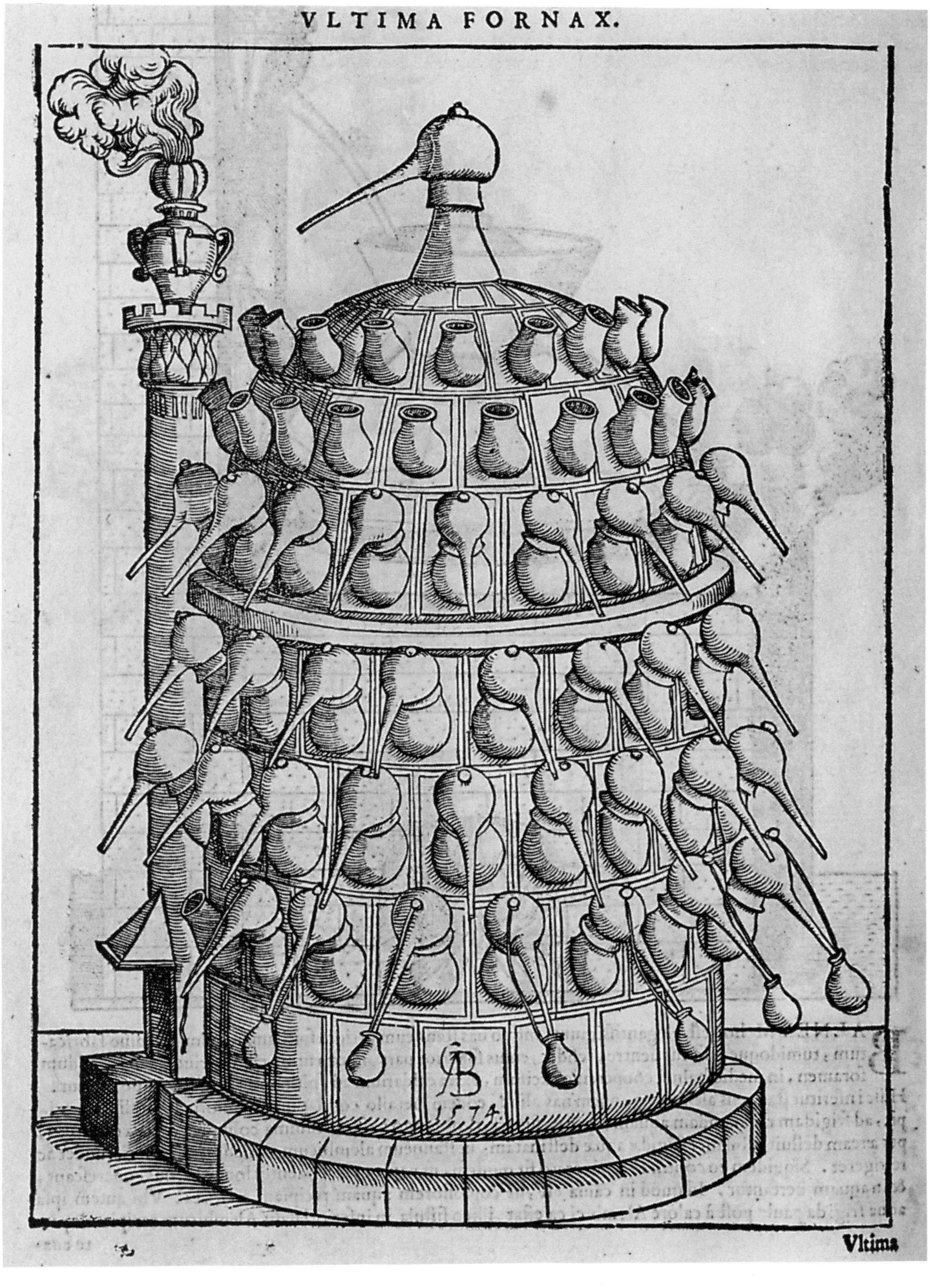

Mattioli's Commentary on Dioscorides contains an Appendix on Distillation illustrated with six large woodcuts. The one above depicts a 'galley' furnace or 'gallery' oven, a distillation tower. Mattioli himself had distilled salt from two human skulls and prepared an oil from scorpions.

The years of scholarship and the countless letters that passed between Mattioli and his co-workers are clearly evident in his commentary. In addition a curious work, the *De ratione distillandi aquas*, was appended at the end, illustrated with striking woodcuts of distilling apparatus.

The success of Mattioli's work was phenomenal, and it was republished many times in various languages until as late as 1744. Altogether at least sixty editions were published. In the preface to the German edition of 1563 it is said that a total of 32 000 copies had been sold. In 1570 Mattioli left Prague and returned to the Tirol. He died at Trento in 1577, a victim of the plague, and is buried in the cathedral.

In the library of the Swedish Pharmaceutical Society there are seven editions. Besides the above Latin edition (Venice, 1570) there is one Italian translation (Venice, 1581), one French (Lyon, 1627), three German of Mattioli's herbal (Frankfurt, 1586, 1600 and Basel, 1678) and Mattioli's *Opera* (Basel, 1674). The German edition of 1600 has all the woodcuts coloured by hand.

MATTIOLI, P. A. & Joachim CAMERARIUS the Younger

Kreutterbuch dess Hochgelehrten unnd weitberühmten Herrn D. Petri Andreæ Matthioli, Jetzt widerumb mit vielen schönen newen Figuren auch nützlichen Artzneyen und andern guten Stücken, zum dritten mal auss sonderm Fleiss gemehret, unnd verfertigt, durch Ioachimum Camerarium . . . Beneben gnugsamen Bericht, von den Distillier und Brennöfen.

Frankfurt am Mayn, printed by Palthenius for Johnae Rosen, 1600.

Folio – *leaf*: 377 *x* 240 *mm. Ff.* [10], 460, [27]. *Title printed in red and black within a large historiated woodcut border. Last page with printer's device. Illustrated with* 1036 *woodcuts of plants and* 7 *of furnaces and distilling apparatus. Title border and all the woodcuts in contemporary hand-colouring. Lacks one gathering* (Kk*) of six leaves (fol.* 193-8) *and fol.* 237. *Eighteenth century half calf, sprinkled boards.*

There are seven old signatures on the title page incl. Montan, Paul Ulrich Paulin *and* J. Fogelberg. *Book-plate:* C.D. Carlsson.

The present edition of Mattioli's herbal (*Kreutterbuch*) is edited by another great herbalist, Joachim Camerarius the Younger (1534–1598) of Nuremberg. He spent some time in Italy and took his medical degree in Bologna before returning to his birthplace, where he kept a botanical garden with many rare plants. Camerarius' *Kreutterbuch*, based on Mattioli, first appeared in 1586 and went through at least four editions up to 1626. Mattioli's German herbal is not to be confused with the Commentaries, as is often the case. The Mattioli/Camerarius *Kreutterbuch* is a mere herbal, a compendium of all the plants known to Mattioli, enlarged with new ones by Camerarius. Its illustrations only correspond with those in the botanical part of Mattioli's *Commentarii*, whereas the text has no bearing on either Dioscorides or Mattioli's Commentaries.

Camerarius' edition is of special interest as it contains illustrations deriving from Conrad Gesner, whose great botanical work, *Historia Plantarum*, was left unpublished. On Gesner's death his material was left to his friend Kaspar Wolf, who in turn sold it to Camerarius. Gesner's already finished wood blocks as well as new ones, cut from his drawings under the supervision of Camerarius, were in part incorporated together with illustrations deriving from the Bohemian edition of Mattioli's herbal of 1596, noted for its fine woodcuts, while the remainder was adapted from the Venice editions of Mattioli's Commentaries, partly copied in reduced size from the finest Venice edition of 1565. In the present copy all the woodcuts are in the original hand-colouring as is the fine title border engraved by 'C S' (Christoph Stimmer) after a drawing by 'I A' (Jost Amman).

Arber, pp. 92-7, 221-6; Greene/Egerton, II, pp. 798-806; Schreiber, p. XLIV; Nissen, BBI, 1304-1315; Hunt I, 59, 90-1, 94, 160; Bruno Zanobio in DSB, IX, pp. 178-80; Anderson, pp. 163-72; Blunt/Raphael, pp. 132-6; Sandra Raphael, 'Mattioli's Herbal' in *The Mattioli Woodblocks* offered for sale by Antiquariaat Junk & Bernard Quaritch; J. Stannard, 'P.A. Mattioli: Sixteenth-Century Commentator on Dioscorides', in *Bibliographical Contributions, University of Kansas Libraries*, I, 1969, pp. 59-81; Waller 6323 (*Commentarii*, Venice, 1558).

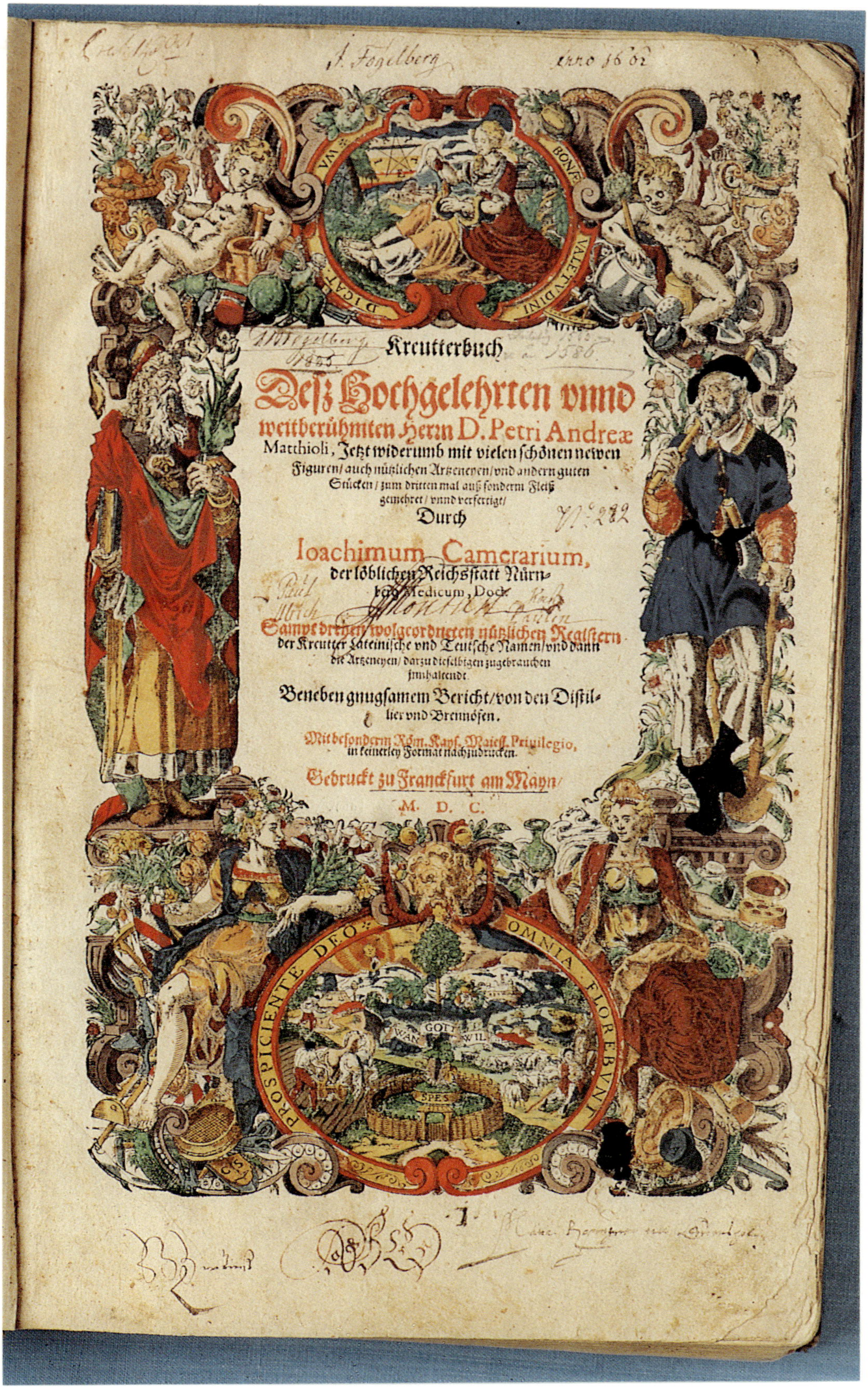
Kreutterbuch
Deß Hochgelehrten vnnd
weitberühmten Herrn D. Petri Andreæ
Matthioli, Jetzt widerumb mit vielen schönen newen
Figuren/ auch nützlichen Artzeneyen/ vnd andern guten
Stücken/ zum dritten mal auß sonderm Fleiß
gemehret/ vnnd verfertigt/
Durch
Ioachimum Camerarium,
der löblichen Reichsstatt Nürnberg Medicum, Doct.
Sampt dreyen wolgeordneten nützlichen Registern
der Kreutter Lateinische vnd Teutsche Namen/ vnd dann
die Artzeneyen/ darzu dieselbigen zugebrauchen
innhaltende.
Beneben gnugsamem Bericht/ von den Distillier vnd Brennöfen.
Mit besonderm Röm. Kays. Maiest. Privilegio,
in keinerley Format nachzudrucken.
Gedruckt zu Franckfurt am Mayn/
M. D. C.
PROSPICIENTE DEO OMNIA FLOREBVNT
GOT WAN WIL
SPES

FIORAVANTI, Leonardo (1517–1588)

A popular Book of Secrets

Del compendio dei secreti rationali libri cinque.
Venice, Andrea Ravenoldo, 1566.

Octavo – *leaf*: 149 *x* 100 *mm. Ff.* [20], 1-112 (113-16 *dropped),* 117-84. *Recto of last leaf has colophon and register [list of signature-letters] with printer's device on verso. Later boards covered with a leaf from a sixteenth century book.*

Book-plate: Ernst Matérn.

Second edition of a popular 'Book of Secrets' that went through numerous editions and translations until the mid-seventeenth century. The first edition was printed in Venice by Vincenzo Valgrisi in 1564. It is a handbook of medicine and pharmacy dealing with 'secrets' and 'mysteries' and is divided into five books devoted to various aspects of medicine, surgery, alchemy, and cosmetics; it contains not only secrets of medicine with the necessary preparation of drugs and remedies, but recipes for several technical purposes as well; in the fifth book Fioravanti describes various methods of making writing ink and printer's ink.

Leonardo Fioravanti was a native of Bologna, where he was known as a celebrated physician, surgeon and alchemist. He studied medicine and practised in Palermo from 1548 to 1550, went with the Spanish fleet to Africa, returned to Naples in 1555, went to Rome, Venice and Bologna, where he was made a doctor, a chevalier and and finally a count. He was one of the few Paracelsists in Italy and has been called a quack. His books have been severely handled by some modern critics. Gnudi and Webster, however, state that Fioravanti 'was one of the clever, dashing figures of the sixteenth century whose unconventional, unacademic approach to medicine, together with his lively curiosity in alchemy and unorthodox remedies, has caused him, perhaps unjustly, to be accused of charlatanery. The boastfulness of his writings and the fact that he unjustifiably claimed a degree from Bologna do, in fact, place him somewhat beyond the pale of respectability, but his quick mind, keen observations and exuberant, often naive spirit endow him with interest to anyone seeking an understanding of his age'. Aldrovandi calls Fioravanti 'Empyricus Venetus' and quotes his notion that the sapphire stimulates gaiety, since it is jovial, and for this reason is a wonderful remedy for all affections of the heart.

Fioravanti was above all a pharmacist, who in his practice put unbounded trust in his specifics. The balsam named after him, which figures in the pharmacopoeias until the beginning of this century, was a very complex mixture. He pretended to give the exact formulas for his various devised 'Nostra', and these were always so complicated that no doubt the rich clients whose patronage Fioravanti cultivated would prefer to buy the remedies readily compounded. His medical advice, though crammed with bombast, was generally sensible, but in all cases he recommended one or another of 'our' remedies, which included 'Balm Artificiall' or 'Baume Fioravanti', which was an alcoholic tincture of canella, cloves, nutmegs, ginger, and other spices, with bay berries, to which were added amber, galbanum, myrrh, aloes, elemi, and other resins, and one-sixth by volume of turpentine. After digestion this mixture was distilled to a yield of about two-thirds of the original bulk. (Wootton)

In his 'Compilation of Secrets' he tells the story that during the war of 1456 both armies consumed human flesh and thus became contaminated. He is perhaps best known for being the first to describe a splenectomy, performed by himself or by a stonecutter, who lifted a hypertrophied spleen from a woman at Palermo in 1549 (nearly 300 years before Quittenbaum) and then had her exhibited publicly in the merchants' square for three whole days. This we can read about in his *Il Tesoro della Vita Humana* (1570), which book is also an important source for the early history of plastic surgery. Fioravanti reports an adventure in Africa: while he was strolling with a Spanish gentleman, Messer Andres Gutiero, his companion encountered a soldier. They drew weapons, and the soldier cut off the Spaniard's nose, which fell in the sand. Fioravanti picked it up, cleaned it by urinating on it, attached it to the Spaniard's face, sewed it on very firmly and bandaged it. After eight days he untied it and found it well attached. 'And this was indeed the truth and Messer Andres can tell of it because he is still alive and healthy' (Gnudi & Webster).

Gnudi & Webster, 116-18; Ferguson I, 278; Schelenz, 454; Partington II, 29; Thorndike VI, 217; Wootton, *Chronicles of Pharmacy* II, 173-5; Waller 3050 (Venice, 1660).

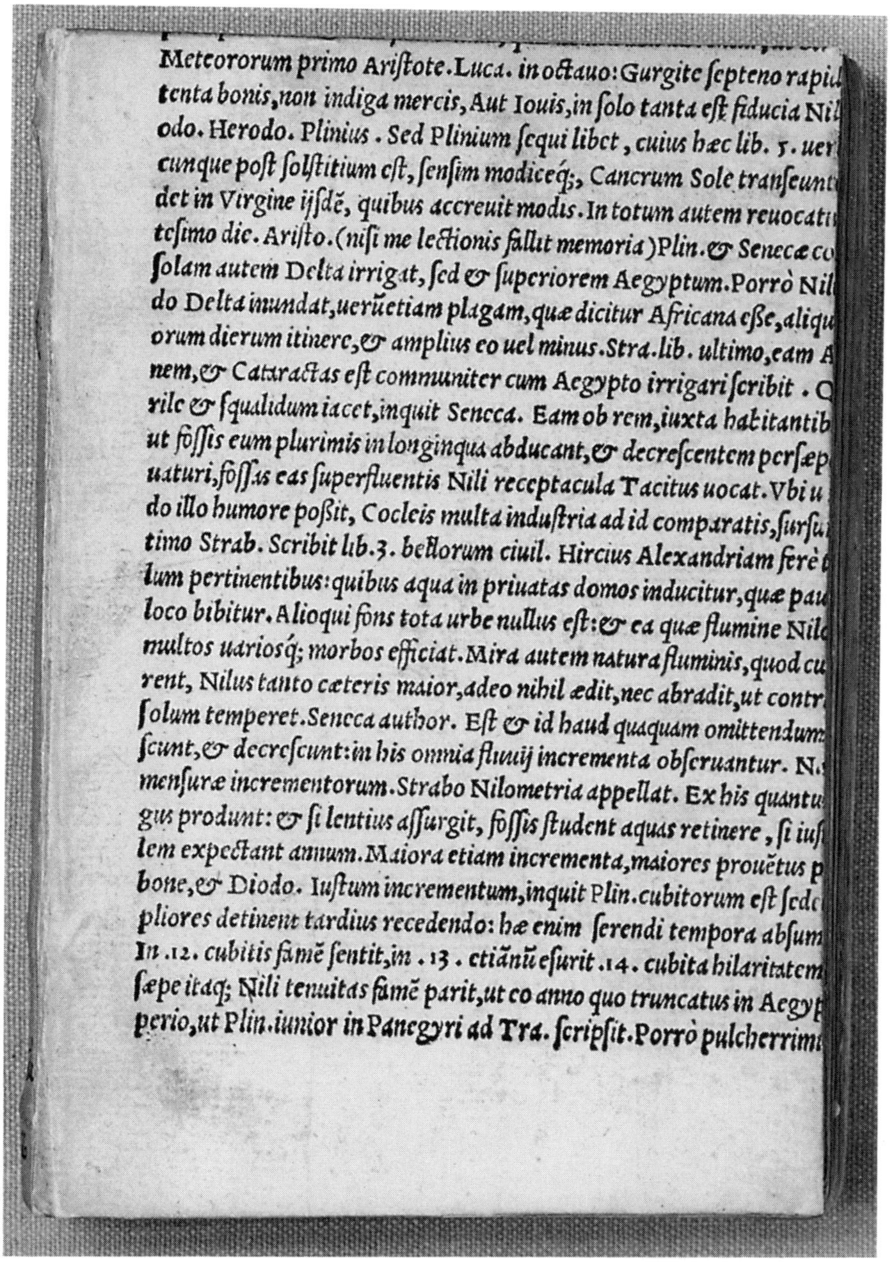

Meteororum primo Aristote.Luca. in octauo:Gurgite septeno rapi
tenta bonis,non indiga mercis,Aut Iouis,in solo tanta est fiducia Ni
odo. Herodo. Plinius. Sed Plinium sequi libet, cuius hæc lib. 5. uer
cunque post solstitium est, sensim modiceq́;, Cancrum Sole transeunt
det in Virgine iisdē, quibus accreuit modis. In totum autem reuocatu
tesimo die. Aristo.(nisi me lectionis fallit memoria)Plin.& Senecæ co
solam autem Delta irrigat, sed & superiorem Aegyptum.Porrò Nil
do Delta inundat, uerūetiam plagam, quæ dicitur Africana esse, aliqu
orum dierum itinere,& amplius eo uel minus. Stra. lib. ultimo, eam A
nem,& Catarractas est communiter cum Aegypto irrigari scribit . C
rile & squalidum iacet, inquit Seneca. Eam ob rem, iuxta habitantib
ut fossis eum plurimis in longinqua abducant,& decrescentem persæp
uaturi, fossas eas superfluentis Nili receptacula Tacitus uocat. Vbi u
do illo humore possit, Cocleis multa industria ad id comparatis, sursu
timo Strab. Scribit lib.3. bellorum ciuil. Hircius Alexandriam ferè
lum pertinentibus: quibus aqua in priuatas domos inducitur, quæ pau
loco bibitur. Alioqui fons tota urbe nullus est:& ea quæ flumine Nil
multos uariosq́; morbos efficiat. Mira autem natura fluminis, quod cu
rent, Nilus tanto cæteris maior, adeo nihil ædit, nec abradit, ut contr
solum temperet. Seneca author. Est & id haud quaquam omittendum
scunt,& decrescunt: in his omnia fluuij incrementa obseruantur. N
mensuræ incrementorum. Strabo Nilometria appellat. Ex his quantu
gus produnt: & si lentius assurgit, fossis student aquas retinere, si iu
lem expectant annum. Maiora etiam incrementa, maiores prouētus p
bone,& Diodo. Iustum incrementum, inquit Plin. cubitorum est sede
pliores detinent tardius recedendo: hæ enim serendi tempora absum
In .12. cubitis famē sentit, in .13. etiānū esurit .14. cubita hilaritatem
sæpe itaq; Nili tenuitas famē parit, ut eo anno quo truncatus in Aegyp
perio, ut Plin. iunior in Panegyri ad Tra. scripsit. Porrò pulcherrim

Fioravanti's Book of Secrets (1566).
Boards covered with a leaf from a sixteenth century book.

Second edition of the Pharmacopoeia Augustana

PHARMACOPOEIA AUGUSTANA 1573.

Pharmacopoeia, seu medicamentorum pro. Rep. Augustana. Cui accessere simplicia omnia officinis nostus usitata, & annotationes in eadem et composita ab Adolpho Occone eiusdem Reip. Medico diligenter congesta.
Colophon: Augsburg, Michael Mangerus for Georg Willer, 1573.

Tall, narrow folio – *leaf:* 290 *x* 98 *mm. Pp.* [2], 391,]1] *errata, [12] index,* [2] *colophon leaf. Nineteenth century paste paper boards. Title within a woodcut border and with the Augsburg* (Augustae Vindelicorum) *coat of arms.*

Provenance: Adalbert Mayrhofer; C.E. Rappaport (*bookseller in Rome*). *From the* Ernst Matérn Collection.

The second edition of the important Augsburg pharmacopoeia, and the first to appear under the name of *Pharmacopoeia.* The first edition of 1564 was entitled *Enchiridion* and appeared without date of publication, name of printer or place of publication; not even the author is mentioned, and the book has no preface. Very few have seen the extremely rare first edition. At the time of Theodor Husemann's excellent account on the various early editions of the *Pharmacopoeia Augustana* in 1892, only two copies could be traced, one in the Augsburg City Library, the other in the University Library of Würzburg. The latter was reproduced in facsimile in 1927. The Swedish Pharmaceutical Society is proud to possess the almost equally rare second edition as well as the successive eleven editions up to the last one in 1734: 3rd ed., 1574, 4th ed., 1580, 5th ed., 1597, 6th ed., 1613, 7th ed., 1622 in folio, 1623 in octavo, 1643, 1646, 1684, 1690 and 1734 – an impressive collection indeed of this important pharmacopoeia, donated by the heirs of Ernst Matérn in the 1950s.

In the sixteenth century three German cities introduced legal standards for compound and simple medicaments. In 1546 Nuremberg became the first to issue an official pharmacopoeia, compiled by Valerius Cordus and approved by the Nuremberg city senate. It was followed in 1564 by Augsburg and in 1565 by Cologne. Although the Nuremberg *Dispensatorium* is the one most often referred to in pharmaco-historical literature, it was the *Pharmacopoeia Augustana* that exerted a much wider influence, appearing in new and improved editions up to the middle of the eighteenth century. Both the Augsburg and the Cologne pharmacopoeias surpassed the work of Valerius Cordus in thoroughness and care. Valerius Cordus was only nineteen years old when he, upon the advice of his uncle, an apothecary, compiled his *Dispensatorium* and submitted it to the Senate of Nuremberg. The compilers of the Augsburg and Cologne pharmacopoeias were physicians of long experience. Unlike Cordus, they had studied not only in Germany, but had acquired their doctor's degree in Italy and there had had access to a number of pharmacological treatises, which presumably were not available to Cordus. In addition, the author of the Augsburg pharmacopoeia had at hand the Occo family library, which, exceedingly rich in treasures, was used and praised by numerous contemporaries. Thus the Augsburg pharmacopoeia is the most learned and thorough of the three city pharmacopoeias of the sixteenth century.

The author of the Augsburg pharmacopoeia was Adolph Occo III, city physician and inspector of the apothecary shops of Augsburg. There were four physicians of the Occo lineage all christened Adolph and differentiated by the designations I, II, III and IV. The second edition is the first to give the name of the author, who has signed the dedication. In it he points out that the first edition had long since been out of print, particularly as a result of demand from abroad. In place of the *Enchiridion* the designation *Pharmacopoeia* appears here for the first time, and the contents are considerably enlarged. The 1573 and the 1597 editions are both in the same tall and narrow folio format commonly used for manuscript recipe books, while the 1574 and 1580 editions are ordinary octavos. All the sixteenth-century editions are associated with the name of Adolph Occo III, and according to Husemann all of them were rare already in 1892. Our copy of the fourth edition of 1580 is in a richly gilt early vellum binding with the signature of *Hieronymi Beck à Leopoldstorf* on the title page and the stamp of *Bibliotheca Conventus,* Vienna.

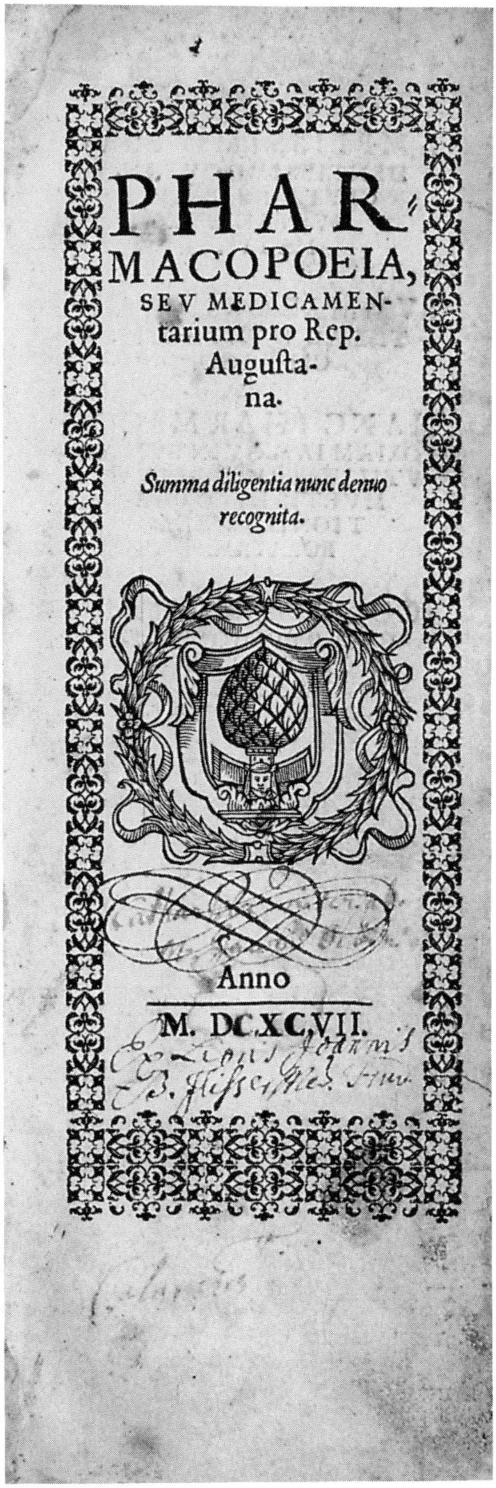

PHAR-
MACOPOEIA,
SEV MEDICAMEN-
tarium pro Rep.
Augusta-
na.

*Summa diligentia nunc denuo
recognita.*

Anno
M. DCXCVII.

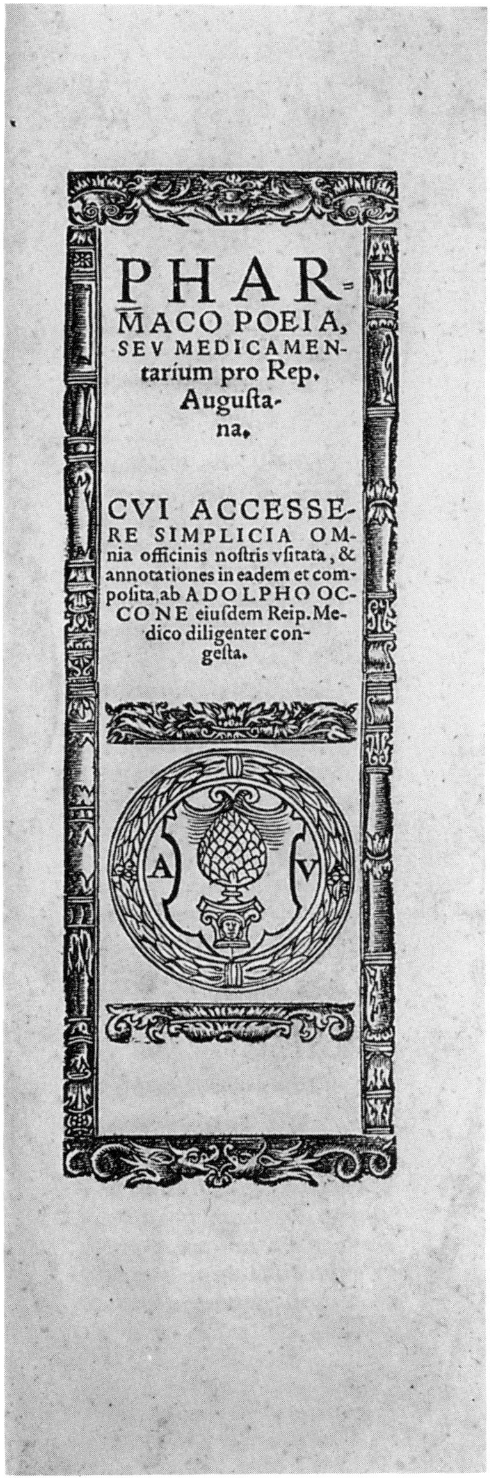

PHAR-
MACO POEIA,
SEV MEDICAMEN-
tarium pro Rep.
Augusta-
na.

CVI ACCESSE-
RE SIMPLICIA OM-
nia officinis nostris vsitata, &
annotationes in eadem et com-
posita, ab ADOLPHO OC-
CONE eiusdem Reip. Me-
dico diligenter con-
gesta.

The second (1573) and the fifth (1597) edition of the *Pharmacopoeia Augustana* with the Augsburg (A[ugustae] V[ndelicorum]) coat of arms: – a pine cone (*Pinus Cembra*).

The first Minderer edition

PHARMACOPOEIA AUGUSTANA 1613.

Pharmacopoeia Augustana. Jussu et auctoritate Amplissimi Senatus a Collegio Medico rursus recognita, ac elaboratior et auctior, nunc sextum in lucem emissa.
Augsburg, Christoph Mang for Johann Kruger, 1613.

Folio – *297 x 195 mm. Pp.* [6], 23, [1], 298, 19, [1]; *Taxa: pp.* [26]. *Engraved title leaf. One (of two) folding tables. The missing table replaced by manuscript in an old hand (this table, however, is present in our second copy from the* C.D. Carlsson Collection). *Contemporary vellum. Signed on the title:* Zacharias Rosenbach . . . 1630. *From the* Ernst Matérn Collection.

The sixth edition of the Augsburg pharmacopoeia, and the first compiled by Raymund Minderer (c.1570–1621), city physician of Augsburg, physician-in-ordinary to Duke Maximillian I of Bavaria and also to the German Emperor Matthias. He was a highly esteemed physician and medical writer, who received from his contemporaries the cognomen 'The Swabian Hippocrates'.

As the five editions of the Augsburg *Pharmacopoeia* of the sixteenth century are associated with Adolph Occo, who represents the orthodox teachings of medicine as contrasted with Paracelsus and his followers, so the four earliest seventeenth-century editions are associated with Minderer. These were the sixth edition (1613) and the seventh edition in folio (1622), reprinted in 1623 in a more convenient, smaller octavo format, of which there also exists a title page edition of 1629. Minderer's first edition (1613) for the most part contains the old, harmless formulas of Occo's *Pharmacopoeia,* but in addition, a considerable number of additional formulas from Paracelsian sources are to be found in the new chapters on extracts. New also is a table of antidotes, which reveals in a drastic manner the very curious opinions held at that time concerning poisons and their antidotes. Minderer still enumerates brain of cat, gypsum, menstrual blood, as well as the sea-hare, which certainly has never injured any Augsburger, as poisons demanding antidotal treatment. The 1613 edition was the first official pharmaceutical standard to list chemicals for internal use. In quite a number of German principalities without a pharmacopoeia of their own, the book was referred to as the one to be followed by pharmacists and it was also used in other countries as a pharmaceutical book of reference until the late eighteenth century.

Minderer is best known to a later generation of apothecaries for a pharmaceutical preparation, the *Spiritus Mindereri,* which has brought his name down to posterity. It was long thought to be identical with ammonium acetate. In *Pharmacopoea Svecica,* 'Minders spiritus' went under the name of *Solutio acetatis ammoniaci* until ed. VIII, 1902. It has, however, nothing to do with ammonium acetate, which is not described in any of the works of Minderer and is not found in any of the editions of the Augsburg pharmacopoeias associated with Minderer. A *Spiritus Mindereri* is first found in the 1643 edition and remained until the last edition of 1734. It is a distillate of several vegetable drugs mixed with *Aqua hirundinum composita major* (the latter is a ridiculous distillate from young swallows (!), *Paeonia, Viscum, Castoreum, Dictamnus*, and other drugs, with the addition of *Spiritus Vitrioli*). It was used in diseases of the eye. Ammonium acetate, i.e. the *Spiritus Mindereri* found in later pharmacopoeias, is found in a different preparation of Minderer, the *Aqua acustica*, introduced into the *Pharmacopoeia Augustana* of 1643. It was poured by its author into the outer ear in cases of deafness. The directions for its preparation are marvellous indeed. No less than sixteen aromatic vegetable drugs, together with castoreum, colocinth, squirting cucumber, cyclamen, and pyrethrum, are infused with a mixture of goat's urine, *Acetum Rutae,* and *Acetum Scillae.* After the addition of the juices of horse-radish and onion, galbanum, and an emulsion of peach kernels, radish seeds, and rue seeds, the decoction is mixed with *Spiritus Juniperi.* From this mixture a distillate is drawn off from a water bath to which is added a small amount of *Spiritus rosarum*. This and other preparations show that Minderer experimented in a chemical way and endeavoured to obtain more potent preparations by distillation. It thus becomes apparent that he used spagyric remedies and no longer represented the point of view of the obstinate Occo III, who until his death ignored the Gregorian calendar as well as the remedies of Paracelsus.

Theodor Husemann, *Die aeltesten Auflagen der Augsburger Pharmkopöe* and *Raymund Minderer und die Augsburger Pharmakopöen von 1613–1629*, first published in a series of articles in *Pharmaceutische Zeitung* in 1892 and 1899, of which an English translation was published as introduction to the *Facsimile of the First Edition of the Pharmacopoeia Augustana,* Madison, Wisconsin, 1927; Waller 7385 (1734 ed.)

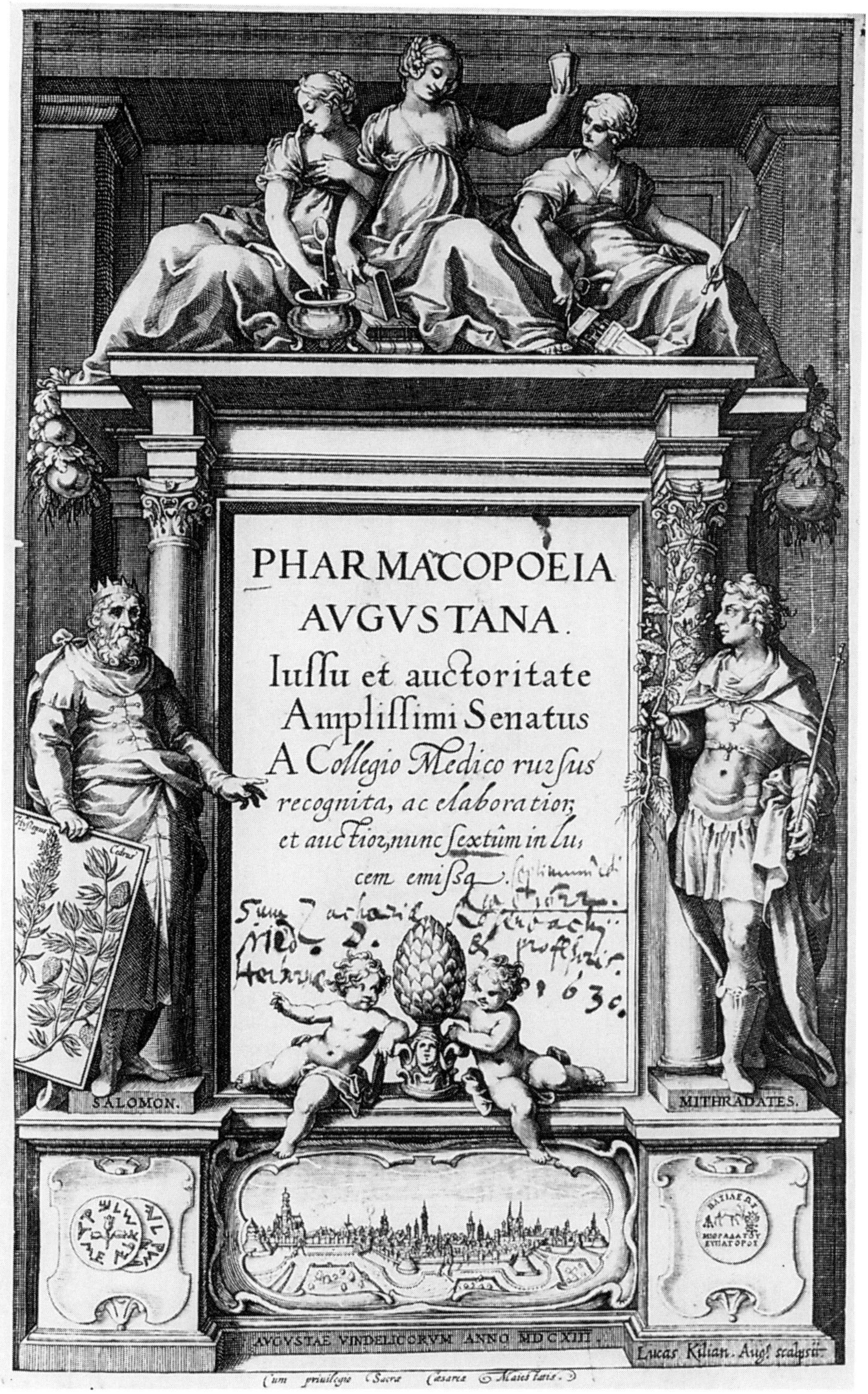

The 1613 edition is the first to have an engraved title page: a triumphal arch, surmounted by three allegorical female figures representing pharmacy, medicine and surgery with their attributes. Beneath the title is the cone of the *Pinus cembra*, the coat of arms of Augsburg, supported by two putti. The shield below bears a view of the city. Leaning against the columns are King Solomon to the left, holding a picture with a spray of cedar and hyssop (*Hyssopus officinalis*), and to the right Mithridates (*Mithridates Eupator*), the great experimenter with antidotes, who in his left hand carries a sceptre and in his right a plant, no doubt intended to represent *Eupatorium*. On both sides of the pedestal are shields with coins. The one to the left shows a sprig of a lily with an ancient Hebraic inscription. Its reverse side reveals the shekel, with value and weight of the coin. To the right is the reverse of a coin of *Mithridates Eupator*, called the Great, with Greek text, a grazing deer, a crescent and star, the symbol of the kings of the Achaemenidae. The engraving is executed by Lucas Kilian, the most illustrious member of the Augsburg family of artists of that name.

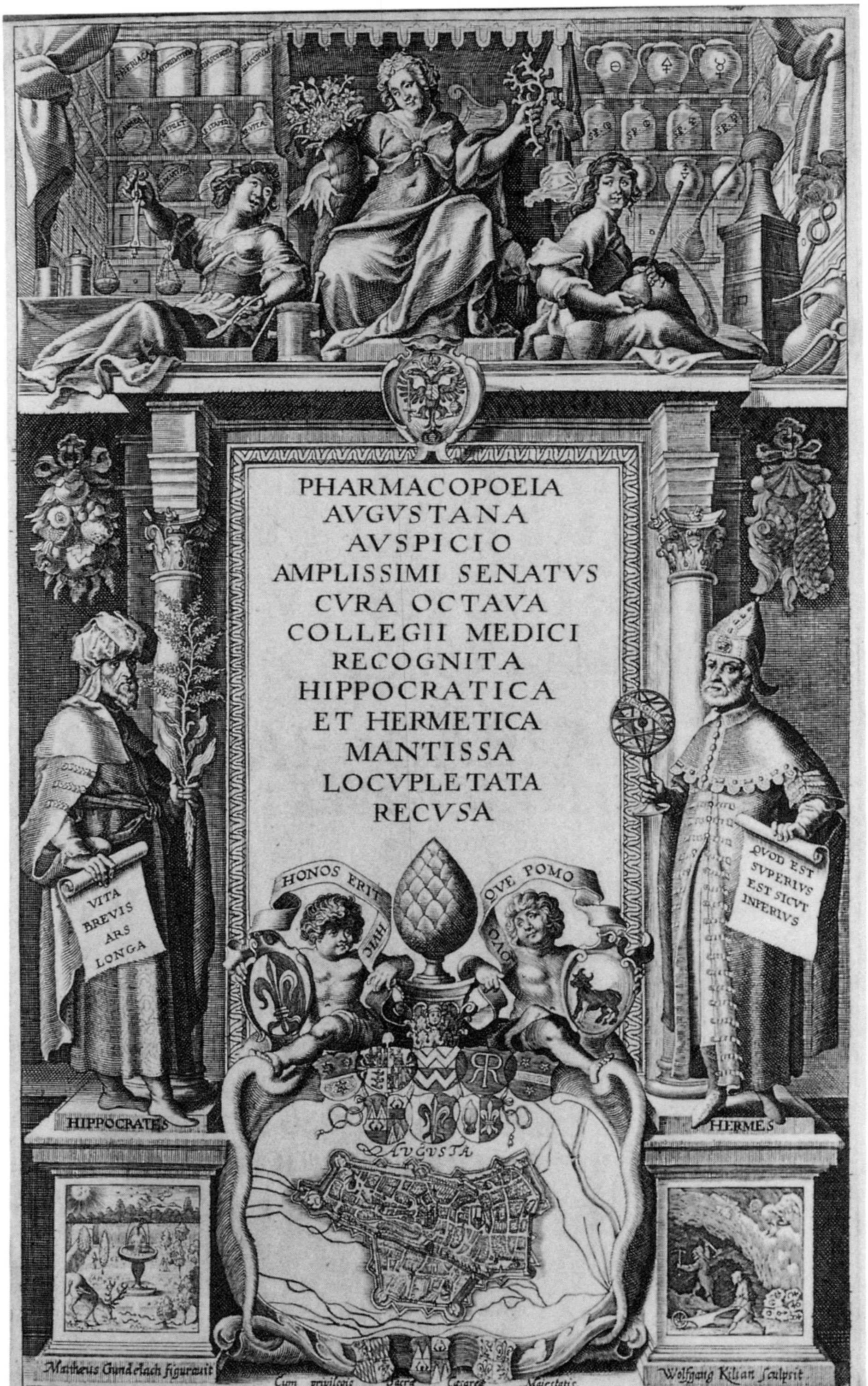

The engraved title page of the above 1643 edition of the *Pharmacopoiea Augustana* is drawn by Mattheus Gundelach and engraved by Wolfgang Kilian. It differs from the 1613 edition in that the female figures are now seated in an apothecary shop. King Solomon and Mithridates are replaced by Hippocrates and Hermes. The former is holding a plant and the latter an armillary sphere. The left pedestal bears a depiction of a garden with a fountain and a deer eating poisonous snakes. Deer were held to be the mortal enemy of the snake. It was thought that they extracted snakes from their holes with the breath from their nostrils, then killed them with their hooves and ate them. This is why so many antidotes for poisons came from the stag's body. The right pedestal, on which Hermes is placed, shows a mine with stones bearing chemical signs.

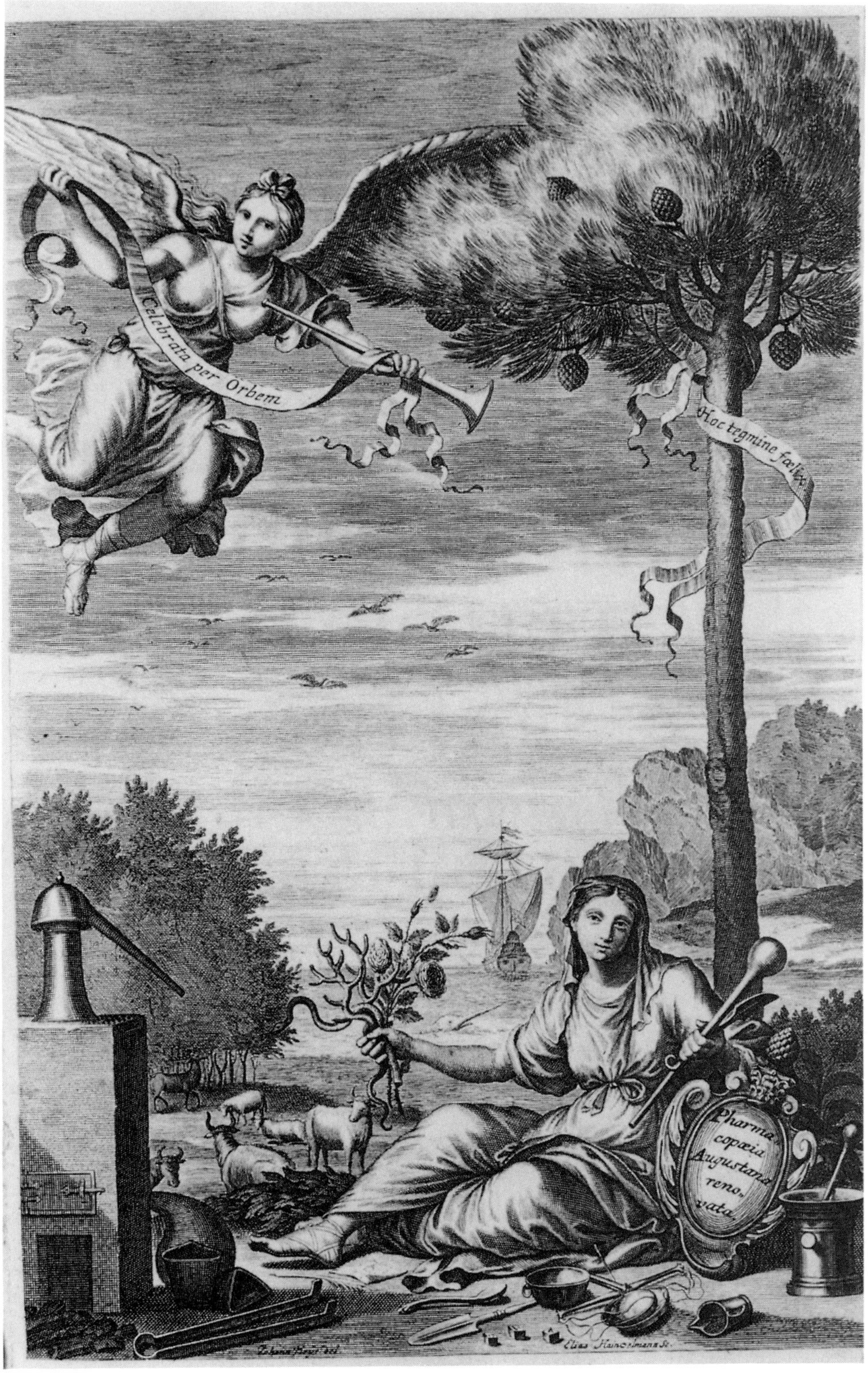

The title page of the 1690 edition of the *Pharmacopoeia Augustana* is drawn by Johann Keys and engraved by Elias Hainzelmann. A furnace and distilling apparatus are placed to the left in a landscape scenery with cattle. A female figure is seated beneath a stone pine bearing cones; the cone of *Pinus cembra* is the coat of arms of Augsburg. She is surrounded by apothecary utensils spread on the ground. In her right hand she holds roses and a snake and in her left a pestle. A ship is bringing exotic medicinal plants from the East and West Indies and in the waves a narwhal is seen with his long spiral tusk (unicorn's horn). The herald angel in the sky brings a banderole with the inscription *Celebrate per orbem Hoc tegmine felix* – Renowned in the World, bringing Fortune under this Sign.

COLOGNE PHARMACOPOEIA 1565

The rare first edition

Dispensarium usuale pro pharmacopoeis inclytae Reipub[licae] Colonien[sis].
Cologne, the heirs of Arnold Birckmann, 1565.

Octavo – *leaf*: 157 *x* 100 *mm.* 212 *leaves, signed* A-Z Aa-Cc[8] Dd[4]. *Title, ff.* 1-198, [199-203], [204-10] *index, last leaf is a blank. One full-page woodcut of a furnace on f.* 65 *recto, and three others on ff.* 181-3. *Contemporary vellum, made up of an old manuscript leaf painted over in black ink. Title page with the Cologne coat of arms with three crowns.*

From the Ernst Matérn Collection.

The extremely rare first edition of the Cologne pharmacopoeia, published within one year after the first Augsburg pharmacopoeia. The first editions of the three official German city pharmacopoeias, including Valerius Cordus' Nuremberg *Dispensarium*, Occo's Augsburg *Enchiridion* and the Cologne *Dispensarium*, are all of the greatest rarity. According to Theodor Husemann (1899), none of the authors who had written about the Cologne *Dispensarium* had ever seen a copy of the first edition and many refer only to the 1627 edition, unaware that it was originally published sixty-two years earlier. Our fine copy, preserved in its original binding, was purchased by Ernst Matérn in 1930 from Gilhofer & Ranschburg, Vienna, for SEK 23.

Towards the middle of the sixteenth century the practise of the apothecaries' art was much in decline in Cologne. The old 1478 decree that placed apothecaries under the authority of physicians was still valid. Physicians were required to inspect the preparation of potent antidotes in person and approve and control the quality and dosage of the ingredients. However, this inspection had with time become insufficient. One critic was Bernhard Cronenburg, who in his comprehensive *Compositione medicamentorum* (1555) decried the poor conditions in the pharmacies.

Thus in 1563 the Cologne Council appointed a committee to prepare for a proper pharmacopoeia for the City of Cologne. The committee, which included no apothecaries, consisted of six persons. Two, however, were professors of medicine (Mauritius Seidel and Hermann Collenberg) and thus members of the medical faculty. The others were the four practising physicians of the city, who besides Cronenburg included Hubert Faber, Johann Echt and Theodor Birckmann. The initiator Cronenburg was beyond doubt the most gifted of the group and the most qualified for the task, a fact of which he was most aware. This contributed to dispute from the very beginning and the early resignation of the two faculty members from the committee. Cronenburg was also soon to depart, but not before fundamental work had been completed on the project.

Once the book had been printed, Seidel and Collenberg claimed that it could not be accepted as an official pharmacopoeia unless it had been approved and issued under the auspices of the Cologne medical faculty. Before this matter was settled, the Council was made to halt distribution by withdrawing all copies. Within a few days the problem was solved. Faber was appointed professor of medicine and thus became a member of the faculty, and the printer, Johann [or Franz] Birckmann, a brother of one of the co-authors, Theodor Birckmann, reset the title leaf, where the four authors' names were given on verso, so that Faber was now given sole authorship and the other three, including Cronenburg, were mentioned only as assistants. The correction was made by substituting the first half (four leaves) of the first gathering, and the first official Cologne pharmacopoeia was finally published in August 1565, bearing on its title page the insignia of the City of Cologne.

Cronenburg, who had not been given the opportunity to read the final proof-sheets after Seidel had made certain revisions and additions, denied all responsibility and accused the printer of including his name among the co-authors without his consent, and moreover misspelling it 'Cronenberg'. The *Dispensarium Coloniense* was valid for more than sixty years up to 1627, when a new revised edition appeared, a splendid folio with a magnificent engraved title page with a view of Cologne.

Husemann, 'Die Kölnischen Pharmakopöen und ihre Verfasser', in *Apotheker-Zeitung*, 14, 1899, in eleven instalments between pp. 403-80; Dann, *Das Kölner Dispensarium von* 1565. Teil I, *Erläuterung*, Teil II, *Faksimile*. Stuttgart, 1969.

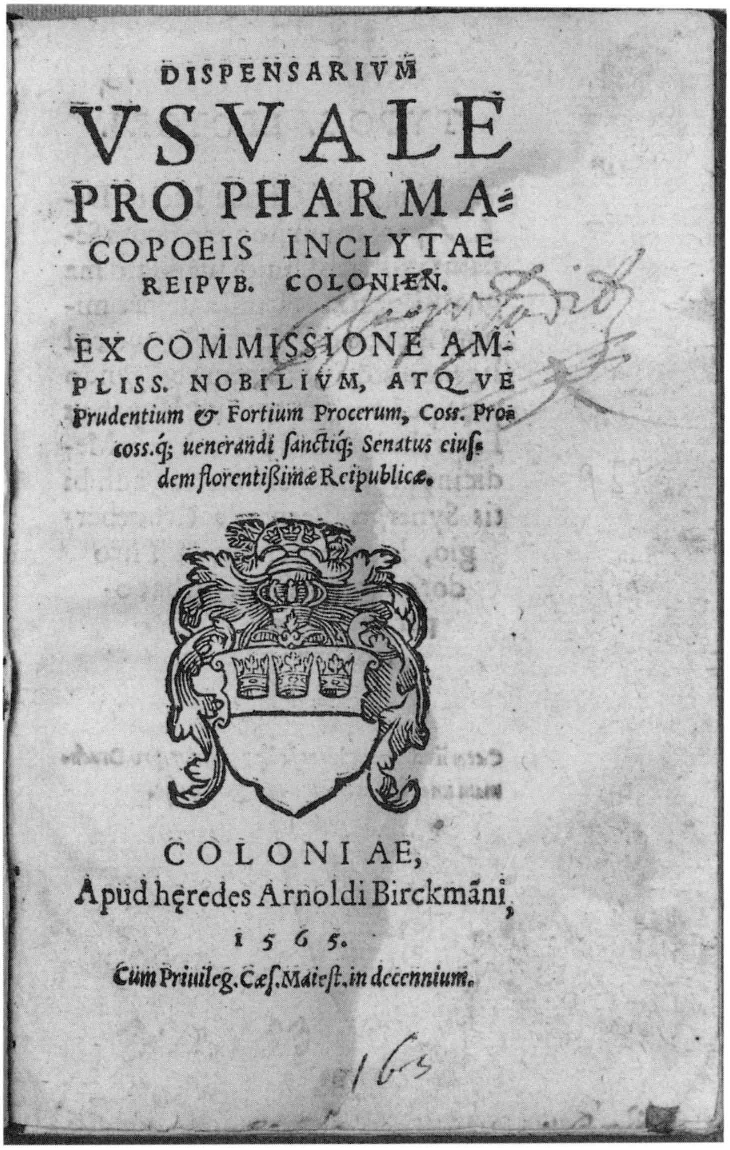

DISPENSARIVM

VSVALE

PRO PHARMA-

COPOEIS INCLYTAE

REIPVB. COLONIEN.

EX COMMISSIONE AM-

PLISS. NOBILIVM, ATQVE

Prudentium & Fortium Procerum, Coss. Pro-

coss.q; uenerandi sanctiq; Senatus eius-

dem florentissimæ Reipublicæ.

COLONIAE,

Apud hęredes Arnoldi Birckmāni,

1 5 6 5.

Cum Priuileg. Cæs. Maiest. in decennium.

The very rare first edition of the Cologne pharmacopoeia (1565).

RONDELET, Guillaume (1507–1566)

Formerly in the Bibliotheca Mellicensis

Dispensatorium sue pharmacopolarum officina.
Cologne, Johann Birckmann, 1565.

Duodecimo – *leaf*: 128 x 70 *mm*. 192 *leaves*: ff. [1]-35, 34-185, [5] *index*. *Sign*.: A-Q12
Printer's device on the title page. Contemporary blindstamped pigskin over wooden boards, two brass clasps. The inner panel with flowers within a frame with medallions of the reformers.

Provenance: *Melk Benedictine Abbey Library in Lower Austria, with two early inscriptions on the title telling that it belongs to the* Bibliotheca Mellicensis. *A later rubber stamp,* Bibliotheca Mellicensis, *is also found on the title and the last page.*
From the Ernst Matérn Collection.

First and only edition of a little-known pharmaceutical work by Rondelet, the famous professor of medicine at Montpellier, among whose students appear such prominent names as L'Ecluse, Platter, Bauhin, L'Obel, Gesner and Belon. He was a good friend of Rabelais, whose character Rondibilis is said to be based on Rondelet. He was a great lover of good food, especially sweets and cakes, was a keen musician and loved dancing, 'very merry and a lover of jokes and fun' (Laurent Joubert). Rondelet's reputation today is mainly built on his great work on fishes and aquatic life, first published in 1554-55, a massive folio of nearly 900 pages with 440 woodcuts. It was the standard reference work on ichthyology for over a century. Rondelet also wrote minor works on *materia medica* and medicine, several of which circulated in manuscript copies or were incorporated in other authors' works.

Rondelet's *Dispensatorium* was published and printed in the very same year as the first edition of the Cologne pharmacopoeia, *Dispensarium usuale pro pharmacopoeias inclytae reipub[licae] Colonie[nse]*, of which a very few copies are known to exist. Rondelet's little book seems to be a great rarity. It is not mentioned by Hirsch or *Biographie Medicale* and is lacking in Waller, Osler, Wellcome and other standard collections. It has also escaped the notice of historians of pharmacopoeias and is not mentioned in Husemann's otherwise scrupulously comprehensive account on the history and authors of the Cologne pharmacopoeia, nor in Dann's introduction to the facsimile edition of the Cologne pharmacopoeia of 1565.

Both of the books are small duodecimos and were printed by Johann Birckmann, the director of the family printing officine at Cologne. Johann was the brother of Theodor Birckmann (c.1534-86), a physician at Cologne, who together with Hupert Faber, Bernard Dessen Cronenburg and Johannes Echt was one of the compilers of the Cologne pharmacopoeia. Theodor Birckmann had studied medicine under Rondelet at Montpellier. The burgers of Cologne regarded him as a 'frivolen Lebemann'. No other medical or pharmaceutical works by Theodor Birckmann are known to have been printed, but his name is immortalized in *Pulvis stomachicus Birckmanni*, a stomach remedy found in the Württemberg pharmacopoeia.

Another pupil of Rondelet was the well-known physician in Basel, Felix Platter, who in his diary (1552-57) tells that Rondelet had presented one of his unpublished manuscripts, probably entitled *De componendis medicamentis*, to two visiting medical students, Valerian Fiedler and Bartholomaeus Wagner. On their homeward journey from Montpellier in 1556, Platter and Birckmann accompanied them as far as Chamberry, where they spent a whole night copying the manuscript. Could that manuscript possibly have any connection with Rondelet's *Dispensatorium*?

The terrible plague that raged in Cologne in the second half of 1564, the worst that the town had ever experienced, could possibly be a reason for the scarcity of these two 1565 Cologne imprints. In a letter Cassander tells: 'Traurig ist der Zustand der Stadt; die Aerzte und Apotheker sind teilsweise geflüchtet, die Plätze sind verödet, die Märkte leer; Gottesdienst wird nur noch von wenigen Geistlichen gehalten: die Priester, deren Mittel es gestatteten, sind geflohen, von dreissigen sind kaum vier zu Hause geblieben. Gerichtssitzungen finden nicht mehr statt; man sagt, dass in diesem Jahre 25000 Menschen in Köln an der Seuche gestorben seien'.

Durling, 3926; Theodor Husemann, 'Die Kölnischen Pharmakopöen und ihre Verfasser', in *Apotheker-Zeitung* (1899), pp.403-06, 412-13, 418-19, 425-7, 435-6, 440-1, 446-7, 456-7, 463-6, 472-5, 477-80; Georg Edmund Dann, *Das Kölner Dispensarium von* 1565, Teil 1, Erläuterung (*Veröff. d. Intern. Gesellschaft f. Geschichte d. Pharmazie,* N.F. vol. 34, 1969); Severin Corsten, 'Unter dem Zeichen der "Fetten Henne" Franz Birckmann und Nachfolger', in *Gutenberg Jahrbuch* 1962, pp. 267-72.

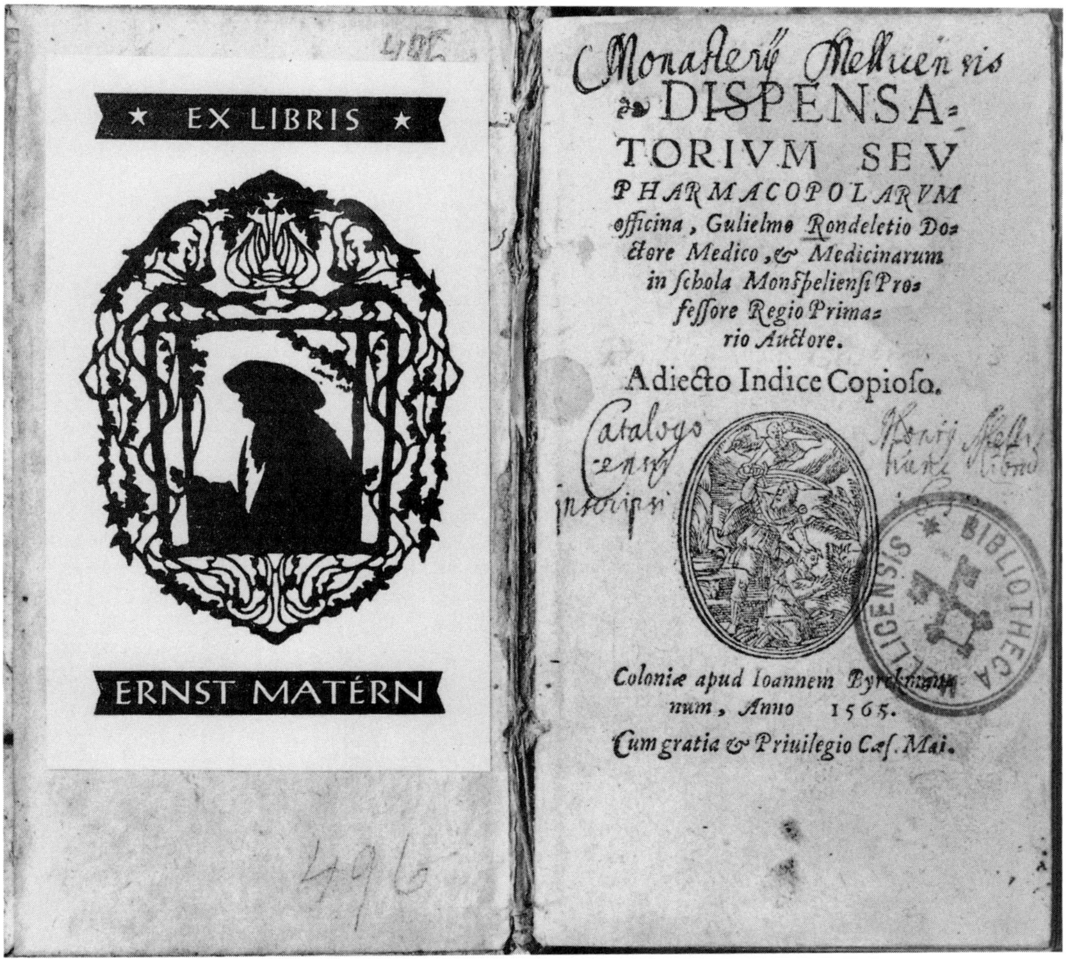

This copy of Rondelet's *Dispensatorium* has for centuries been housed in the Library of the Benedictine Abbey at Melk in Lower Austria. The title page has two early inscriptions stating that it belongs to the *Bibliotheca Mellicensis* together with a rubber stamp from the beginning of this century also found on the title and the last page. The old medieval monastery buildings were demolished in the early eigthteenth century to be replaced by its present block of buildings. The library is famous for its most magnificent Baroque interior. In 1926 they had to dispose of books, among others a Gutenberg Bible, which went to the USA for £ 21.000. The present copy of Rondelet's *Dispensatorium* was purchased by Ernst Matérn in December, 1928, from *L'Art Ancien,* Lugano, Switzerland. He paid SEK 23.00, and it is most probably the same copy they had listed in their *Bulletin* XVI, item 1544. It bears Matérn's book-plate, a silhouette figure designed by Johan Leksell in 1925.

One of the great pre-Linnaean botanists

L'OBEL, Matthias de (1538–1616) in collaboration with **Pierre PENA** (c. 1535–1605)

Nova Stirpium Adversia, . . . Quibus accessit Appendix cum Indice variarum linguarum locupletissimo . . . Additis Guillielmi Rondelletti aliquot Remediorum formulis, nunquam antehac in lucem editis. Antwerp, Christopher Plantin, 1576

Folio – *leaf*: 280 *x* 190 *mm. Pp.* [4], 471, [1] *blank,* Rondelet*: pp.* 1-15, [1] *blank. Sign.*: π² A-Z Aa-Pp⁶ Qq-Rr⁴ †-††⁴. *With* 300 *woodcuts of plants in the text. This copy does not have the* 20 *leaves at the end with* 36 *pages of indices and* 3 *pages of added illustrations (sign.: *-*****⁴). Lower margin of the title leaf shaved. Rebound in nineteenth century brown half calf, richly gilt spine with four raised bands.*

Book-plate: C.D. Carlsson.

This is actually the second issue of *Stirpium adversia nova,* first published by Thomas Purfoot in London, 1570-71, of which Plantin in Antwerp bought 800 copies for 1200 florins. He replaced the original title leaf with a new one, bearing his own imprint, added 36 leaves of new material at the end and published the whole as *Nova Stirpium Adversia* in 1576. The new material was Lobel's *Appendix*, Rondelet's *Formulae Remediorum*, Lobel's new indices, and three pages of new illustrations of plants. It was issued separately as above and also formed the second part of Lobel's *Plantarum sue stirpium historia,* the first part of which contains 646 pages with 1473 woodcuts of plants, printed by Plantin in the same year. Later Plantin also bought 250 of the 272 wood blocks that Purfoot had made, and used them for the Flemish edition of *Plantarum sue stirpium,* which appeared in 1581 under the title of *Kruydtboeck.*

The *Stirpium adversia nova* (1570) is one of the milestones of modern botany and was, next to William Turner's herbal (1551-62), the most important botanical book published in England. Lobel was one of the great pre-Linnaean botanists. Prior to any contemporary botanist he divided the plants into groups according to the form of their leaves. It seems that he had an inkling of natural families and that he attempted to use, if not the terms, at least the concepts of genus and family. Linnaeus honoured his forerunner by giving the name 'Lobelia' to a genus of aquatic plants.

Neither of the two authors, who were both physicians, was a native of England. Pierre Pena was born at Jouques in Provence, and Matthias Lobel (L'Obel), latinized Lobelius, was a native of Lille in Flanders. Pena's name appears first on the title page and evidently his contribution was substantial. The customary attribution of the work mainly to Lobel seems to have arisen because he continued to work and publish in botany, whereas Pena turned to a successful medical career, including his position as physician to King Henry III of France. Pena had travelled widely in Europe before arriving at the University of Montpellier in 1565. There he met Lobel, who had been travelling in Germany and Italy, and both became pupils of the celebrated physician and naturalist Guillaume Rondelet (1507–1566). United by a common interest in botany they became close friends and went on botanical excursions together. When Rondelet died in 1566 he bequeathed to Lobel, his favourite pupil, all his botanical manuscripts.

In the autumn of the following year the two friends left Montpellier for England. Their joint botanical work was already partly completed, and they now decided to have it published in England. They arrived in London in December of 1569 and after having botanized throughout the British Isles, which enabled them to add a number of plants unknown to Turner, the book appeared in 1570-71, dedicated to Queen Elizabeth I. After the publication of the book, both authors returned to the Continent. Pena became a prosperous and successful medical practitioner in France. In Antwerp Lobel saw many subsequent publications through the Plantin Press and became physician to William of Orange, *Stadtholder* of the Low Countries. Following the assassination of William in 1584, Lobel returned to England, his wife's native country, where he remained for the rest of his life. In 1607 he was appointed royal botanist to James I.

Hunt I, 127; Johnston, *Cleveland Herbals,* 114; Henrey, I, pp. 26-31; Sorgeloos, *Labore et Constantia,* 310; Durling, 2829; DSB, VIII, 435-6; Greene /Egerton, II, pp. 877-937.

270 *STIRPIVM aduerſaria noua*

luteouirentes Elatines, ſiue Veronicæ fœminæ pares & ſimiles. Illic Pharmacopœi, penuria & ignoratione Cotyledonis veri, miſcent Populneo vnguento.

SMILACIS ASPERÆ, & SALSÆPARILLÆ
figuræ & naturæ diſcrimen.

SMILAX ASPERA.

DIFFERT hæc à læui vuis foliis, ſpinis, radice, floribus, viticulis, atque viribus, denique natalibus. Quippe non niſi montoſis & collibus feruidiorum tractuum, Romaniæ, Hiſpaniæ, Linguagotię, vbi plurima, horridis aduncisque crebribus ſpinis, Rubi ritu, implicat mordicus proxima quæque; aſſurgitque vltra ſupraq; parietes & ſepes vicinos. Folia Hederacea, longiora, Bryoniæ nigrę ambitu & ſuperficie: non inciſa, ſed lęuia, & in medio, ſecundum ſtrias neruulorum, ſpinulas habentia atrouirentia, acinosq; rubros, racematim copioſos, Ribes magnitudine & modo: nec flores diſsimiles Ribes vtriuſuis racemoſi, ſed albi. Radices tametſi longius excurrãt ſubter humum, ternis aut quaternis vlnis longiores, non tantæ tamen cum Salſa-parilla ſimilitudinis ſortitas ſcimus, quantum hactenus perſuaſum doctis quibuſdam fuit: qui ſcriptis mandarunt Salſæparillæ eandem planè eſſe: cuius tamen conſpicuæ intuenti patent, à Smilacis radicibus, differentiæ. Siquidem Smilacis geniculatæ, articulatis ſegmentis radices, candidæ, foris nitentes, Graminis carnini, aut Harundinis valatorii.

SALSA-PALLA.

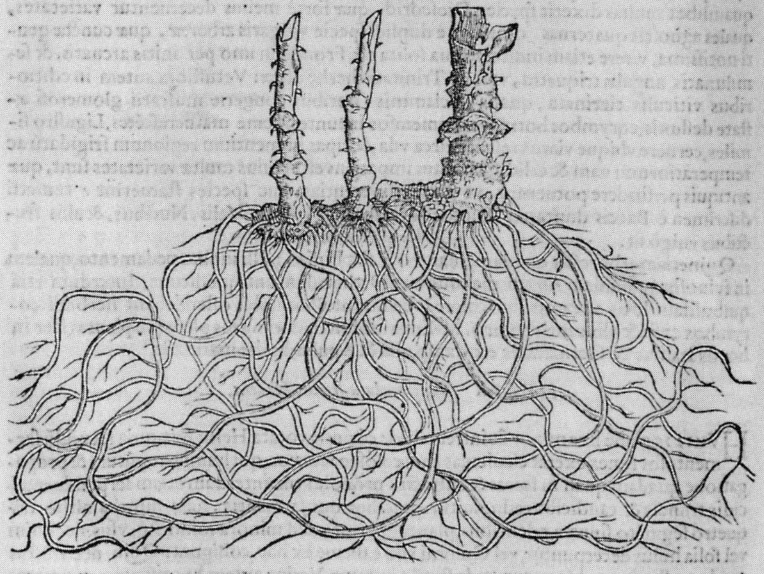

At Parillæ crebris loris prolixiſsimis, ab vno trunco radicis magno, pręduro, ſtrumoſo rugoſiſque capitibus, hinc inde ſubtus, vt in Aſparago, vel Ruſco, oriuntur numeroſi concolores lori, æquabiles & ſine geniculis vel nodis; recti, flexiles, cortice duriuſculo, pullo, rugis ſtriato in longitudine, quam vicenum pedum interdum metiti ſumus. Intus farinacea medulla, non ita ingrata, ſed viſcida, nonnihil ęmplaſtica, amaricante, nec tamen calorem prodente. Eapropter perſpicuum eſt, non magis eſſe Smilacis, Rubi, aut Clematidis alteræ Viorna dictę, quàm ſint Cinnamomi, & nonnullæ arbores, tum

Sarsaparilla, a popular drug, prepared from the long fibrous roots of several species of the genus *Smilax*. Sarsaparilla was first introduced to Seville from New Spain about 1535 and was used as an excellent medicine in the treatment of syphilis.

A monument of human stupidity and folly

CARRICHTER, Bartholomaeus (c. 1507–1573)

Horn des Heyls menschlicher Blödigkeit, oder Gross Kräuter Buch dess Edlen und Hochgelehrten Herrn Bartholomaei Carrichters, . .. darinn die Kräuter dess Teutschlands, auss dem Liecht der Natur, nach rechter Arth der himmlischen Einfliessung beschrieben. Nicht allein allen Medicis, Pharmacopaeis und Chirurgis zu gutem in Truck gegeben, sondern auch allen Liebhabern . . . Hier ist zu Ende beygefügt das Menschliche Kräuter-Bild, Nach denen zwölff himmlischen Zeichen und vier Elementarischen Complexionen auff die innerliche und äusserliche Glieder dess menschlichen Leibes gerichtet: zusammen getragen auss obgedachten Auctoris Schrifften von Theophilo Krafften, von Gladenbach auss Hessen.

Frankfurt am Main, Thomas Matthias Götzen's heirs, 1673.

Quarto – *leaf*: 208 *x* 173 *mm. Pp.* [36], 1-352, 351-374, [16]. *One large folding leaf* 'Homo Herbaceaus' [550 x 600 *mm*] *with table within a fine typographical border. With* 58 *woodcuts of plants in the text. Title page printed in red and black with printer's device. Contemporary vellum over wooden boards.*

Signature inside the front cover: A. Rumplow [?], *dated Copenhagen,* 1694.

The herbals of the German Renaissance by scholars like Brunfels, Bock, Fuchs and Valerius Cordus, were 'too scientific, too rational, to satisfy a large part of the German public whose minds were corrupted by astrological fancies and needed some kind of "astrological botany" (Sarton). Carrichter's *Horn des Heyls menschlicher Blödigkeit,* which title reveals its occult tendencies, is an example of that astrological thinking which practical scientists had fought against for hundreds of years. The belief in astrology probably began with the Chaldeans, had influenced even such men as Hippocrates and Galen, and became almost universal during the Middle Ages.

The first edition of this remarkable herbal was published in 1576 under the pseudonym of Philomusus Anonymus and printed by Christian Müller in Strassburg. Another of Carrichter's books, *Kräuterbuch* (cf Pritzel, No. 1541), had appeared in 1575, and both these astrological herbals went through many editions, the last appeared as late as 1739. The present edition of 1673 is enlarged by Theophil Krafft and has the same number of woodcuts as the first, all of which are in fact copies of those in the small edition of Fuchs' herbal. The authorship has been doubted and according to some sources, a certain Melchior Schönfeldt was hidden under the anonymous 'Philomusus'. Carrichter's works, which also include a *Practica* (1575, 1579), were published posthumously, edited by Michael Toxites, the wandering supporter of Paracelsus, who was also a friend of Carrichter.

In the astrological herbals of Carrichter 'the plants are arranged according to the signs of the Zodiak, but the principle on which the allotment is made remains mysterious to the lay mind. Much stress is laid upon the hour at which the herbs ought to be gathered, particular attention being paid to the state of the moon at the time' (Arber). In our library is also the second edition of Carrichter's *Neuaufgerichtete Stadt- und Land-Apotheke* (Nürnberg, 1677), edited by Johannes Hiskias Cardilucius, a thick octavo of over 1200 pages.

Very little is known about Carrichter. He was born in Reckingen on the Rhine (at the south end of the Black Forest) and served as physician-in-ordinary to the Holy Roman Emperors Maximilian II and Ferdinand I, who suffered literally from a lack of medical attention at the hands of such quacks as he and his contemporary Thurneysser. According to Sarton, Carrichter was accused of having caused the death of Ferdinand I in 1564 through malpractice. The *Nouvelle Biographie Universelle* says of Carrichter's herbal that it is a monument of human stupidity and folly.

Hirsch I, 840-1; Hunt, 123 (first edition of 1576); Krivatsy (NLM), 2183 (wanting the folding-leaf '*Homo Herbaceaus*'); Arber, p. 258; Nissen, BBI, 332; Pritzel, 1542; Waller 1786 (*Stadt- und Land-Apotheke*).

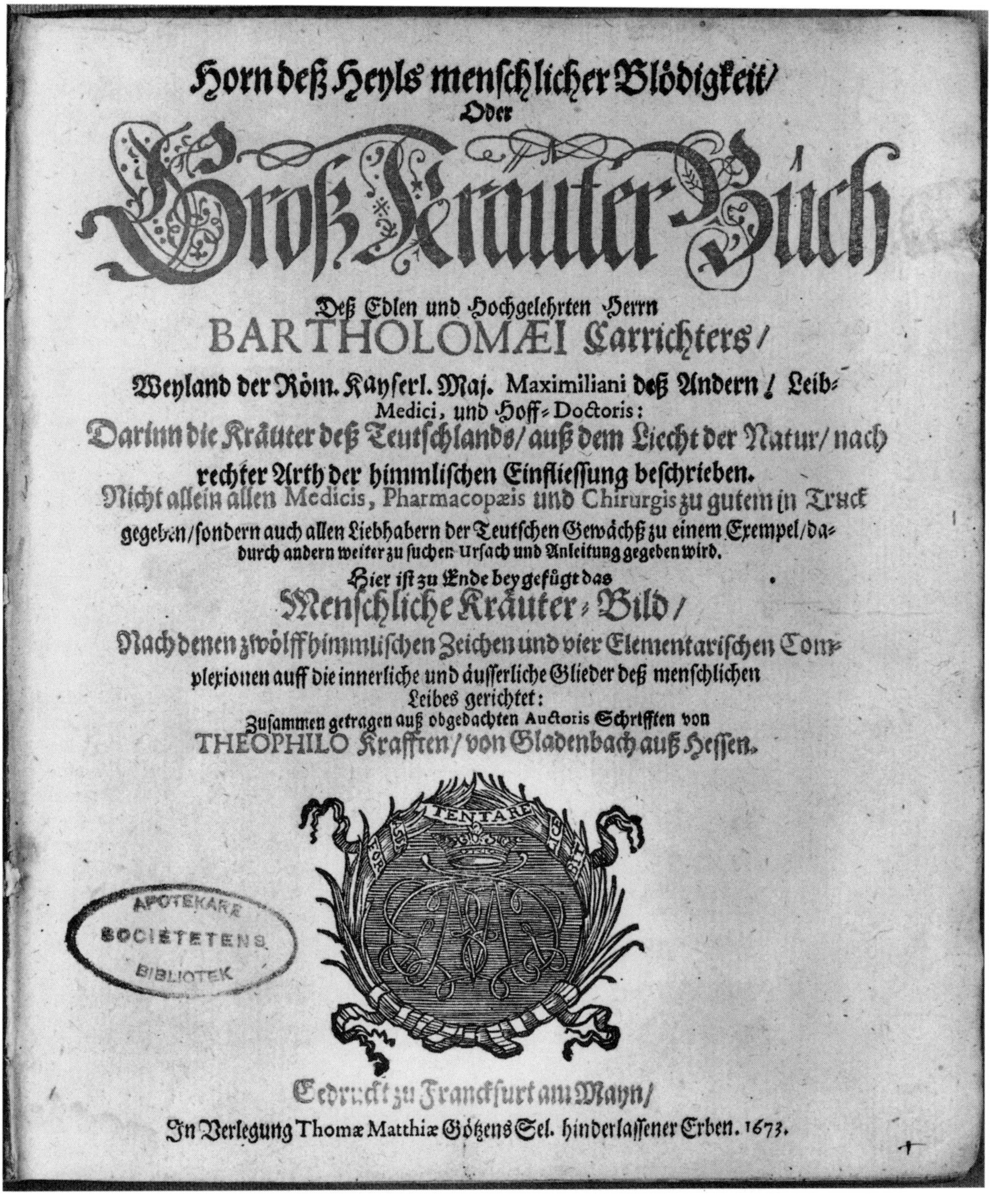

Horn deß Heyls menschlicher Blödigkeit/
Oder
Groß Kräuter-Buch
Deß Edlen und Hochgelehrten Herrn
BARTHOLOMÆI Carrichters/
Weyland der Röm. Kayserl. Maj. Maximiliani deß Andern/ Leib-
Medici, und Hoff-Doctoris:
Darinn die Kräuter deß Teutschlands/ auß dem Liecht der Natur/ nach
rechter Arth der himmlischen Einfliessung beschrieben.
Nicht allein allen Medicis, Pharmacopæis und Chirurgis zu gutem in Truck
gegeben/ sondern auch allen Liebhabern der Teutschen Gewächß zu einem Exempel/ da-
durch andern weiter zu suchen Ursach und Anleitung gegeben wird.
Hier ist zu Ende beygefügt das
Menschliche Kräuter-Bild/
Nach denen zwölff himmlischen Zeichen und vier Elementarischen Com-
plexionen auff die innerliche und äusserliche Glieder deß menschlichen
Leibes gerichtet:
Zusammen getragen auß obgedachten Auctoris Schrifften von
THEOPHILO Krafften/ von Gladenbach auß Hessen.

Gedruckt zu Franckfurt am Mayn/
In Verlegung Thomæ Matthiæ Götzens Sel. hinderlassener Erben. 1673.

THURNEYSSER ZUM THURN, Leonhard (1531–1596)

A 16th-century master of the 20th-century art of public relations and image-making

Historia sive descriptio plantarum omnium, tam domesticarum quam exoticarum: . . .
Berlin, Michael Hentzke for Thurneisser, 1578

Folio – *leaf:* 375 *x* 250 *mm. Pp.* [12], 156, [20]. *Title within an elaborate woodcut border, portrait of the author within a pompous frame, which is found repeated a few pages further on with the author's portrait replaced with that of the Lord our Father, 36 woodcuts of plants, numerous smaller woodcuts in the text of apparatus, animals, human figures and astrological diagrams. Final leaf with printer's device and colophon. Original brown calf with five raised bands, gilt (faded) ornamental border around sides within blind fillets, fleurons at outer corners of inner frame. Oval centrepiece with Thurneysser's device and his motto:* FESTINA LENTE. *New endpapers.*

Bookplate: C.D. Carlsson.

First Latin edition of this remarkable herbal, published in the same year as the German edition. It is the first and only part of a prospected ten-volume project in which Thurneysser intended to set out the occult nomenclature and virtues of all known plants, illustrated with woodcuts made after specimens in his own large collection, with diagrams showing the conjunctions of the heavenly bodies under which each plant should be picked, prepared, and used. This first part deals with the *Umbellifers*, which were regarded as being under the dominion of the Sun and Mars. In Wilfrid Blunt's opinion this foolish book, directed at the credulous, is illustrated with better woodcuts than it deserves. The present copy is, except for new endpapers, in its original binding with Thurneysser's device and motto.

The intent of the publication of the *Historia plantarum*, printed at the author's own press, was to impress, deceive, and sell. Thurneysser, 'Geheimmittelschwindler und Zauberarzt' (Ferchl), was a sixteenth-century master of the twentieth-century art of public relations and image-making. 'Gifted with a quick, perceptive mind, he learned quite soon in life that there were many gulls waiting, in fact longing, to be duped, and so he settled on his road to fortune' (Anderson).

Thurneysser was the son of a goldsmith and took up his father's profession. He never attended a university but was employed by Johann Huber, a physician, to collect plants and to read aloud to him from the works of Paracelsus. In 1547 he set off on his *Wanderjahre* to England and France. Back in Germany, he in 1551 joined the troops of Margraf Albrecht of Brandenburg and fought at Sievershausen in 1553, where he was taken prisoner by the Saxon army. On his release he returned to Basel and married a wealthy widow, Margarette Müllerin. He soon fell in the hands of Jewish moneylenders, and tried to remedy the situation by selling gold-plated lead as pure gold. When this was discovered in 1558, Thurneysser was forced to flee Basel and went to Russia, leaving his wife behind. He then worked as a miner, smelter, mechanic and goldsmith in Nuremberg, Strassburg and Constance, where he met Anna Hüetlin, who became his second wife. He became inspector of the mines at Tarrenz, in Tyrol, and also started a smelting works of his own. He now came under the patronage of Archduke Ferdinand, on whose instructions he made journeys to the Orkney Islands, Spain and Portugal, and later down to Egypt, Greece, Italy, and Hungary, everywhere to acquaint himself with metallurgical methods and medicine. He collected recipes, books, plants, minerals and other rarities and tried in vain to find out the secret of the highly coveted 'Philosopher's Stone', thought by alchemists to be capable of transmuting base metals into gold.

In 1571 Thurneysser moved to Frankfurt an der Oder, where he had a work printed, entitled *Pison*, after the river that flowed through Eden. *Pison* concerns hot and cold waters, mineral deposits, plants and planets. This tome attracted the attention of the inhabitants of Brandenburg since Thurneysser in one of its chapters states that their land should contain vast deposits of gems, minerals, amber and spas, and that the river Spree contain gold dust. The young Elector of Brandenburg, Johann Georg, who had good reason to improve the financial state of his land, had long sought a gold-maker and now contacted the talented author, who showed him extracts from *Pison*. Following that, Thurneysser was entrusted with the care of the chemical laboratories of Berlin and Halle. Schelenz considers *Pison* to be Thurneysser's most important contribution in the history of pharmacy.

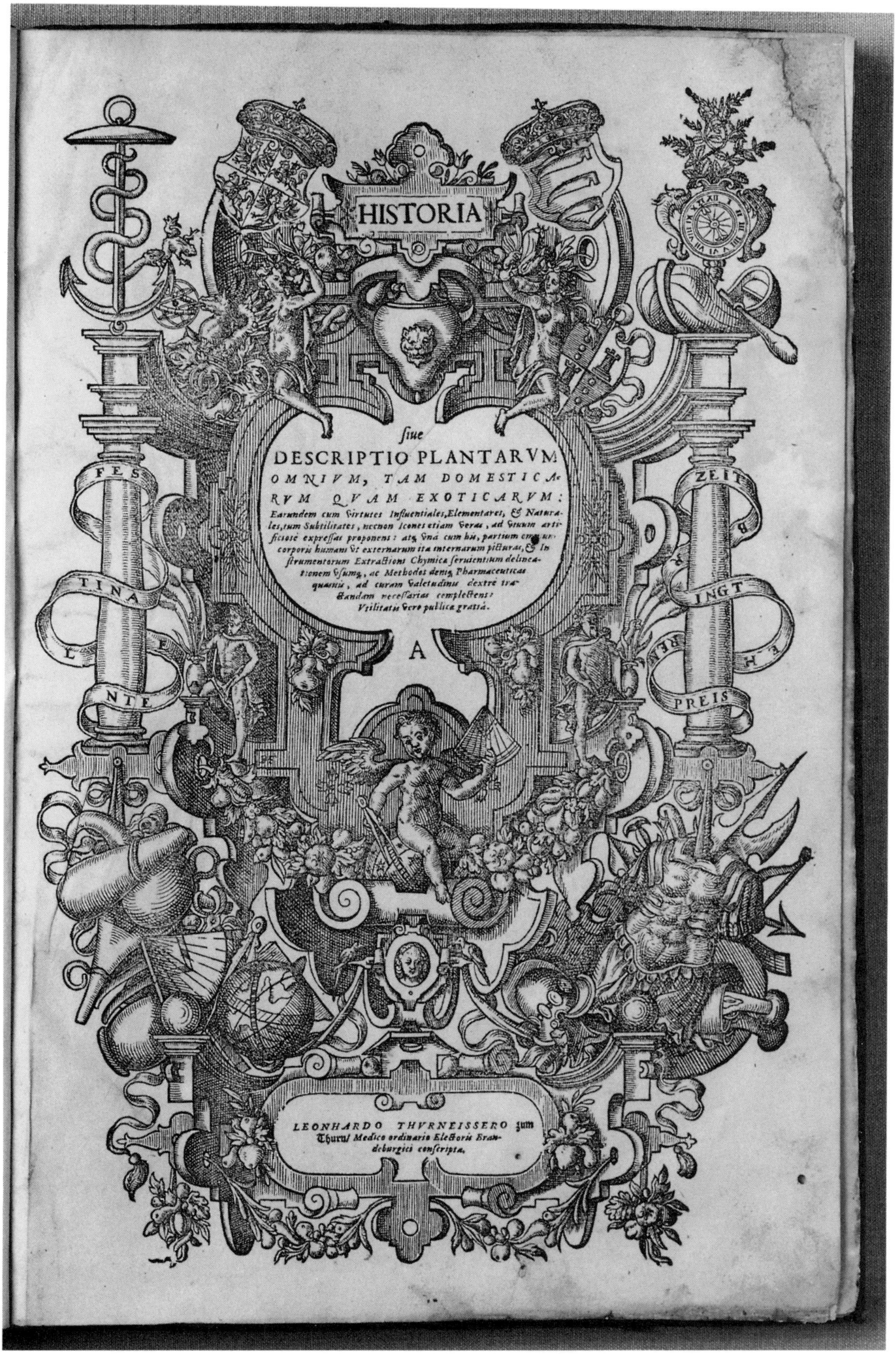
HISTORIA
sive
DESCRIPTIO PLANTARVM
OMNIVM, TAM DOMESTICA-
RVM QVAM EXOTICARVM:
Earundem cum Virtutes Influentiales, Elementares, & Naturales, tum Subtilitates, necnon Icones etiam Veras, ad Viuum artificiosè expressas proponens: atq; Vnà cum his, partium corporis humani Vt externarum ita internarum picturas, & Instrumentorum Extractioni Chymicæ seruientium delineationem Vsumq;, ac Methodos deniq; Pharmaceuticas quasuis, ad curam Valetudinis dextrè tractandam necessarias complectens:
Vtilitatis Vero publicæ gratiâ.
A
LEONHARDO THVRNEISSERO zum Thurn/ Medico ordinario Electoris Brandeburgici conscripta.
FES
TINA
LENTE
ZEIT
INGT
PREIS

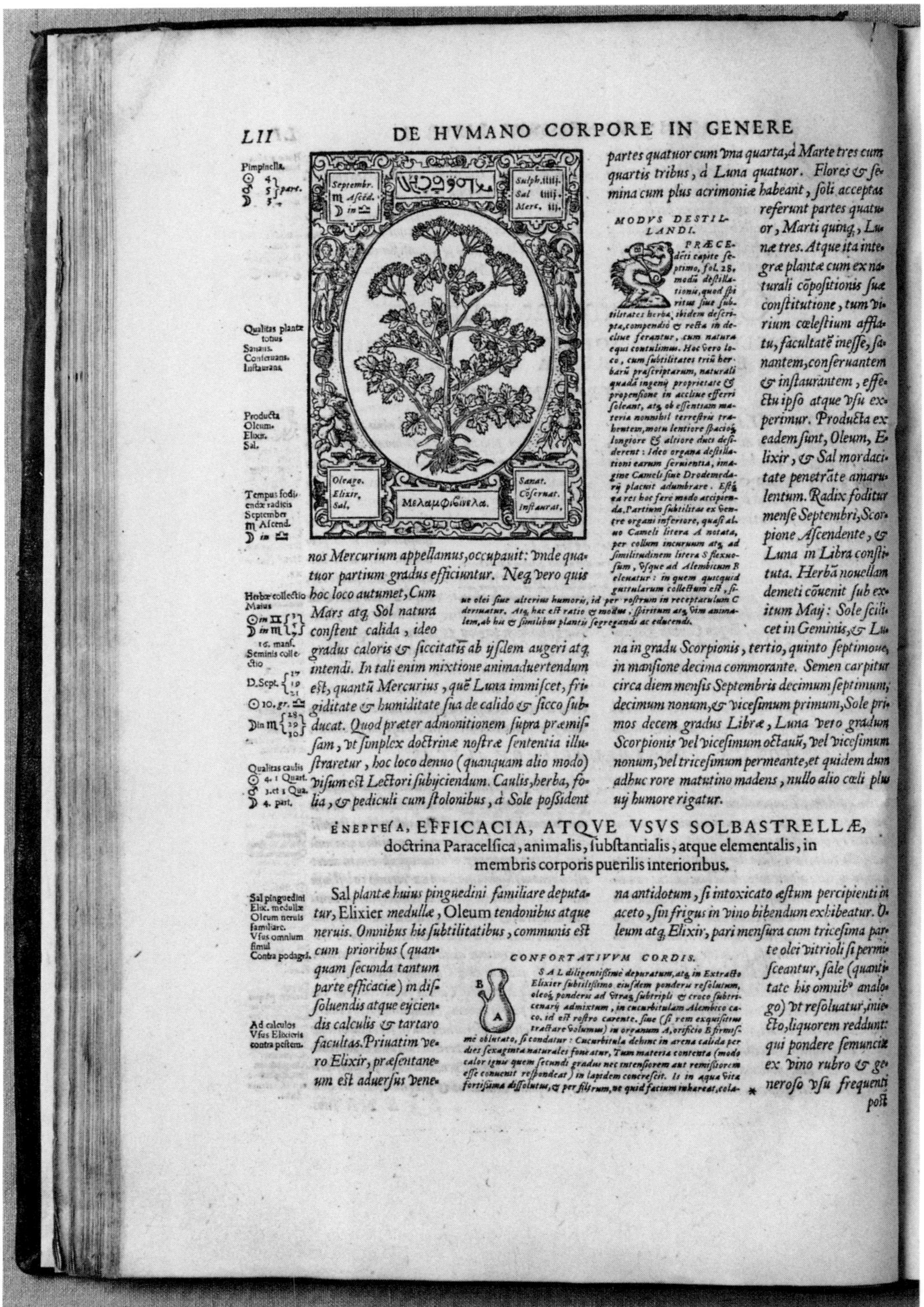

One of the pages in Thurneysser's *Historia Plantarum* with a picture of a plant with mystifying text written in many foreign languages and adorned with astrological symbols. At the end of the book are indices of plant names in different languages including numerous Oriental typefaces, followed by indices of places, persons, anecdotes, parts of the body, constellations, diseases, and medicaments. 'Thurneysser konnte sich rühmen, in einem einzigen Buche Wörter aus 32 europäischen und 63 asiatischen Sprachen untergebracht zu haben' (*Aventur und Kunst* (1940), p. 111). Many of the figures were cut by the artist Peter Hille of Frankfurt.

Thurneysser was summoned to the Elector's court, where he succeeded in making the right diagnosis on, and even cure, Johann Georg's wife, Sabina. This awarded him the unlimited confidence of the Elector, who made Thurneysser his physician-in-ordinary. This was the start of a fourteen-year influential period of an extraordinary career.

In the capital, Berlin, he was granted the use of a part of the *Grauen Kloster*, a former Grey Friar monastery, where he took up lodgings and started to build up an imposing enterprise. In his laboratory, indeed a factory, he made potable gold, tincture of rubies, amulets and talismans, and cosmetics, which he sold at high prices. He taught boys chemistry for high fees, and practised astrology. In his great medical practice he developed his own method of making long-distance diagnosis as an uroscopist. Servants of rich people soon travelled all over the Holy Roman Empire with their masters' sealed urine jars along with at least 10 Thalers each for the payment of Thurneysser, and when returning they brought back the prescribed drug, with costly-sounding names, such as *Aurum potabili, Bernstein-Essenz, Rubinen-Tinktur, Destilliertes Amethysten-wasser*, etc., prepared in Thurneysser's laboratory and sold at exorbitant prices. 'He established and reorganized alum and saltpetre works and, in order to obtain apparatus, introduced improvements in glass factories. In this way he certainly laid the foundations of the chemical industry in Prussia' (Partington).

He even founded his own printing press, from which he published his astrological calendars, prognostications, alchemical and medical tracts, and a wide variety of polemics. In order to have easy access to Greek, Arabic, Syrian, Hebrew and Chaldean type faces he also founded his own letter foundry and had a staff of over two hundred people including printers, bookbinders, artists, woodcutters, engravers, translators, secretaries for his large correspondence, etc. He soon became a wealthy and famous man who appeared in princely dress of black silk and velvet, with golden necklaces. When touring in his four-in-hand carriage he was accompanied by two servants on horseback and when walking, by two page-boys. As a man of property he built up a great library, a magnificent *Wunderkammer* with shells, stones, a herbarium, portrait pictures, silver, weapons and he kept a menagerie, Berlin's first Zoo. He had agents in a number of German and Polish cities, who advertised his wares and sold his drugs, cosmetics, and amulets to the gentry and wealthy burghers of Germany, Poland and Denmark. Thurneysser also conducted a sort of school of alchemy, which numbered the distinguished apothecary Michael Aschenbrenner among its students.

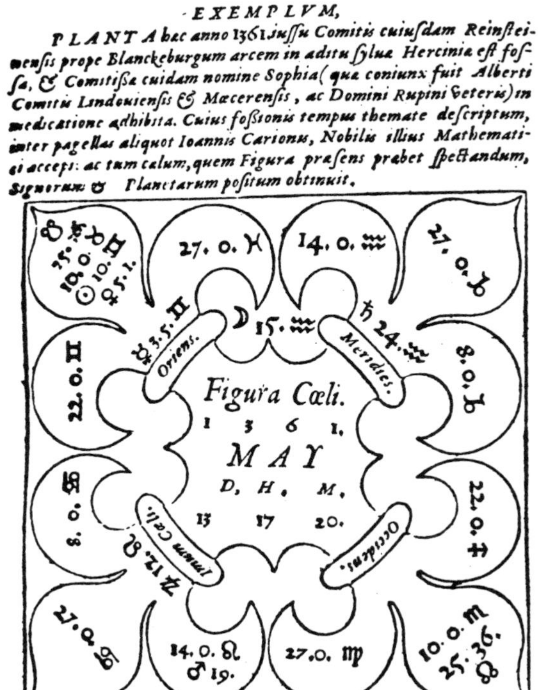

Thurneysser's *Historia Plantarum* has numerous horoscopes with astrological arcane symbols, whose major purpose was to baffle the uninitiated.

In 1577 Thurneysser had a stroke, sold his printing office to his typesetter, Michael Hentzke, and moved back to Basel and there married his third wife, which was a disastrous mistake. He had brought a considerable amount of his wealth to Basel. In divorce proceedings two years later, the Basel town council made over all of his remaining wealth to his wife, terms against which Thurneysser railed in a pamphlet, directed 'an alle Stände der gantzen Christenheit'. He had now lost all his money, lived in Berlin and was, according to unverified statements, forbidden to leave the service of Johann Georg until he had succeeded to transmute a large quantitity of silver into gold. In 1584 he left Berlin in secrecy and went directly to Rome, where he remained for six years and became physician-in-ordinary to Cardinal Marx Sittich II of Hohenems, Bishop of Constance. In Frascati, outside Rome, he acquired a beautiful country estate, 'Belvedere', which he rebuilt at great expense. He returned to Germany and died in obscurity in Cologne. This amazing personality who had lived in great splendour asked in his will to be buried beside Albertus Magnus, a wish that was never granted.

Thurneysser's name did appear in more serious circumstances. Partington credits him with laying the foundations for Prussian chemical industry; he founded the first zoo in Berlin and contributed to fighting the plague by advising on public hygiene, and is also credited with being the first to study birds' migration by ring marking.

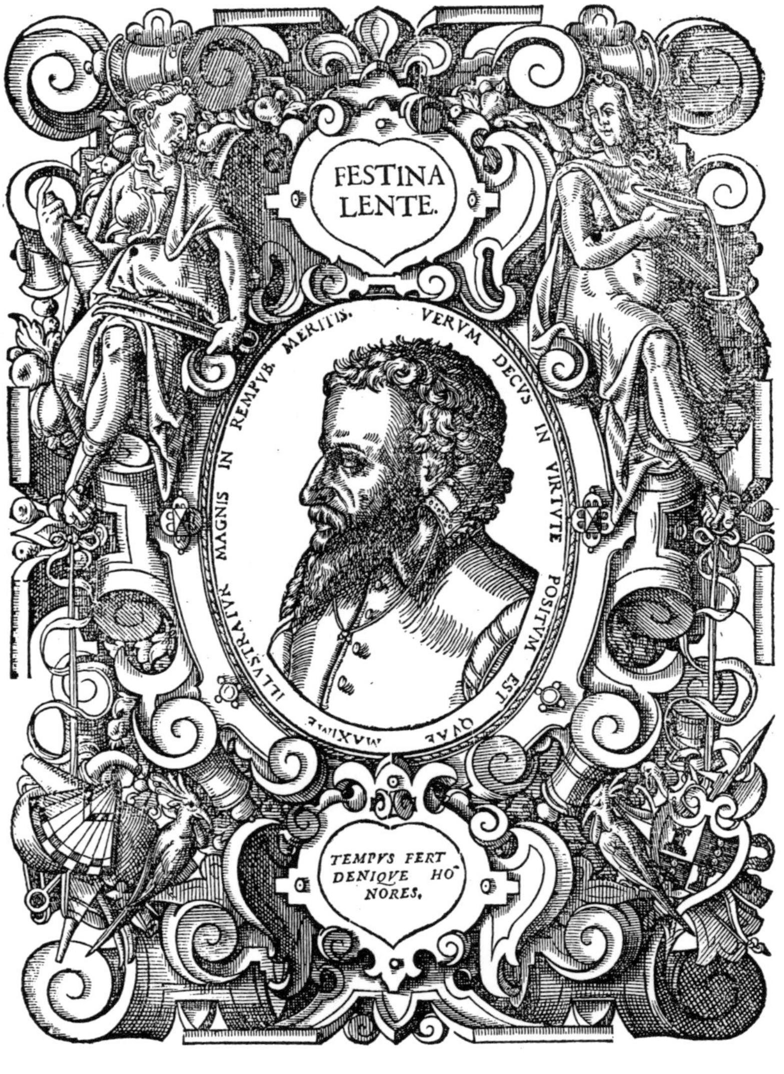

The portrait of Thurneysser within an elaborate border in his *Historia Plantarum.* A few pages later, the same border encloses the portrait of the Lord our Father himself, whose physionomy is very similar to that of Thurneysser. – 'Who could doubt the merits of a man whose portrait is so impressively presented?' (Anderson). Woodcut by Jost Amman.

Thurneysser's *Historia Plantarum* is an elaborate typographical production, with printed annotations in the margins, blocks of text inserted within other textual matter, lavish use of Greek and Hebrew characters, plus a host of astrological symbols, diagrams, and plant illustrations. The descriptions of distillation methods are illustrated with horses, giraffes, fish, bulls, ostriches and other animals which often merge with the distilling apparatus itself. Plants are classified as male, female, and children, depending upon the degree of strength and activity they manifest. Herbs used to cure males are to be gathered when the sun or moon is in Sagittarius, Aquarius or Leo. Those intended to cure women are to be plucked preferably in Virgo, Taurus or Cancer. All is murky, written in lofty phrases intended to mystify. Thurneysser purported himself to be a follower of Paracelsus, but although he frequently quoted from him, he often invented the passages himself. Many of his books contain words in languages that he did not know. Some of the magic spells and terms that he gave have been identified as common Hungarian swearwords. His works were severely criticized by other physicians, and he was publicly accused of harbouring in his inkpot a devil who dictated to him. The *Historia Plantarum* is dedicated to the King of Poland, Stephan IV Bàthory, but when the king paid him less money than he felt was his due, he later dedicated the German edition to Frederick II, King of Denmark.

Gabriele Spitzer, . . . *und die Spree führt Gold. Leonhard Thurneysser zum Thurn, Astrologe – Alchimist – Arzt und Drucker im Berlin des 16, Jahrhunderts*. Berlin, 1996; Paul H. Boerlin, *Leonhard Thurneysser als Auftraggaber. Kunst im Dienste der Selbstdarstellung zwischen Humanismus und Barock* (1976); Moehsen, *Leben Leonhard Thurneisser zum Thurn*, Berlin, 1783 (Facs. 1976); Partington, II, 152-5; DSB, XIII, 396-8; Ferguson, II, 4505; Anderson, 181-6; Hunt, I, 135 (German ed.); Mellon Collection, 45 (German ed.); Forbes, 151-2; Schelenz, 402-03; Waller 9578.

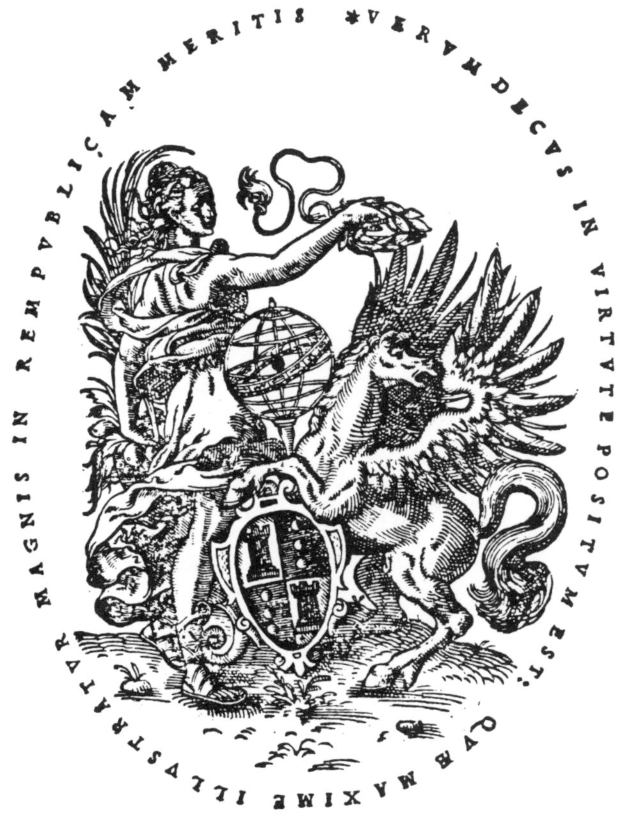

Thurneysser's printing device with Pegasus, with his arms and an armillary sphere. In 1580 he purchased an estate in Basle called 'Zum Thurn', which enabled him to style himself grandly as Leonhard Thurneysser zum Thurn. Woodcut by Jost Amman.

Early work on cosmetics

NOSTRADAMUS [Michel de Notre Dame] (1503–1566)

Michaelis Nostradami. Dess Weitberümbten, Hocherfarnen, Philosophi, Astrologi, und Medici, zwey Bücher, darinn wahrhafftiger, gründtlicher, und volkomner bericht gegeben wirt, wie man erstlich einen ungestalten Leib, an Weib unnd Manns personen auswendig zieren, schön, unnd junggeschaffen machen, unnd allerley wolreichende, köstliche, krefftige wasser, pulfer, öl, seyffen, rachkertzlin, bisamkugeln, zu mancherley gebrechen dienstlich, artlich zubereyten. Und wie man folgents allerley frücht auff das künstlichest, und lieblichest, in zucker einmachen, und zur notturfft auff behalten soll. Erstlich in Frantzösicher sprach von ihme beschriben: Nun aber, unserem Vatterlandt zu gutem, in das gemain Teutsch auff das trewlichst verdolmetscht, durch Hieremiam Martium, bestelten Doctorn der Artzney zu Augspurg.

Augsburg, Michael Manger, 1589.

Octavo – *leaf*: 152 *x* 100 *mm. Pp.* [16], 206, [10]. *Title page printed in red and black. Bound with a similar work by Albertus Magnus, the latter of which is richly illustrated with small woodcuts, but lacking the first gathering incl. title* (colophon: *Frankfurt, Christian Egenolph*, 1585). *Contemporary panelled vellum, triple fillets, inner panel with fleurons in outer corners, repeated as centrepiece, and with the initials* 'CE' *and the date* 1592.

A rare book on cosmetics by the famous French astrologer, better known for his prophecies and prognostications, which have frequently been reprinted well up to the present day. According to the preface the first French edition appeared in 1552. The first German edition, translated by Jeremia Martin, who published many other popular medical works of the same character, was first printed in 1572, of which the above 1589 edition is a re-issue with the date on the title page changed from M.D.LXXII. to M.D.LXXXIX.

Nostradamus, the assumed name of Michel de Notre Dame, of Jewish origin, was born at St Rémi in Provence. After receiving his early education in the liberal arts at the University of Avignon, he proceeded to the University of Montpellier, and was officially matriculated in 1529. He was, however, labelled an apothecary, accused of having slandered doctors, and was struck from the list of students by Guillaume Rondelet, who was the procurator of students during that year. After quarrelling with his unfriendly colleagues, Nostradamus left Montpellier in 1532 and became a wandering physician. He settled in Agen and in 1544 established himself at Salon near Aix in Provence. Both at Aix and at Lyon he acquired great distinction by his labours during the outbreaks of the plague.

'More than any writer in modern times Nostradamus knew how to titillate the deep-seated craving, felt by potentate and plebeian alike, to foresee the future, near and remote . . . Wrapping himself in the mantle of the ancient Hebrew prophets, to whose religion his ancestors had adhered . . . and claiming divine inspiration for his astrological forecasts', Nostradamus published in 1555 the first edition of his Centuries, a book of rhymed prophecies, which secured him the notice of Catherine de Medici, as well as of Henry II and in 1564 of King Charles IX. '. . . the adversaries and supporters of Nostradamus have continued until our time respectively to denounce him as a charlatan and to predict retrospectively such portentous crises as the French Revolution and World War II' (Edward Rosen).

Less known are Nostradamus' pharmaceutical writings published between 1555 and 1557. This German version of his works on cosmetics and on sweets and other confections is divided into two books: 'the first contains a series of pharmacological recipes for the preservation of youth and the maintenance of a fair complexion, including instructions for dyeing hair black, bleaching skin, concocting toothpaste, mixing facial pomades, and blending beauty aids from gold. The second book offers over thirty recipes for the candying or preservation of various fruits and nuts, and directions for making marzipan; whereby the manufacture of brandy is not neglected either.' (Jörg Schäfer)

Edward Rosen in DSB, X, pp 152-3; Hirsch, IV, pp. 386-7; Vicaire, col. 627-30.

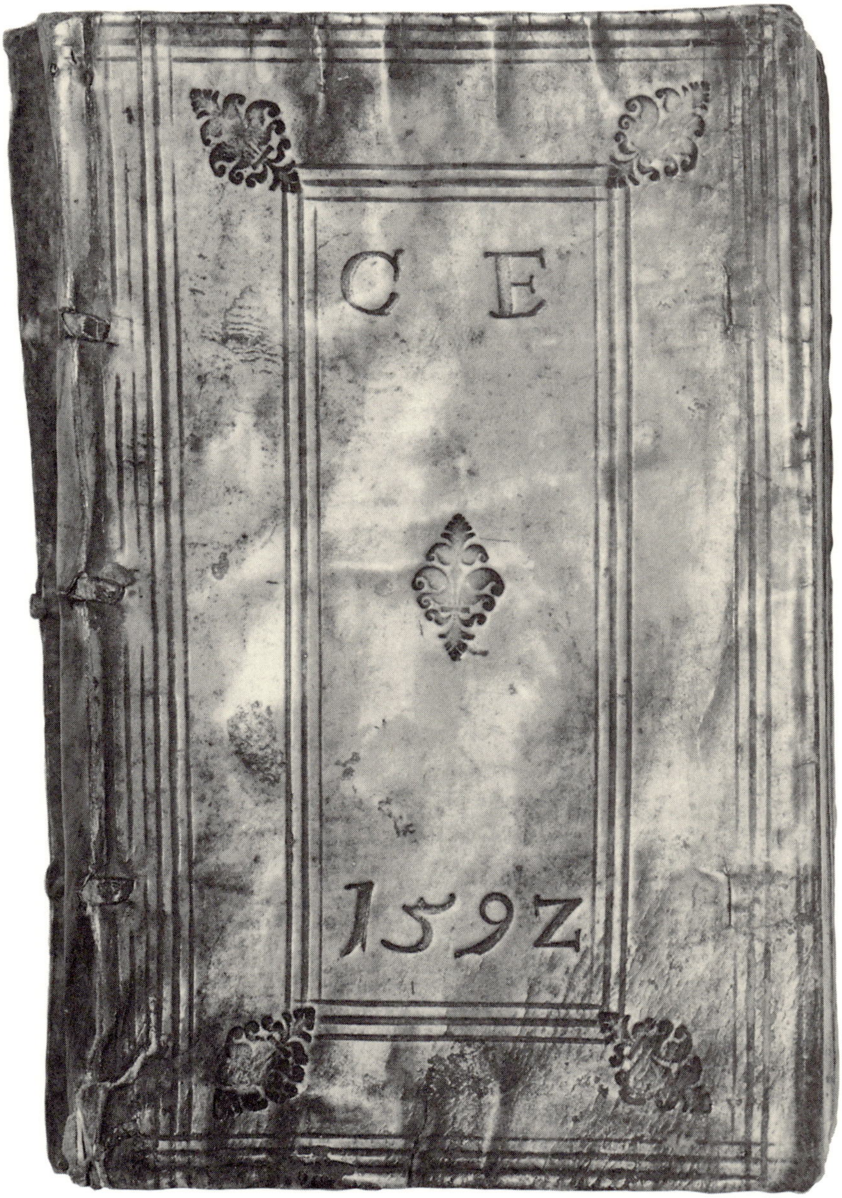
C E
1592

The Doctrine of Signatures

PORTA, Giovanni Battista della (1535–1615)

Phytognomonica. Octo libris contenta; in quibus nova, facillimaque affertur methodus, qua plantarum, animalium, metallorum; . . . Accedunt ad haec confirmanda inifinita propemodum selectoria secreta, . . .
Frankfurt, Johann Wechel & Petrus Fischer, 1591

Octavo – *leaf:* 190 *x* 120 *mm. Pp.* [16], 552, *one blank leaf. Title printed in red and black with printer's device. Woodcut portrait of the author on verso of the title leaf and* 32 *woodcuts in the text. Contemporary blindstamped pigskin with four bands. Front and back cover with the arms of Strassburg,* INSIGNA REIPUBLICA ARGENTORATINEIS. *Signature on the title page:* Joh. Danielis Widt, Med. Doc.

From the Ernst Matérn Collection *with his book-plate.*

In his *Phytognomonica*, first published in Naples in 1588, here in its second edition published by Wechel in Frankfurt for the market in northern Europe, Porta was the first ecologist, grouping plants according to their geographic locale and distribution. In this work he presents the Doctrine of Signatures – the idea that the external form of a plant indicates its medicinal properties. By its likeness to human members the plant indicates which disease it will heal. In their movement, colour and figure, plants are associated with different stars, metals and gems, and share their respective virtues. Each part of the world produces flora and fauna according to the qualities of the local sky and earth.

According to the Doctrine of Signatures, plants were supposed to be marked by some natural sign or symbol which indicated the particular medicinal use to which they could be put. Both in ancient China and in the West the notion that God had marked certain things in ways that indicated their therapeutic value was generally accepted. Plants were divinely 'signed' for the treatment of diseases of the organs of the human body that they resemble in shape, colour or general appearance. Plants with similar leaves possess like virtues, as do plants with similar odours. Plants of yellow colour are to be used for jaundice; peaches, lemons, and certain bulbous roots proclaim themselves as remedies for heart troubles because of their resemblance to a heart; plants of dark colour generate melancholy; milky plants are good for the milk; bony plants heal the bones; long-lived trees promote longevity. The most beautiful plants aid in the generation of beautiful offspring. Herbs growing in the clefts of rocks are suited to break the stone in human bodies; a walnut can cure head ailments as is made evident by its resemblance to the human brain; digitated herbs are good for the fingers; scaly things such as pine cones, thistles, and the overlapping skin on lily bulbs cure scaly conditions of the skin. The human shape of the mandrake or mandragora spurred many superstitions.

Porta's *Physiognomonica*, which offered a simplified method of selecting appropriate remedies quickly, gained popular acceptance and was also meant to serve the apothecary. The book was popular and re-published several times up to the middle of the seventeenth century.

Porta enjoyed a great reputation through another of his books, the *Magia Naturalis* (on Natural Magic), which went through some thirty editions and translations. It is an extraordinary hodge-podge of material representing a unique combination of curiosity and credulity in the late Renaissance. In it he was the first to describe the pinhole camera (camera obscura). He also wrote a famous book on human physiognomy, on plants, on physics, mathematics, and other topics. In 1560 he founded the first scientific society, the *Accademia Secretorum*, a forerunner to both the *Accademia dei Lincei* (of which Porta was Vice-President and Galilei the most illustrious member) and the *Royal Society*. The members met in Porta's house in Naples to discuss and study the secrets of nature. The Society soon roused the suspicions of the Inquisition and Porta was summoned to the Pope in Rome to explain the reports of witches' salves and necromantic arts. He was released on condition that he dissolve the Society and ceased to study dangerous sciences. After 1592 Porta's works were prohibited by the Inquisition, a ban not lifted until 1598.

M.H. Rienstra in DSB, XI, pp. 95-8; Thorndike, VI, pp. 422-3; Anderson, *Herbals*, Chapter 25; Ferguson, II, p. 216; Mortimer, *Italian*, II, 399 (1588 ed.); Hunt, I, 158 (1588 ed.); Waller 7568 (1588 ed.).

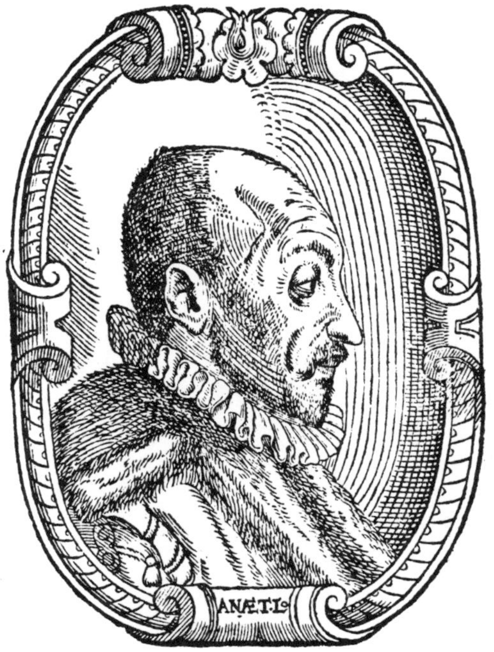

Woodcut medallion portrait of Giovanni Battista della Porta.

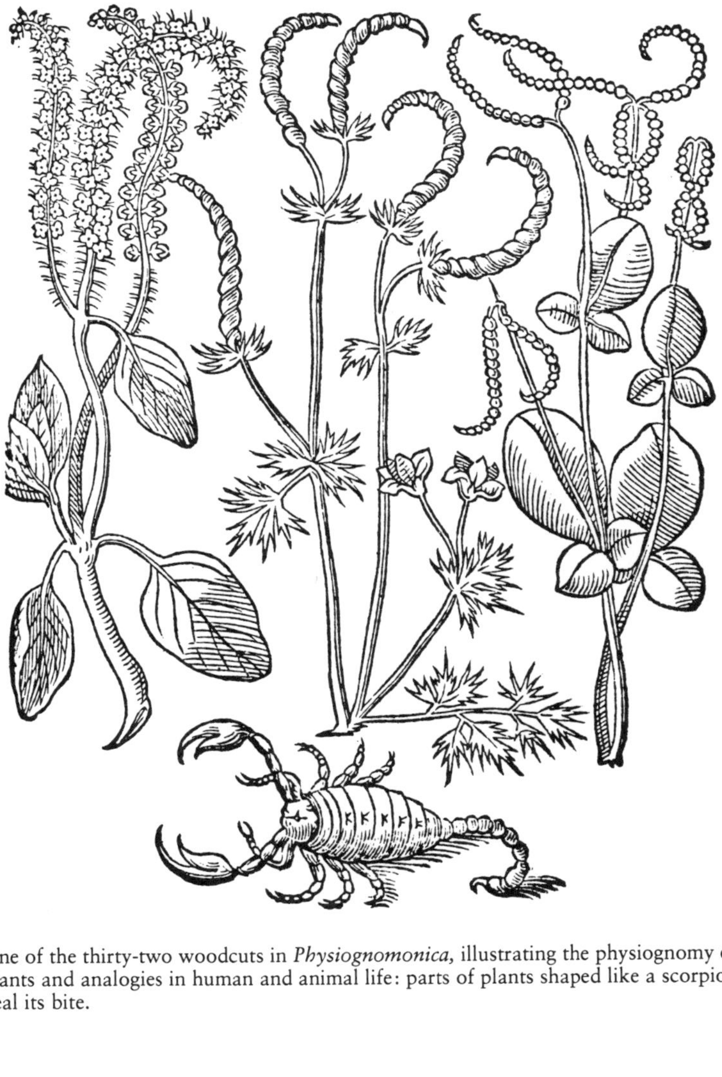

One of the thirty-two woodcuts in *Physiognomonica,* illustrating the physiognomy of plants and analogies in human and animal life: parts of plants shaped like a scorpion heal its bite.

The great centre of botanical information

CLUSIUS, Carolus (Charles de l'Ecluse) 1526–1609

Rariorum Plantarum Historia.
Antwerp, Johann Moretus at the Plantin Press, 1601.

Folio – *leaf*: 340 *x* 218 *mm. Liber* I-III: *pp.* [12], 364; Liber IV-VI *&* Appendix: *pp.* I-CCLX; Fungorum: *pp.* CCLXI-CCXCV, (1) *blank*; Epistola: *pp.* CCXCVII-CCCXX; Pona: *pp.* CCCXXI-CCCXLVIII, [12] *index. Engraved title page. Issue lacking* *1, *with the original* *2-5, *and* *6 *in the second form of the cancellans with, on verso, a poem by Joannes ab Hogheland headed* 'IN EANDEM', *preceded by a poem by Bon. Vulcanius headed* 'IN EFFEGIEM'. *The engraved portrait of the author, separately printed as an insert, is not present in this copy. With over* 1100 *woodcuts of plants in the text. Contemporary vellum.* Ms *title on the upper spine, the rest of the spine painted in orange-red. Upper cover with gilt arms and the letters* 'I.G.P.' *and the date* 'M.DC.XXXV'. *Early inscription of the Capuchin Monastery in Munich on the title. From the* C.D. Carlsson Collection.

Exoticarum libri decem: quibus Animalium, Plantarum, Aromatum, aliorumque perigrinorum Fructuum historiae describuntur: item PETRI BELLONI Observationibus, eodem Carolo Clusio interprete.
Antwerp, Raphelengien at the Plantin Press, 1605.

Folio – *leaf*: 353 *x* 220 *mm. Pp.* [16] *incl. engraved title,* 378, [8] *index,* [2] *errata & register,* Monardes: *pp.* 52; Altera Appendix: *pp.* [28]; Belloni: *pp.* [12], 1-2 (= *last pages of index*), 3-242, [2] *errata. With c.*275 *woodcuts of plants and animals. Early issue without the two extra inserted leaves with poems, printed c.*1607. *Contemporary vellum, spine divided into six compartments with double gilt fillets, Ms title in black ink, covers with gilt fillets around sides and a gilt arabesque oval centrepiece. This copy formerly belonged to the Royal Pharmaceutical Institute, now in the Scheele-room, Biomedcial Library, Faculty of Pharmacy, Uppsala University.*

These two volumes form the first collected edition of the works of Charles de l'Ecluse, better known to botanists under the latinized name of Clusius. His books were printed at the famous Plantin press in Antwerp, who published the numerous illustrated herbals of the greatest botanists of their day: Dodoens, De l'Obel (Lobelius) and De l'Ecluse. Their intimate friendship allowed them to work side by side without rivalry, and use each other's observations and figures in their books.

After studying at various universities l'Ecluse went to Montpellier and was, like l'Obel before him, received in the house of the famous physician Guillaume Rondelet, who was also an able botanist. Rondelet not only cured l'Ecluse of a severe illness, but also awakened in his pupil an interest for botany, which was to be his ruling passion for the rest of his life. Like many of the inquiring minds of the Renaissance l'Ecluse travelled widely in various parts of Europe. A journey to Spain, during which he discovered two hundred new species of plants, resulted in his first important work, *Rariorum aliquot stirpium per Hispanius observatorum historia* (Plantin, 1576). In 1573 l'Ecluse was invited to Vienna by the Emperor Maximilian II and remained there for some fourteen years. This gave him the opportunity to explore the mountain flora of Austria and Hungary, described in a book published by Plantin in 1583, in which he also included an account of various oriental plants which had reached Vienna through Constantinople. His gift for languages was of great service for botany, for besides translating the Flemish herbal of Dodoens into French, he made Latin versions of the Portuguese work of Garcia de Orta, and the Spanish writings of Christoval Acosta and Nicolas Monardes, as well as publishing the *Antidotarium* (1561), being his Latin translation of the first European pharmacopoeia, the *Ricettario Fiorentino.*

Crippled and aged sixty-six he was in 1593 appointed to the chair of botany at the University of Leiden to succeed Dodoens. There he took charge of the botanic garden, which within a year had over a thousand species and varieties, mostly medicinal, growing there. His enthusiastic cultivation of foreign plants, particularly those from Turkey and the Levant, prepared the way for the splendid gardens of seventeenth-century France, Germany, Austria, Flanders and Holland. He was the chief founder of the bulb culture which has played so conspicuous a part in the history of the Netherlands.

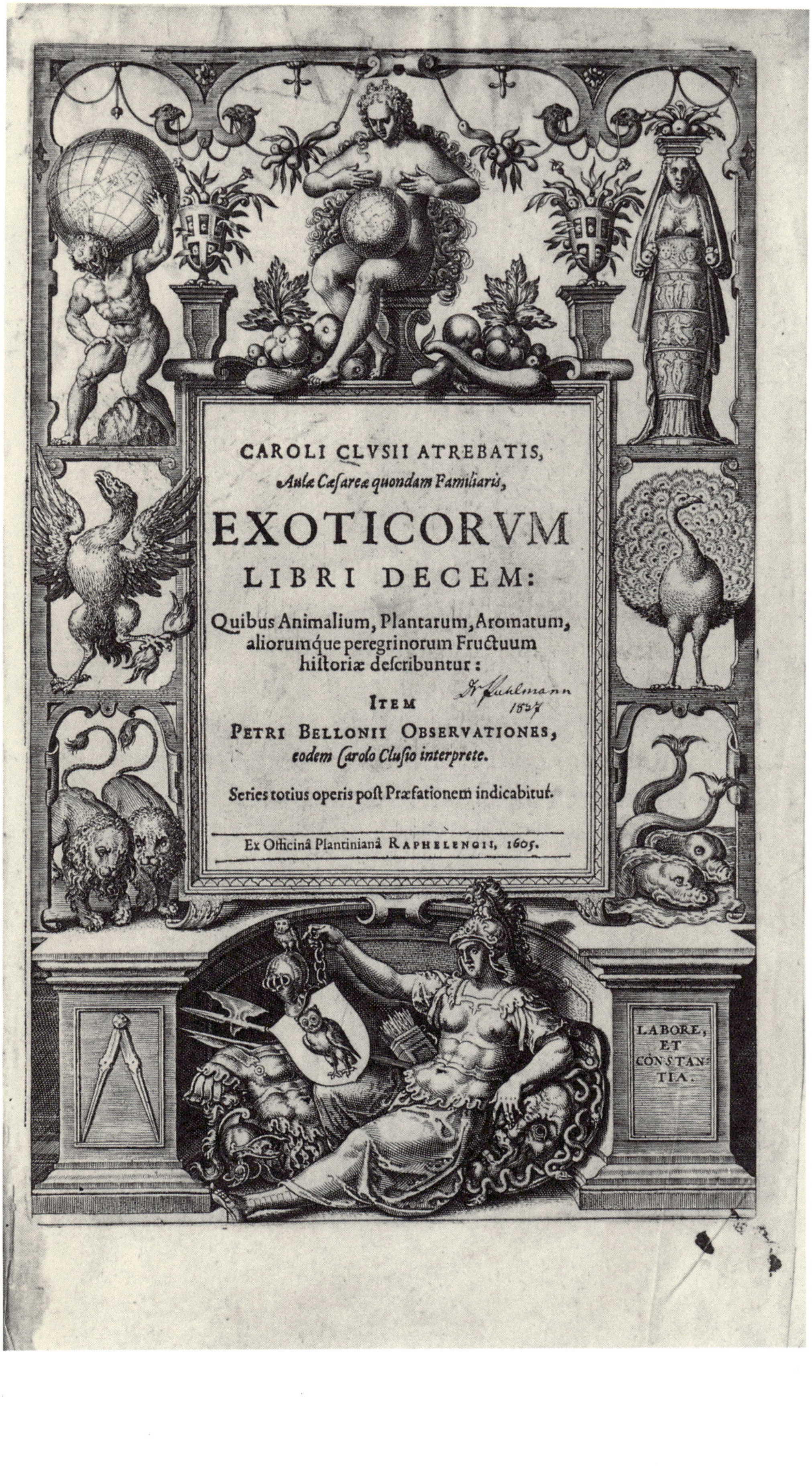
CAROLI CLVSII ATREBATIS,
Aulæ Cæsareæ quondam Familiaris,
EXOTICORVM
LIBRI DECEM:
Quibus Animalium, Plantarum, Aromatum, aliorumque peregrinorum Fructuum historiæ describuntur:
ITEM
PETRI BELLONII OBSERVATIONES,
eodem Carolo Clusio interprete.
Series totius operis post Præfationem indicabitur.
Ex Officinâ Plantinianâ Raphelengii, 1605.
LABORE, ET CONSTANTIA.

L'Ecluse, we are told, 'charged such an extortionate price for his tulips that no one could procure them, not even for money'. Of more practical importance to the common people was his introduction of potatoes into the Low Countries. During the latter part of his life he was the great centre of botanical information. The fine botanical woodcuts illustrating his books were executed under the direction of l'Ecluse, many of them by Pieter van der Borcht, one of the most gifted of all the artists employed by Plantin. A massive two-volume biography by F.W.T. Hunger (1927-42) provides the most detailed account of the eventful life of this distinguished man.

In his two books, the *Rariorum* and the *Exoticarum*, l'Ecluse has collected the most important results of his labours. The *Rariorum* contains material from his works on the floras of Spain, Austria and Hungary and is divided into six books: the first treats of trees and shrubs, the second of bulbous plants, the third of sweet-smelling flowers, the fourth of flowers without smell, the fifth of poisonous, narcotic, and acrid plants, and the sixth of those that have milky juice, the *Umbelliferae*, ferns, grasses, etc. This is followed by the first edition of *Fungorum Historia*, the first monograph on fungi with numerous and excellent woodcut illustrations of mushrooms. At the end are letters to l'Ecluse from Honorius Bellus and Thobias Roelsius and finally, with separate title leaf, a treatise by the Veronese apothecary Giovanni Pona on the medicinal plants of Monte Baldo near Verona.

PARADISEA AVIS *majoris generis.*

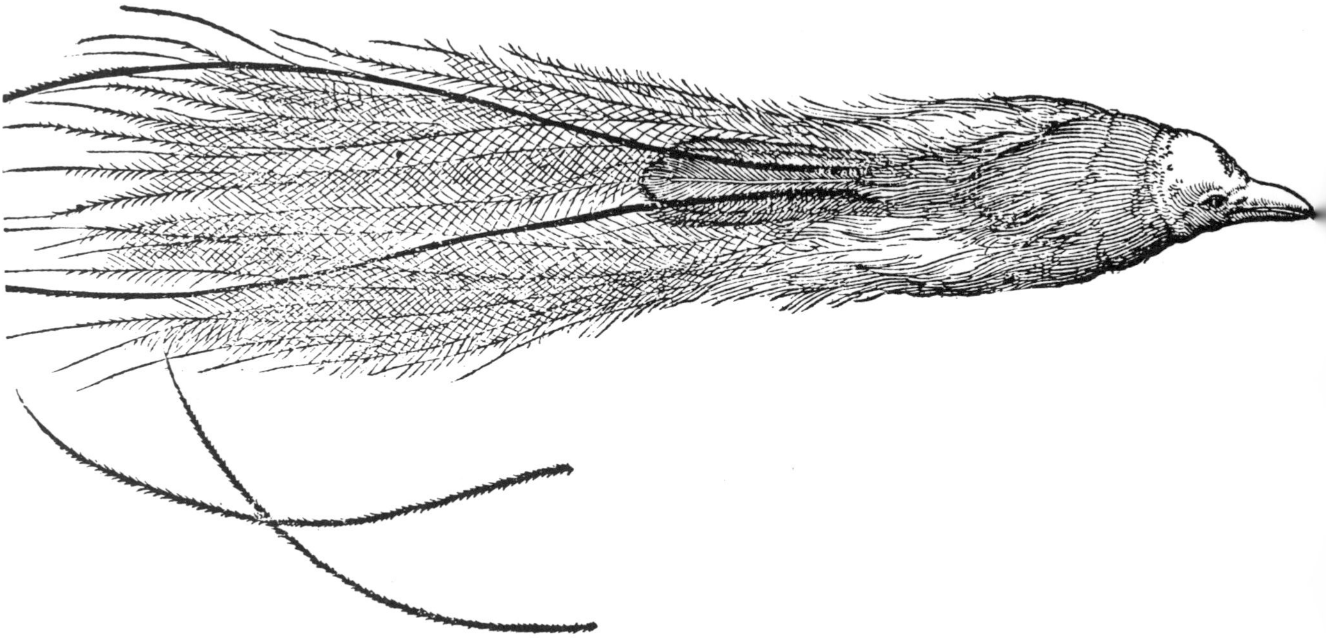

The birds of Paradise were known to seafarers and oriental traders for centuries before any Westerner found their home. Their bright plumage was used by the natives of New Guinea in trade, and they prepared specimens by skinning the body, cutting off the legs, and then drying the skin. When such skins first reached Spain in 1522 from the Magellan circumnavigation, it was thought that they lacked feet, were obliged to fly continuously and therefore lived in the highest sky far above the range of human vision and that they required no other food or drink than dew from Heaven. As late as 1760 Linnaeus named the principal species *apoda* or 'footless', as no perfect specimen had been seen in Europe. Already in the fifteenth century, the élite corps of the Ottoman Sultan's army wore Bird of Paradise plumes in their ceremonial headgear. Women's hat trade of the late nineteenth century finally converted feather hunting into big business. At the height of the trade, between the 1880's and World War I, up to 80 000 birds were killed and exported from Dutch New Guinea every year.

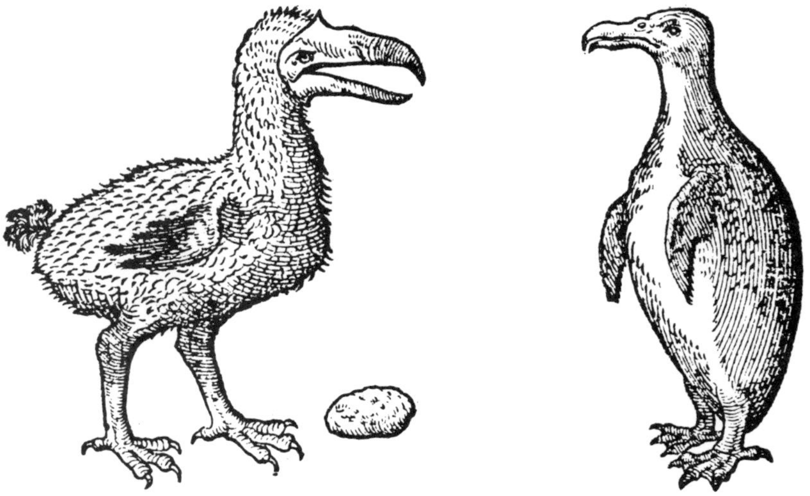

L'Ecluse presented plants and animals unfamiliar to Europeans, many brought home from the New World. In his *Exoticarum* Europeans got the first glimpse of a dodo and a penguin.

The *Exoticarum* is divided into ten books. Libri I-VI contain new material, Libri VII and VIII contain l'Ecluse's abridgement and translation, with his own comments, of Garcia da Orta's *Coloquios dos simples e drogas,* which was the first account of Indian *materia medica* written by a European; the original Portuguese edition was printed at Goa in 1563, and is a priceless book. Liber IX contains l'Ecluse's Latin translation of Cristoval Acosta's illustrated Spanish version of Orta's *Coloquios*, and Liber X contains l'Ecluse's translation of Nicolas Monardes' *Simplicium Medicamentorum,* the first treatise on Central American drugs, and for many years the most important work on the medicinal plants of the New World. These are followed by Monardes *Libri tres* [*De Capite bezaar & herba scorzonera, De ferro,* and *De nive*] and Monardes' *Libellus de rosa* and *Dissertatiuncula de citriis.* At the end, with separate title-leaf, is the Latin version of Pierre Belon's account of his exploring voyage to the Middle East and of the plants of the Near East. In the *Exoticarum* 'we can read the accounts which early Spanish or Portuguese travellers and residents in the East or West Indies had given of the fruit-eating bat, three-banded and six-banded armadillos, the sloth and pangolin, the sperm-whale, the manatee, the cassowary, dodo and penguin, hummingbirds and birds of Paradise, the chimæra, diodon, tetrodon and ostracion, the king-crab and gorgonia, the banyan, mace, nutmeg, spice-clove, cinnamon, pepper, lac, the Egyptian lotus, the coco-nut, pine-apple, vanilla, arnotto, capsicum, copal and tobacco, besides foreign drugs, such as aloes, assafetida, sarsaparilla, balsam of tolu, castor-oil and opium' (Miall). The descriptions are accompanied by woodcuts, many of which depict these exotic creatures and plants for the first time in a European book.

Hunt, I 182; Arber, pp. 229-30; Johnston, *Cleveland Herbal Collection,* 149 & 151; Miall, *The Early Naturalists* (1912), pp. 72-3; Blunt/Stearn, pp. 82-4; Blunt, *Tulipomania,* p. 9; Colin Clair, *Christopher Plantin,* pp. 116, 187-8; Hunger, F.W.T. *Charles de l'Ecluse* (*Carolus Clusius*) *Nederlandsch Kruidkundige,* 1526-1609. The Hague, 1927-42; Waller 11556 (*Rariorum* only)

A giant herbal with nearly 2400 illustrations

TABERNAEMONTANUS, Jacob Theodor (1520–1590)

New vollkommen Kräuter-Buch, darinnen uber 3000. Kräuter, mit schönen und kunstlichen Figuren, auch deren Underscheid und Wirckung, sampt ihren Namen in mancherley Spraachen, beschrieben: Dessgleichen auch, wie dieselbige in allerhand Kranckheiten, beyde der Menschen und des Viehs, sollen angewendet und gebraucht werden, angezeigt wird. Vormals durch D. Casparum Bauhinum . . . gebessert. Jetzt widerumb auffs newe übersehen, mit nutzlichen Marginalien, Synonimis . . . und anderm vermehret durch Hieronymum Bauhinum.

Basel, Jacob Werenfels for Johann König, 1664.

Folio – *leaf*: 380 *x* 250 *mm. Pp.* [16], 663, [1]*; part* II *and* III*: pp.* [4], 665-1529, [1] *blank,* [132] *index,* [2] *list of authors quoted. Lacks the engraved title leaf, the sub-title leaf to part* II *and one leaf in the index* (8F1)*. Printer's device on the printed title page, more than* 2400 *woodcuts in the text. Contemporary richly blindstamped pigskin over wooden boards (restored). The three parts bound in one very thick volume. The device on the printed title page and the woodcuts on the first* 600 *pages are coloured by a contemporary hand.*

Gift from A. Wiström.

This new and enlarged edition of Tabernaemontanus' *Kräuter-Buch* is a massive and copiously illustrated herbal. With its nearly 2400 woodcut figures of plants it is one of the most voluminous herbals ever printed. Its lasting popularity is attested by the fact that the last edition appeared as late as 1731. It was much used by pharmacists, physicians and botanists. Linnaeus owned a copy of the 1664 edition.

Jacob Theodorus took the name Tabernaemontanus, which is Latin for Bergzabern, his birthplace in Zweibrücken. He was closely connected to the German Fathers of Botany having been the pupil of Otto Brunfels already as a boy and afterwards working as an assistant to Hieronymus Bock, whom he called 'mein lieber Praeceptor'. Medicine and pharmacy were his professions and he worked in a pharmacy in Weissenburg before he began to study medicine in France. After graduating as M.D. he became town physician in Worms and later physician-in-ordinary to the court of the elector in Heidelberg and to the bishop of Speyer.

Tabernaemontanus devoted all his time gathering material for his herbal and he spent what he could on it, but the total cost was beyond his means. The eventual printing of the book, after he had worked upon it for thirty-six years, was due in part to the generosity of Count Palatine Frederick III, and of the Frankfurt publisher Nicolaus Bassaeus. The first edition, and the only its author saw in print, appeared in two volumes in 1588-91. Although it was richly illustrated, a special edition in oblong quarto, *Eicones plantarum,* appeared in 1590, with 2255 woodcuts of plants only and with no other text than the Latin and German names. Most of the pictures were copied from the herbals of Bock, Fuchs, Mattioli and from the many botanical works published by the Plantin press in Antwerp. This great collection of wood blocks became familiar in England a few years later when they were acquired by John Norton, printer to the Queen, who used them to illustrate Gerard's *Herball* (1597).

Tabernaemontanus' herbal was revised and enlarged by the famous physician and botanist Caspar Bauhin, whose *Pinax* was one of the most used reference works for plants before Linnaeus. Bauhin's edition was published in three volumes in 1613 with a new edition in 1625. The herbal was later even further revised and enlarged by Bauhin's grandson, Hieronymus Bauhin, whose edition is the present one of 1664. It went through two more editions, in 1687 and 1731. Next to Thomas Johnson's enlarged edition of Gerard's herbal (1633-36) it is the bulkiest herbal ever printed.

The book was evidently a great success for the publisher and was recommended to 'allen Aertzten, Apoteckern, Wundärtzten, Schmieden, Gärntnern, Köchen, Kellners, Hebammen, Hausvättern, und alle andern Liebhabern der Artzney'. Himself an author of popular medical works, Tabernaemontanus zealously warns people of the fatal and destructive methods of his rivals: 'Juden, Barbierer, Baderknechte, Zahnbrecher, Spinnenfresser und dergleichen Landfahrer'.

Nissen, BBI, 1931; Arber, p.76.

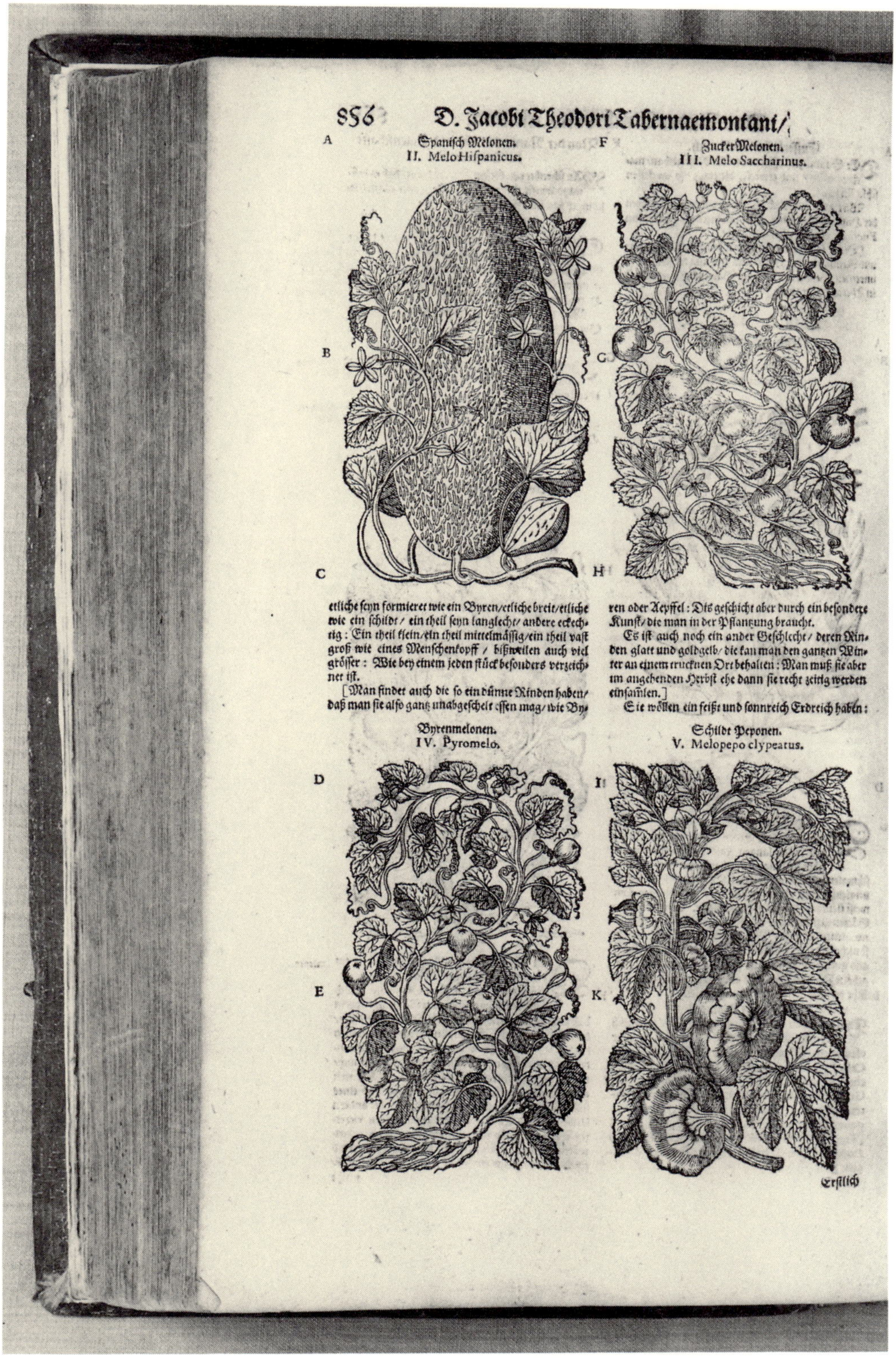

Bauhin's enlarged edition of Tabernaemontanus' *Kräuter-Buch*, with its nearly 1700 pages and 2400 woodcuts, is one of the bulkiest herbals ever published.

AGRICOLA, Johann Georg (1558–1633)

The Deer, an animal rich in medicaments

Cervi exoriati et dissecti in medicina usus. Das ist: Kurtze Beschreibung welcher gestalt dess zu gewisser zeit gefangenen Hirschens fürnembste Glieder in der Artzney zugebrauchen: Und Erstlich: Was massen dass abgenommene und zubereite Geweyhe in mancherley dess Leibs beschwerungen beyzubringen. Dann zum Andern: Wie die ybrigen stück in ander wege mögen genossen und applicirt werden. Mit besondern fleiss auss vieler Alten und anderer fürnemer Medicorum Bücher, und durch erfahrung zusamb getragen.

Amberg, Michael Forster, 1603.

Quarto – *leaf*: 182 *x* 140 *mm. Pp.* [24], 120, [4]. *Title page in red and black within a pictorial woodcut border. Old half vellum, marbled boards. Title leaf shaved in outer margin affecting the printed border.*

Book-plate: Rud. Ferber, Med. Dr. (*Germany*); C.D. Carlsson.

The very rare first edition of one of the earliest works exclusively devoted to the natural history of the deer and its medicinal use. A greatly expanded edition (244 pages) was issued in 1617 by the same publisher. This first edition is dedicated to Prince Georg Ludwig of Leuchtenberg with his full-page woodcut arms on verso of the title leaf. The fine title border has pictures of deer and deer hunting, deer horns, on one side the goddess of the chase, Diana (Artemis), armed with bow and arrows and with a crescent on her head; on the other side is Actaeon, the famous hunter, who, having accidently seen Diana while she was bathing, was transformed by her into a stag and torn apart by his own fifty dogs.

Johann Georg Agricola, physician-in-ordinary to the Elector of Amberg, is not to be confused with Johann Agricola, the alchemist, who lived about the same time. The book has two parts, the first is divided into four chapters dealing with the natural history of the stag, and especially with its horn's preparation for use in medicine. The second part has 21 chapters, each dealing with a separate part of the animal, discussing its preparation and use in various diseases and human ailments. There are chapters on the deer's flesh, blood, teeth, heart, stomach, lungs, skin, hooves, its short tail, excrements, the stag's sperm, the hind's uterus, bones and marrow, tallow, kidneys, genitalia, etc.

Of special value was a kind of bezoar stone made of the congealed humour distilled from the eyes of deer when standing in water up to their lips in order to suffer no ill effects from the poison of the snakes which they have eaten in order to free themselves from worms. It was thought that deer extract snakes from their holes with the breath from their nostrils, then kill them with their hooves and eat them. That is why so many antidotes for poisons come from the stag's body. Pliny tells 'that the deer, as everybody knows, is the mortal enemy of the snake'. Practically every part of the animal was said to possess valuable medicinal properties. The most highly esteemed was the bone, or rather cartilage, of the stag's heart, which the hunters call the heart's cross on account of its shape, which was administered in the form of powder for heart troubles.

One of Linnaeus' most devoted pupils, the Swiss-born Friedrich Ehrhart, who spent several years at Uppsala and was employed at the university pharmacy, reproduces in his *Beiträge zur Naturkunde,* vol. v, (1790), the prescription for *Spirit. destill. cum Corde Cervi* ('Hiorthiertewattn') administered to the King of Sweden 'pro Serenissimo Rege', adding sarcastically that 'a slice of roast deer probably would have had a better result' (Fries, *Linné,* II, pp. 174-5).

The deer has always had a reputation as an animal rich in medicaments, which is also why the representation of a deer at an early date came to adorn a well-assorted apothecary's shop.

All the following have the second edition of 1617 only: Waring 322; Schwerdt, I, 7; Souhart, 5; Jeanson Sale (Sotheby's), 8; *Deliciae Cobresianae*, 3; Schelenz, 501.

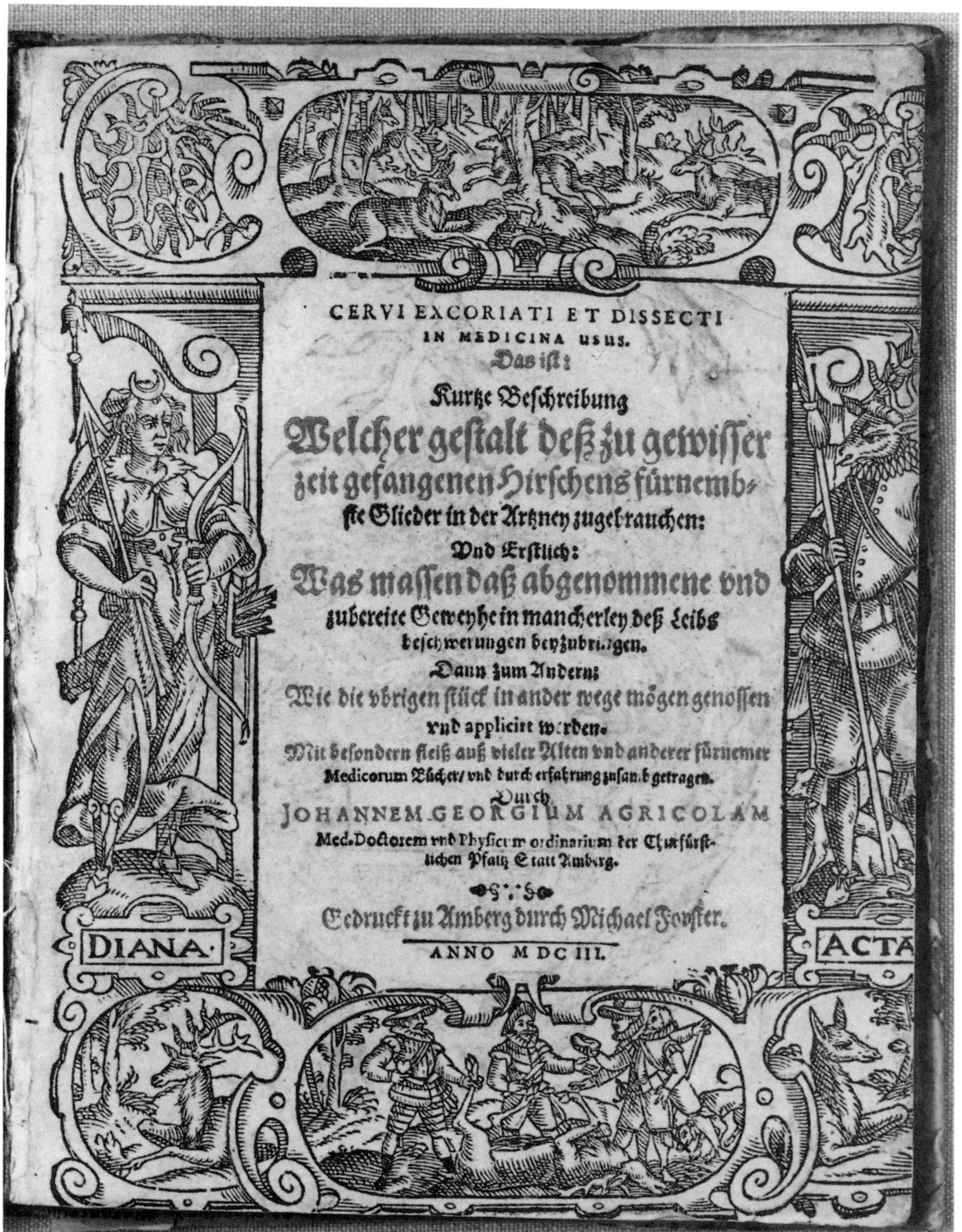

CERVI EXCORIATI ET DISSECTI
IN MEDICINA USUS.
Das ist:
Kurtze Beschreibung
Welcher gestalt deß zu gewisser
zeit gefangenen Hirschens fürnemb-
ste Glieder in der Artzney zugebrauchen:
Und Erstlich:
Was massen daß abgenommene vnd
zubereite Gewehe in mancherley deß Leibs
beschwerungen beyzubringen.
Dann zum Andern:
Wie die vbrigen stück in ander wege mögen genossen
vnd applicirt werden.
Mit besondern fleiß auß vieler Alten vnd anderer fürnemer
Medicorum Bücher/ vnd durch erfahrung zusamb getragen.
Durch
JOHANNEM GEORGIUM AGRICOLAM
Med. Doctorem vnd Physicum ordinarium der Churfürst-
lichen Pfaltz Statt Amberg.

Gedruckt zu Amberg durch Michael Forster.
ANNO MDCIII.

The greatest work on chemistry of the 17th century

LIBAVIUS, Andreas (c.1540–1616)

D.O.M.A. Alchymia . . . recognita, emendata, et aucta, tum dogmatibus & experimentiis nonnullis; tum Commentario Medico Physico Chymico: qui exornatus est variis Instrumentorum Chymicorum picturis; . . .
Frankfurt, Johannes Sauer for Petrus Kopff, 1606.

Folio – *leaf*: 340 x 210 *mm. Pp.* [20] *incl. engraved title leaf,* 196, [12]; Commentarius I: *pp.* [10], 402; Commentarius II: *pp.* 192, [19]. *The two parts of commentary with separate title pages. With c.*200 *woodcuts in the text. Contemporary vellum, blind-stamped into panels with floral borders within fillets, arabesque centrepiece, spine divided into six compartments with floral decoration. Remnants of leather ties.*

From the Ernst Matérn Collection.

This is the first illustrated edition of Libavius' main work, which had appeared in a shortened form in German as: *Alchymistische Practic: Das ist, von künstlicher Zubereitung der vornembsten Chymischen Medicinen* (1603). The *Alchymia* (1606) is significantly enlarged, with commentary added, and is considered the greatest and, due to the numerous illustrations, the most beautiful of all books on chemistry of the seventeenth century. It is a splendid folio volume with more than 200 woodcut illustrations of various sorts of chemical glassware, vessels, apparatus, and furnaces, as well as an architectural plan of a large chemical laboratory or institute, which includes bathrooms, a museum, wine cellars, covered walks and gardens.

Andreas Libavius, the son of a poor linen weaver, was born at Halle in Saxony. The exact date of his birth is unknown. After a period of study in philosophy, history and medicine at the University of Jena he became a teacher at Ilmenau and Coburg. In 1588 he graduated M.D. at the University of Basel and in the same year was appointed town physician in Rothenburg and inspector for schools. From 1607 until his death in 1616 he was director for the newly founded Gymnasium Casmirianum Academicum in Coburg. He took a keen interest in chemistry and composed a large body of work on this subject besides several schoolbooks and works of philosophy, etc.

Libavius' main value to science consists in his extraordinarily voluminous alchemical works, which represent a compendium of the chemical knowledge of the time. His *Alchymia* is often regarded as the first real textbook of chemistry in the modern sense. Partington considers it an excellent practical textbook. Its author shows a full mastery of his sources and a clear, concise, and sensible style, entirely different from the rambling, bombastic, and obscure verbosity of Paracelsus or other alchemical authors.

The *Alchymia* is a mixture of alchemical and chemical learning and illustrates a transitional phase of chemical science. Although Libavius presents much rational material, he also admits the possibility of the transmutation of base metals. In his attempt to systematize chemistry, Libavius uses a terminology which sounds strange today, though in its own setting is clear and logical. He uses the word *alchemia* in the sense in which we now use the word *chemistry*. He subdivides the science into *encheria*, which deals with chemical methods, and *chymia*, which concerns substances and their properties. *Magisteria* is a term which denotes not only chemical substances but also their properties and the forces which they produce. In all practical recipes Libavius' style is extremely clear. It becomes obscure in the sections dealing with the Philosophers' Stone. He tried to penetrate and understand works on the Philosopher's Stone, and commented broadly in his own way. He declared that the mysterious alchemical substance called 'azoth' was really 'liquor [or spiritus] sublimati' (stannic chloride), later known as 'spiritus fumans Libavii'.

Libavius has been called the first chemist of note in Germany who stood up manfully against the excesses of Paracelsus and who vigorously combatted the defects of his doctrine, the obscurities in his writings, his fantasies and sophisms, and the employment of 'secret remedies'. This does not mean that he was opposed to alchemy and iatrochemistry. He defended the art of alchemy against the censure of the Parisian medical faculty.

W. Hubicki in DSB, VIII, pp. 309-12; Partington, II, pp. 244-67; Thorndike, VI, pp. 238-53; Ferguson, II, p. 31; Duveen, p. 357.

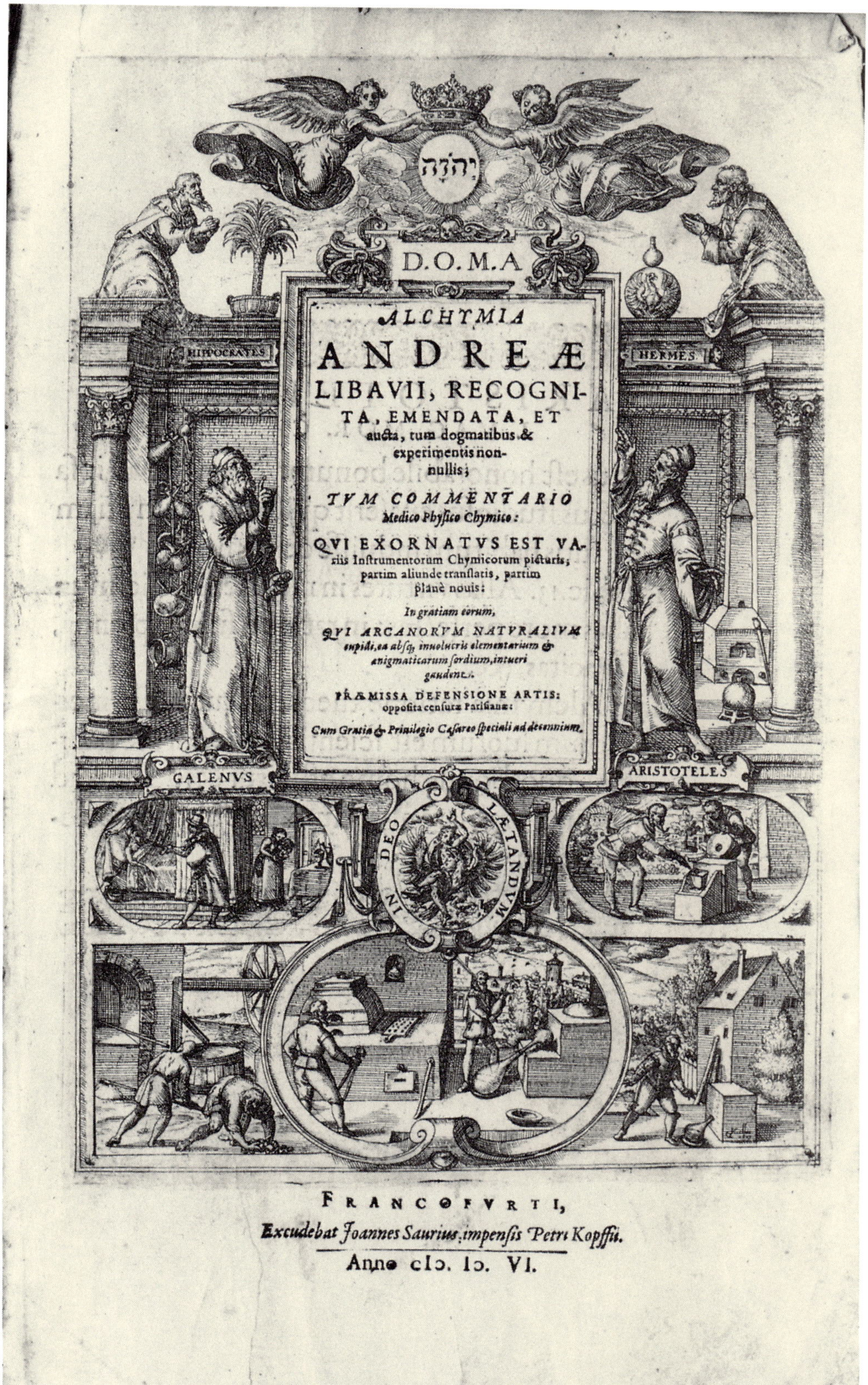

יְהֹוָה

D.O.M.A

ALCHYMIA
ANDREÆ
LIBAVII, RECOGNITA, EMENDATA, ET
aucta, tum dogmatibus & experimentis nonnullis;

TVM COMMENTARIO
Medico Physico Chymico:

QVI EXORNATVS EST VAriis Instrumentorum Chymicorum picturis; partim aliunde translatis, partim planè nouis:

In gratiam eorum,

QVI ARCANORVM NATVRALIVM cupidi, ea absq; inuolucris elementarium & ænigmaticarum sordium, intueri gaudent.

PRÆMISSA DEFENSIONE ARTIS:
opposita censuræ Parisianæ:

Cum Gratia & Priuilegio Cæsareo speciali ad decennium.

HIPPOCRATES

HERMES

GALENVS

ARISTOTELES

IN DEO LÆTANDVM

FRANCOFVRTI,
Excudebat Joannes Saurius, impensis Petri Kopffii.
Anno clɔ. Iɔ. VI.

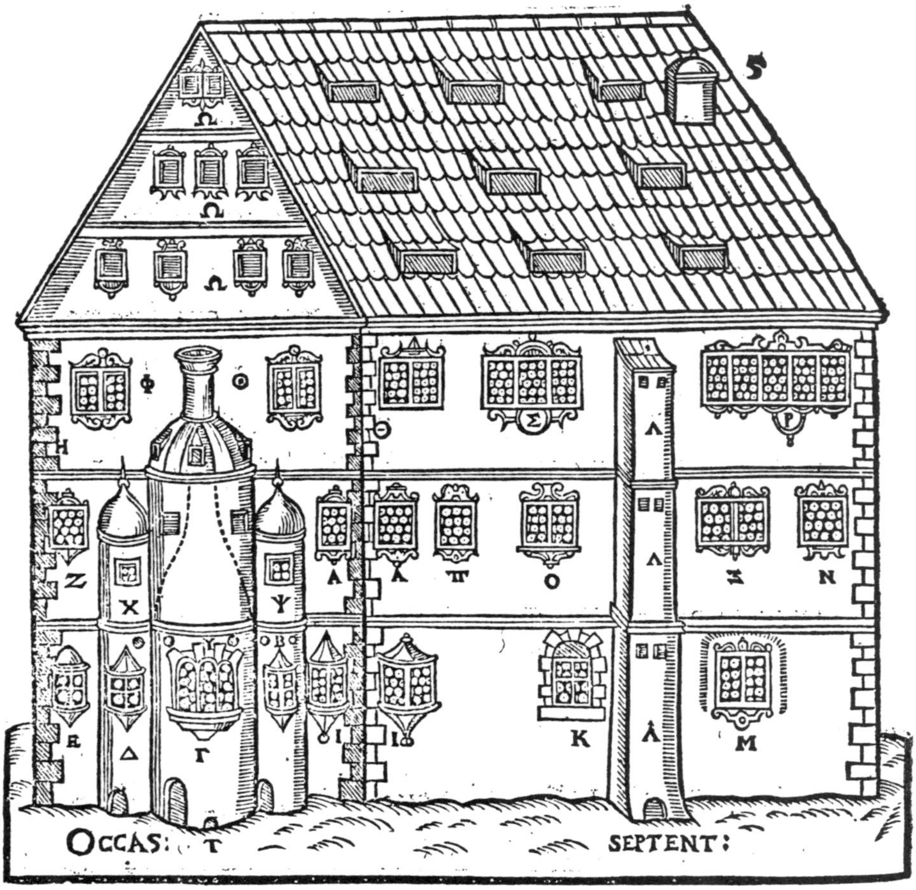

Libavius' *Alchymia* contains a remarkable plan of a Utopian chemical institute, which goes far beyond the laboratories of the alchemists or apothecaries that existed at the time. It is a building for the experimenter and research worker of the future. Besides areas with apparatus for distilling, for analytical weighing, for crystallizing, for the work of the chemical apothecary, and so on, it also includes a secret laboratory with a gold-maker's furnace, to which one gains access by a narrow spiral staircase, as well as a museum, bathrooms, wine cellars and covered walks and gardens – delightful features unhappily overlooked by the modern architect of chemical laboratories.

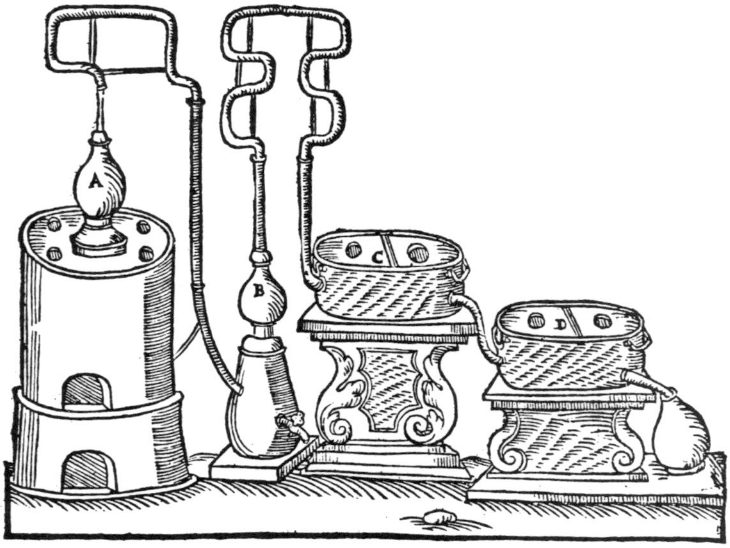

There are hundreds of woodcuts in the *Alchymia* depicting equipment in a chemical laboratory including several distilling apparatus. The still above is with condenser and double cooler.

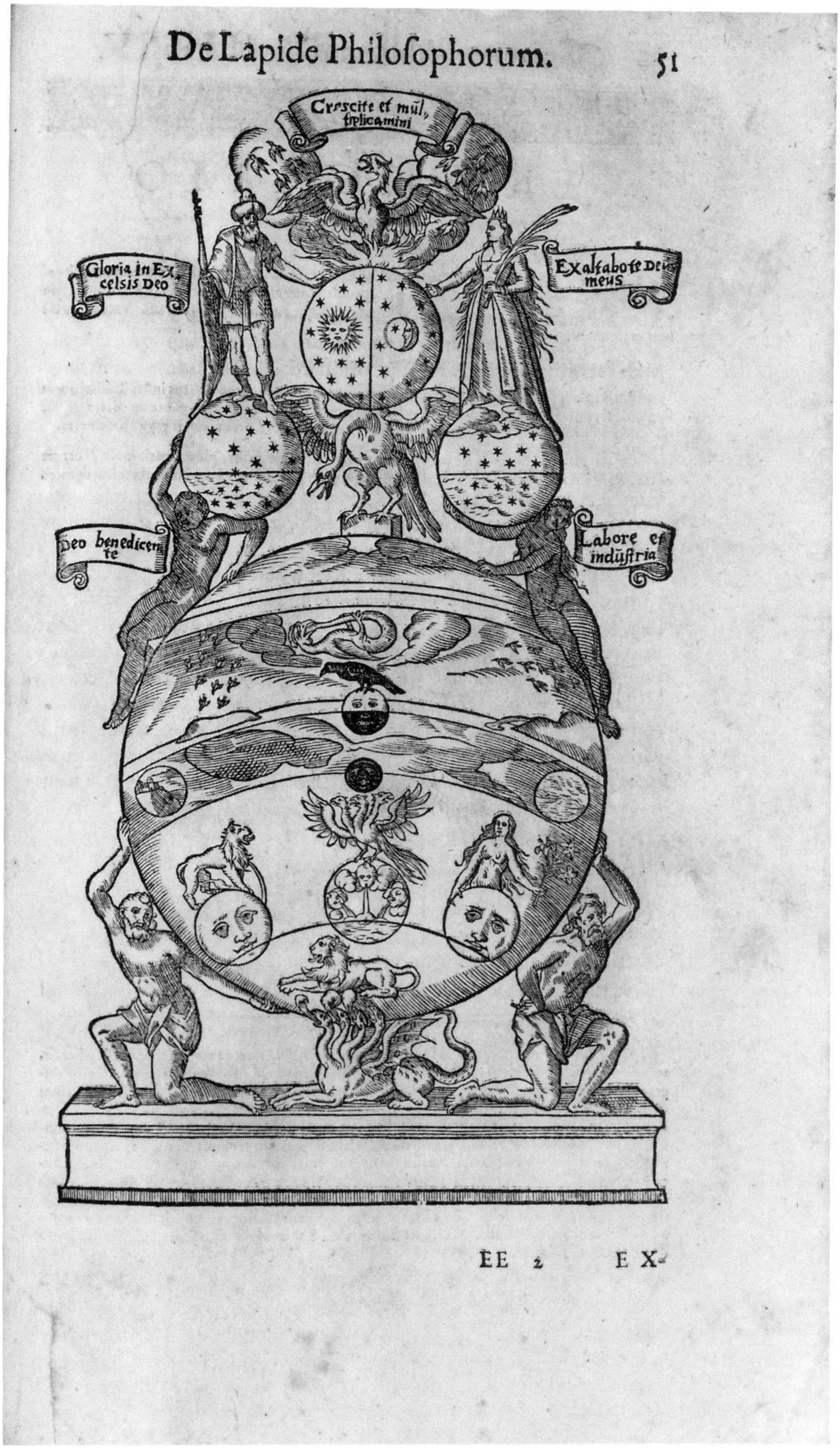

One of the three full-page woodcuts in Libavius' treatise on the Philosopher's Stone in his *Alchymia*. – 'The conception of the Philosopher's Stone was the mainspring in alchemy. It provided an unexampled motive power, a kind of alchemical perpetual motion, which animated some forty generations of alchemists. The story of this imagined Stone and the allied Elixir of Life is the most enduring and romantic epic to be found in the whole history of science.' (John Read, *Through Alchemy to Chemistry* (1957, p. 28).

The standard scientific work on iatrochemistry

CROLL, Oswald (c. 1560–1609)

Basilica Chymica oder Alchymistisch Königlich Kleynod: Ein Philosophisch, durch sein selbst eigne erfahrung confirmirte und bestättigte Beschreibung und gebrauch der aller fürtrefflichsten Chimischen Artzneyen so auss dem Liecht der Gnaden und Natur genommen in sich begreiffent. Beneben angehengtem seinem newen Tractat von den innerlichen Signaturn oder zeichen der dinge.
Frankfurt, Gottfried Tampachen, (1629?)

Bound with: D.O.M.A. Hermetischer Wunderbaum, worinnen zu ersehen, wie die Wunderbahre Wercke Gottes, von Liebhabern warhaffter Chymischer Artzney, recht zu verstehen unnd zu erkennen; . . . Aus dem grosen [*sic*] Hermetischen Lustgarten zusamen [*sic*] getragen und in sieben Büchlein abgetheilet. Durch ANONYMUM [*sic*] Feldtaw.

Frankfurt am Main, Anthoni Hummen for Johann Gottfried Schönwetter, 1635.

Quarto – *leaf*: 210 x 170 *mm. Pp.* [8] *incl. undated engraved title* (*no letterpress title*), 248, [16]; Tractat von den innerlichen Signaturn, *with separate title leaf, dated* 1629: *pp.* 72, [8]; Hermetischer Wunderbaum: *pp.* [8], [4], 1-66. *With* 26 *engravings in the text* (*two full-page and some with numerous figures*). *The two conjugate leaves following the first gathering of four preliminary leaves consist of a variant title leaf followed by one leaf,* 'ad Momum & Zoilum', *with errata on verso; this second title has the same reading as the first one, except for one line added at head before* 'Hermetischer Wunderbaum' *reading* 'D.O.M.A. CROLLIUS REDIVIVUS Das ist', *and with the misprints in the first title* ('grosen', 'zusamen', *and* 'ANOYMUM') *corrected. The verso of the last leaf* [(:)4] *in the preceding gathering has the catchword* 'D.O.M.A'.

From the Carl Hyltén-Cavallius Collection (1842), *bound for* (*or by*) *him in dark violet boards, orange spine label. Early signature on the title*: Hans Bach. *Numerous annotations by an early hand in the margins and on the back free endpaper.*

The first German edition of Croll's *Basilica Chymica*, the standard scientific work of iatrochemistry. Whether Croll lived to see the first Latin edition (1609) is uncertain. This celebrated work was republished several times and was also translated into German, French and English. This German edition has no letterpress title, just the engraved allegorical title without date. The appendix, the Treatise on Signatures, has a separate title leaf dated 1629. It seems that most copies were issued with the *Crollius Redivivus* (1635). In the Duveen copy the name of the anonymous *von Feldtaw* is given as Abraham von Franckenberg in an old hand.

Oswald Croll, or Crollius, was born in Wetter, near Marburg. He studied at Marburg, Heidelberg, Strassburg and Geneva, receiving his M.D. about 1592. He travelled frequently in Italy, France and Germany and after 1593 in eastern Europe as a physician. Prague became his permanent place of residence from 1602. He was the physician of Prince Christian I of Anhalt-Bernburg (to whom de dedicated his *Basilica Chymica*) and afterwards to the Emperor Rudolph II.

'Croll complained that most medical books and students were overburdened with a mass of false and idle recipes which he refused to accept. Instead he had thoroughly tested by his own manual experience the Spagyric arcana, which he could not learn by hearsay or from old writings but had won partly by prayers, partly by payment and exchange, from iaotrochemists of vast experience during almost twenty years of laborious travel through France, Italy, Germany, Bohemia, Hungary and Poland. These precious remedies he now proposed freely to reveal for the poor sick and the public good, although many would be angry with him for breaking the Hermetic seal and revealing such secrets. One is a compound of a dozen ingredients. Another is salt of pearls. Others are seals, amulets or pentacles formed in accordance with the constellations. Another is *mumia* prepared from the corpse of a red-headed man 24 years old who has suffered a violent death, cut into bits, sprinkled with powder of myrrh and aloes, soaked in alcohol, suspended in air and dried, and so on' (Thorndike).

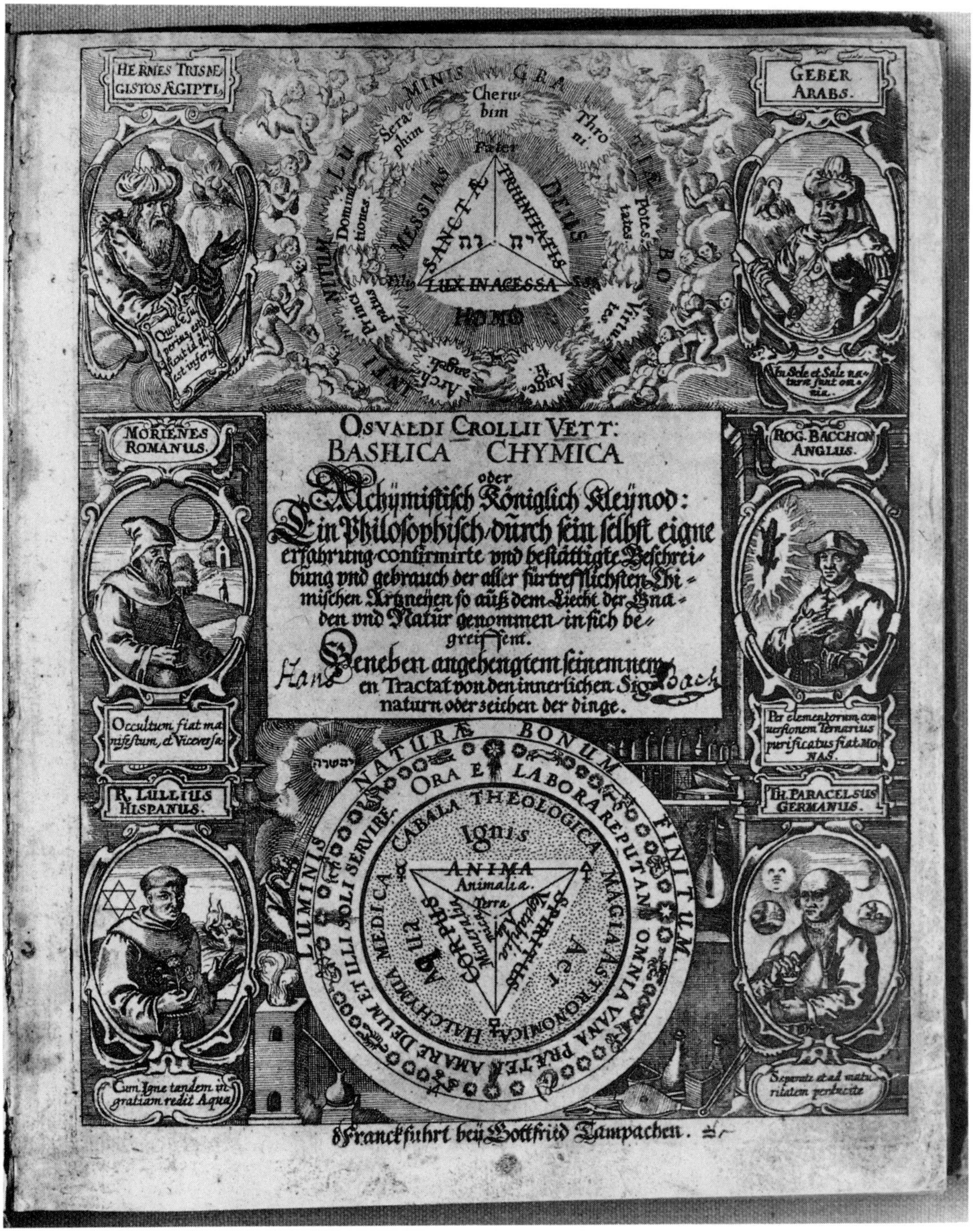

The engraved title of Croll's *Basilica Chymica* pictures the mysterious symbolism of alchemy. There is the celestial and the terrestrial sphere, and within the latter the four Aristotelian elements (fire, air, earth and water) have found their place as well as the symbols of the Paracelsic three essential substances, sulfur, mercury and salt. The men portrayed are: Hermes Trismegistus, Geber, Morienes, Roger Bacon, Ramon Lull and Paracelsus.

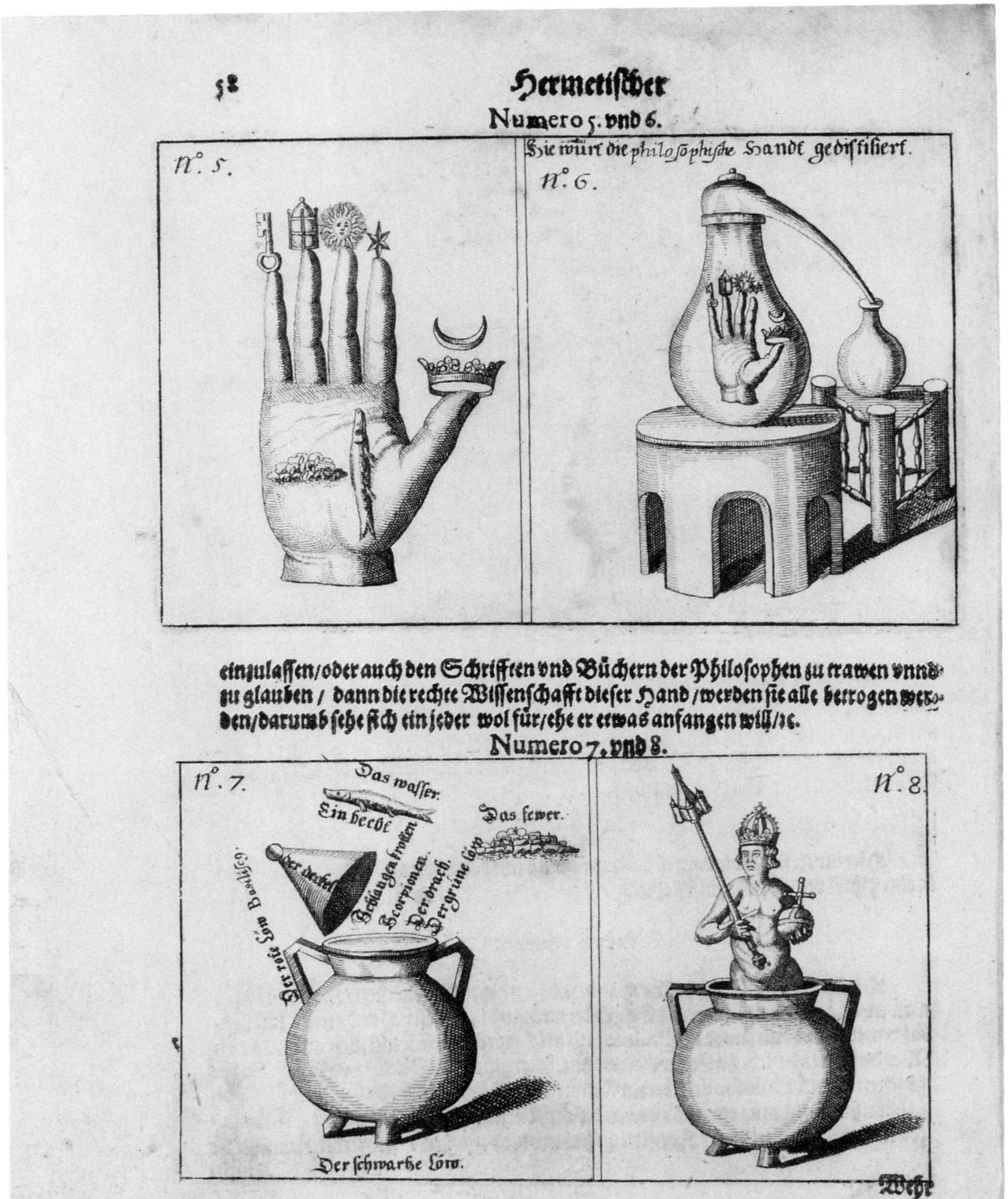
52 Hermetischer

Numero 5. vnd 6.

einzulassen/oder auch den Schrifften vnd Büchern der Philosophen zu trawen vnnd zu glauben / dann die rechte Wissenschafft dieser Hand /werden sie alle betrogen werden/darumb sehe sich ein jeder wol für/ehe er etwas anfangen will/ꝛc.

Numero 7. vnd 8.

Mehr

Crollius Redivivus, *Hermetischer Wunderbaum* (1635).

The *Basilica Chymica* was Croll's principal work, in which he recorded his knowledge, his experiments, and his theoretical views. It contains an exposition of the teachings of Paracelsus and a collection of recipes, or *materia medica*. The appendix is a treatise on signatures in which he describes himself as *Medicus et Philosophicus Hermeticus*. He assumes that medicinal plants or other sources of medicine bear some symbol or sign of their curative value in their colour, shape or other visible characteristic, intended by God as markings to make them known to those expert and wise in their interpretation. The *Basilica Chymica* also deals extensively with the influence of the heavenly bodies on substances of animal, vegetable, and mineral origin. As an example, walnuts have the complete signature of the head. From the shell, therefore, a salt can be made of special use for wounds of the pericranium. The inner part of the shell will make a decoction for injuries to the skull; the pellicle surrounding the kernel makes a medicine for inflammation of the membrane of the brain; the kernel itself nourishes and strengthens the brain.

'Paracelsus gave impetus to a trend, in evidence since the time of the Arabs, that saw the art of pharmacy become increasingly associated with alchemy and hence with chemistry. The Paracelsians developed distillation techniques that were suitable for volatile substances, and thereafter the use of alcohols, spirits, essences, and oils increased significantly. Strong mineral acids were also discovered, among them oil of vitriol and aquafortis. Finally metallurgical advances provided supplies of mercury, antimony, and lead, and lesser amounts of arsenic, iron, gold, copper, cobalt, bismuth, and zinc. From these were produced new compounds like corrosive mercuric sublimate and calomel.

The advances in pharmaceutical chemistry had to be taught to the physicians who were to use the new drugs and, especially, to the pharmacists who were to prepare them. Several works provided the needed instruction. One was the *Basilica chymica* of Oswald Croll. This influential volume, which contained a strong defence of Paracelsus, included an essay on the doctrine of signatures. It also listed drugs and gave directions for their preparation' (Cowen & Helfand).

Croll states that Paracelsus wrote for experts in a magic style and not for the vulgar, that he concealed his mysteries under a varied nomenclature, using magic words that few understand. In sharp contrast with Paracelsus' vagueness, Croll describes in detail the individual preparations, their composition, and their application. His recipe for the *Sympathetic Unguent* was as follows:

'It consists of four ounces of aged wild boar fat and four of bear fat, boiled half an hour in red wine, then poured on cold water and the fat collected which floats on the surface. Then one adds a powder of earthworms which have first been washed, the brain of a boar, red sandal wood, *mumia*, *haematites*, each an ounce, with one dram of scrapings from the cranium of a man violently slain. This last is to be gathered under a waxing moon in a good astrological house, with Venus, if possible, certainly not Mars or Saturn, in conjunction. Unless a nerve or artery has been severed, this concoction is guaranteed to cure any wound, provided the weapon which inflicted the wound is anointed with it. This weapon should be kept in pure linen and in a place which is not too hot, or the patient may suffer injury. Caution should further be taken that no dust gets on it and that it is not in a cold wind, or the patient will be sore afflicted. If the wound has been made with the point of a sword, the sword should be anointed downward to the tip. If the weapon is not to be had, a stick dipped in the blood from the wound may do. The healing is worked by identity of balsam or spirit thereof in the patient and the blood.' (Thorndike)

Upon Croll's death iatrochemistry lost one of its great exponents, for he is credited with gaining academic recognition of the medicinal value of many previously rejected remedies. The *Basilica Chymica* became the standard scientific work of iatrochemistry. Johannes Hartmann (1568–1631), the first professor of iatrochemistry and the first professor of chemistry in Europe, used it as a practical textbook. Thorndike concludes his section on Croll: 'It is hard for us today, accustomed as we are to the precise and objective methods of the laboratory and their expression in emotionless scientific terminology and mathematical formulae, to realize that such discoveries might be made by a person so given to pious and mystical lingo, and so creduously as to occult influences, as Croll. But the truth may be that just such a person was the most likely to make them in his day and generation.'

Duveen, pp. 150-1; Ferguson, I, pp. 185-7; DSB, III, pp. 471-2; Wootton, I, pp. 185-6; Partington, II, pp. 174-7; Thorndike, V, pp. 649-51, VIII, p.89; Cowen & Helfand, p. 60; Waller 11107 (Latin ed.)

The *materia medica* of Brazil

PISO, Willem (1611–1678) & **Georg MARGGRAF** (1610–1644)
Historia Naturalis Brasiliae . . . in qua non tantum Plantæ et Animalia, sed et Indigenarum morbi, ingenia et mores describuntur et Iconibus supra quingentas illustrantur,
Leyden & Amsterdam, Fr. Hack & L. Elzevir, 1648.

Folio – *leaf*: 390 *x* 250 *mm. Pp.* [12], Piso: *pp.* 1-122, [2]; Marggraf: pp. [8], 293, [7]. *Engraved pictorial title page and 540 woodcuts in the text, of which 300 are of plants and the rest of animals and Indians, and three tables. Contemporary calf with six raised bands, double gilt border around sides.*

Book-plate: C.D. Carlsson.

First edition of this fundamental and important work on diseases, medical plants and the natural history of Brazil. Until the publication of the results of the great expeditions of the nineteenth century, the *Historia Naturalis Brasiliae* was the only illustrated work on the natural history of Brazil. Luxuriously printed by the Elzevier press, it is one of the most beautiful books on Brazil in existence. The book comprises two distinct works: Piso's *Medicina Brasiliensi* in four parts, and Marggraf's *Historiae rerum naturalium Brasiliae* in eight parts with an appendix on the Tapoui Indians and Chile, adorned with a full-page woodcut of the llama of Peru.

This first edition was printed in Holland during Piso's stay in Brazil under the editorship of Johannes de Laet. Piso disliked the manner in which de Laet edited the work, which contained many errors, and decided to re-organize it entirely and publish it anew with the addition of Bontius' work on the *materia medica* of the Dutch East Indies. That enlarged 'second' edition, *De Indiae utriusque re naturali et medica,* has the same engraved title but the female Brazilian native is replaced by an East Indian, and the old man lying down in the foreground is replaced by a Babirura pig and a panther. In the background the dancing natives are replaced by an East Indian rhinoceros and a Dodo-bird from Mauritius.

Willem Piso (or Pies) practised medicine in Amsterdam until his departure for Brazil to substitute for Count Johann Mauritz Nassau's physician, who died upon Piso's arrival in the mid 1630s. Piso seems not only to have served the Governor of Dutch Brazil but was also chief of a scientific mission, sent out by the West India Company at Nassau's request, to investigate the natural resources and *materia medica* of Brazil. Georg Marggraf was his assistant. Piso was a pioneer on tropical medicine. He studied the medical lore of the Brazilian natives very closely and recommended their methods if they proved effective. He was the first to point out that the health of Europeans in the tropics is best preserved by adopting the way in which the natives live. His work was intended to be a handbook on tropical medicine and pharmacology. He was the first to separate yaws from syphilis (page 35 in *Medica Brasiliensi*) and to bring the ipecacuanha root to the attention of the Western medical world with a depiction of the plant (1658 edition), of which he noticed the existence of two varieties.

The premature death of the notable scientist Georg Marggraf at the age of 34 in Africa, before he could return to the civilized world, constitutes an irreparable loss. Many of his papers were lost, including the diary of his voyages to northeastern Brazil. Marggraf wrote all his studies in an alphabet of his own invention – a ciphered language probably intended to avoid the utilization of his notes by others. Marggraf's brother vehemently accused Piso of plagiarizing and withholding the former's name from many descriptions of new species. Count Nassau gave the papers referring to natural history to de Laet for publication, who published them in the *Historia Naturalis Brasiliae.* Laet writes in the preface that it took pains to decipher the manuscript and put the author's notes in order. The first three of the eight parts or books are on plants, the fourth on fish, the fifth on birds, the sixth on quadrupeds and serpents, the seventh on insects, and the last one on the northeastern region of Brazil and its inhabitants together with a treatise on the natural history of Chile and, added at the end, a treatise on the Tapuia Indians, taken from an account written by Jacob Rabbi, a famous interpreter in Dutch service.

The book is copiously illustrated throughout with 540 excellent woodcuts of plants and animals, many of which are here depicted for the first time and designed by Marggraf himself.

Borba de Moraes, 152-4; DSB, x, 621-2; Hunt, 1, 280; Garrison-Morton, 1825, 2263.1, 5303; Waller 7472 (2nd ed., 1658).

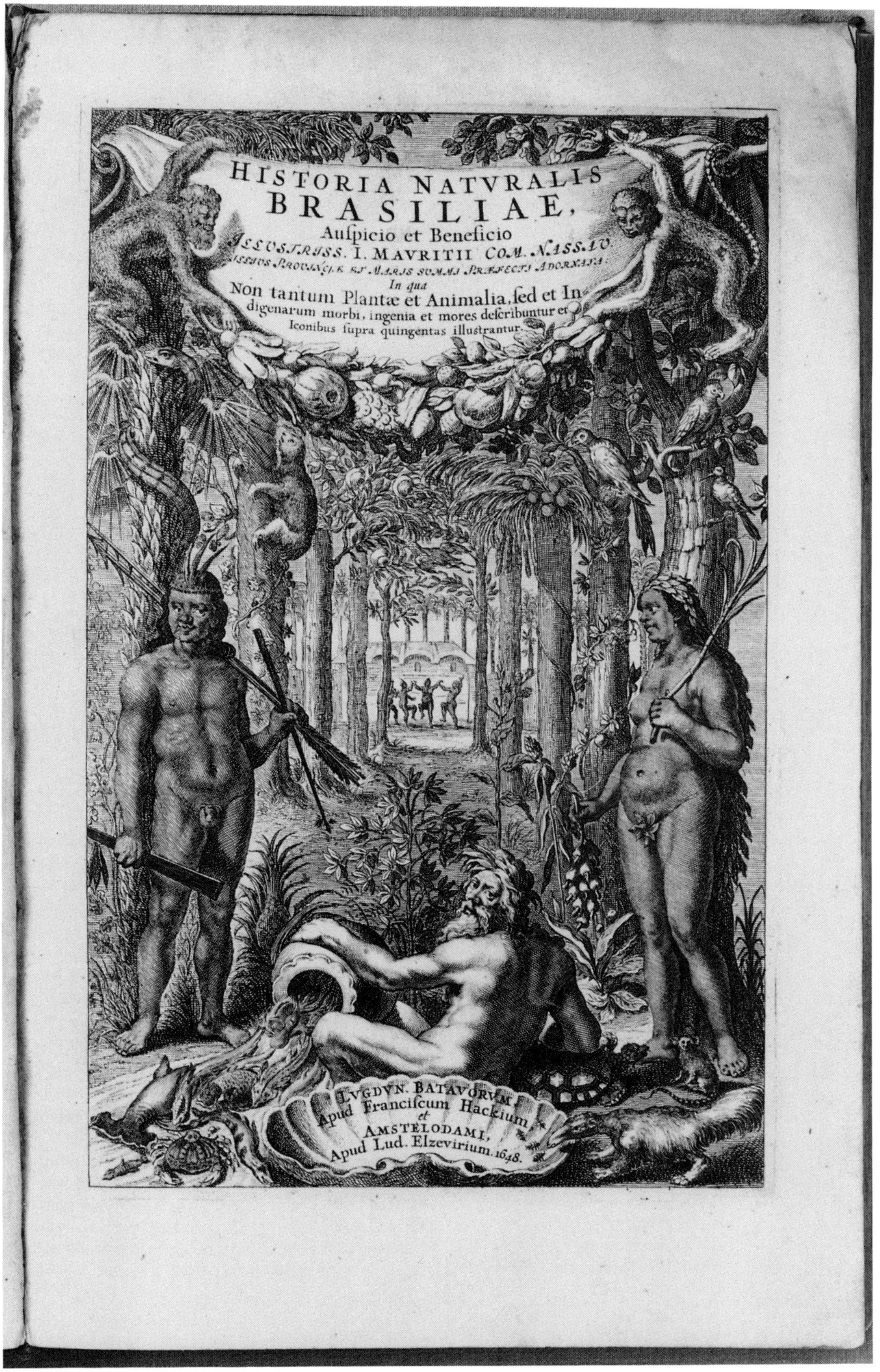

HISTORIA NATVRALIS
BRASILIAE,
Auspicio et Beneficio
In qua
Non tantum Plantæ et Animalia, sed et Indigenarum morbi, ingenia et mores describuntur et
Iconibus supra quingentas illustrantur.
LVGDVN. BATAVORVM,
Apud Franciscum Hackium,
et
AMSTELODAMI,
Apud Lud. Elzevirium. 1648.

The first printed Swedish herbal

MÅNSSON, Arfvid (17th century)

En myckit nyttigh Örta-Book, Om the herlige örter, som uti thet höghberömde Konungarijket wårt käre Fädernesland Swerige åhrligen wäxa. Såsom ock, Om några Uthländska örter, huruledes som the emoot monge bådhe inwertes och uthwertes Kranckheeter och Siukdomar brukas skola. Medh itt Register på the Örter och Kranckheter som uti thenna Book beskreffne och antecknade äre. Aff Latiniska och Tydska Böcker in på wårt Swenska Tungomål affsatt, aff ARVIDH MÅNSON Rydaholm. Och uthi Ordning satt, aff PETRO JONAE Ang.[ermannus] Wex. Ep. Sampt En Ny Trägårdz Book widh Endan tilsatt och aff Trycket uthgången.

Stockholm, Ignatius Meurer, 1654.

Octavo – *leaf*: 150 *x* 95 *mm. Pp.* [16], 268, [10]; Trägårdz Book: *pp.* [2], 36, [2]. *Lacks the final leaf with colophon. Old half calf.*

Purchased at 16 sk.B. *by H. Norman Tingstadius,* 8 *September,* 1816.

Among the few books studied by Linnaeus as a young boy back home at the vicarage at Stenbrohult in Småland was Månsson's *Örta Book* (herbal), which he 'pored over day and night to the point of knowing it like the back of his hand' but in mature years condemned as wretched guidance. It is the first printed herbal in Sweden.

The first edition, printed by Christopher Günther at Kalmar in 1628, is an extremely rare book that few have seen. Even the following two editions (1637 and 1641), printed by Günther since he had moved to Linköping, are very rare. Following the publication of the book in Stockholm in 1642 it became very popular and went through many editions. The above is the tenth and last edition, which is a reprint of the 1642 edition, with a gardening manual (*Trägårdz Book*) added at the end, the same edition as Linnaeus studied, a gift from his father.

Arfvid Månsson, latinized Arvidi Magni Rydaholmensis, was born about 1590 in the small parish of Rydaholm in Småland, not far from Linnaeus' birthplace, and like his later successor he was a son of the local vicar, Magnus Arvidi. Månsson was an autodidact, the only education he received was at lay schools, among others in Växjö. Nevertheless he seems to have practised medicine and refers to himself as *Medicus* in the preface to his *Practica* on blood-letting (1642). As there was no physician in that district of Småland at the time, not even in the city of Växjö, Månsson became a charlatan of repute much in demand among maids and peasantry as well as the gentry and clergy. It is rumoured that he even cured Queen Christina of an ailment. His practice lasted for nearly fifty years. The date of his death is not known but he was certainly dead in 1666.

His little herbal lists some 150 plants, mainly indigenous to Sweden, with a short description of their preparation and use. Each plant has a number of virtues: nettles for instance can be used for 41 ailments including rabies, intestinal worms, swollen feet, cronic coughing, etc. For retention of urine he gives no less than 34 remedies. Some material was of a particularly sensitive nature, such as lewdness, and these passages are written in German. For several cures he adds: this is proven.

According to the title page the contents is taken from old German and Latin books, and as was often the case most of the material was just translated from various foreign books, e.g. Henrik Smid's Danish *Laegebog* and others.

Arfvid Månsson was generally held as a quack but he was never brought to trial, either for sorcery or failed cures, which in many cases were punishable by death. He was obviously a clever practitioner, who had close connections with the Church and especially with the Bishop of Växjö, who not only paid for the printing and wrote a short preface, in which he salutes the pious reader, but seems also to have helped Månsson in writing the text or 'put it in order' as is stated in the title.

Krok, pp. 516-17; SBL, II, pp. 324-5 under Arvidi Magni Rydaholmensis; Inge Nilsson, 'Arvid Månssons örtabok' in Landsbibliotekets gamla samlingar. *Om handskrifter och böcker ur Landsbibliotekets i Växjö gamla samlingar* (Växjö,1994), pp. 27-31; Collijn, 633; Waller 6231.

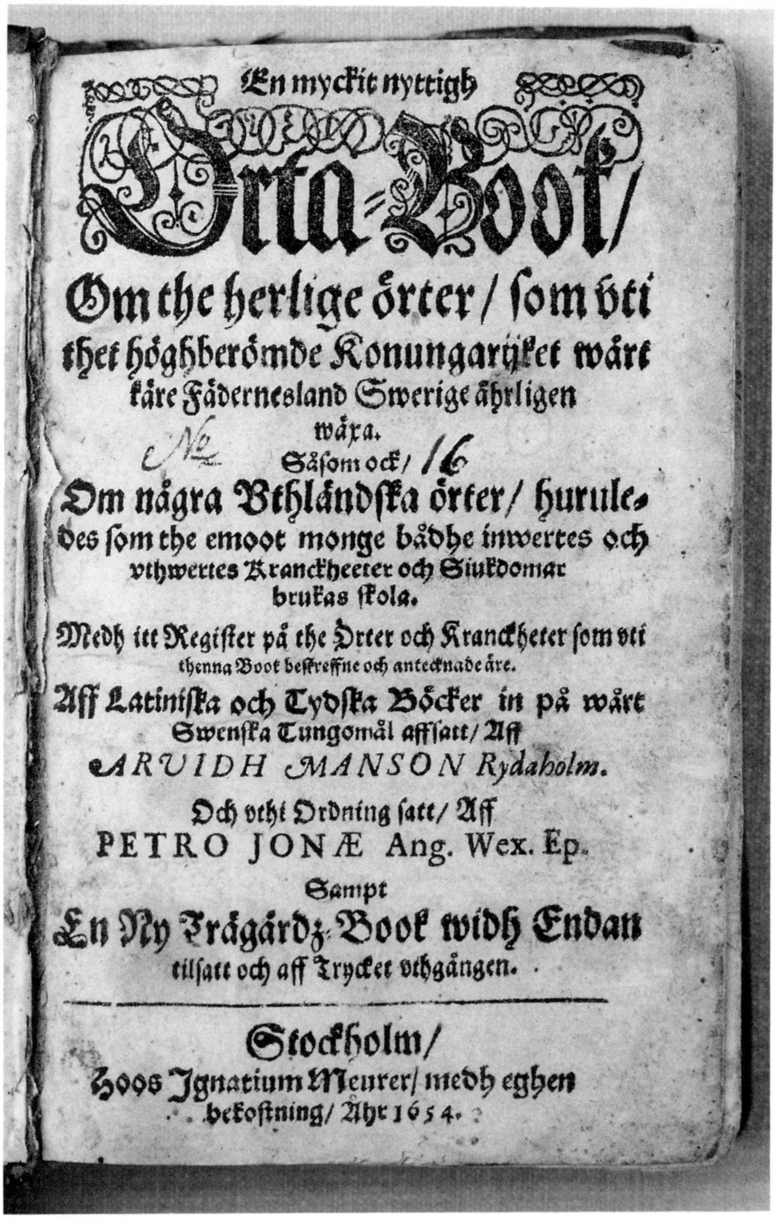
En myckit nyttigh

Örta-Book/

Om the herlige örter/ som vti thet höghberömde Konungarijket wårt kåre Fädernesland Swerige åhrligen wäxa.

Såsom ock/

Om några Vthländska örter/ hurule-des som the emoot monge bådhe inwertes och vthwertes Kranckheeter och Siukdomar brukas skola.

Medh itt Register på the Örter och Kranckheter som vti thenna Book beskreffne och antecknade äre.

Aff Latiniska och Tydska Böcker in på wårt Swenska Tungomål affsatt/ Aff

ARVIDH MANSON Rydaholm.

Och vthi Ordning satt/ Aff

PETRO JONÆ Ang. Wex. Ep.

Sampt

En Ny Trägårdz-Book widh Endan tilsatt och aff Trycket vthgången.

Stockholm/

Hoos Ignatium Meurer/ medh eghen bekostning/ Åhr 1654.

The first illustrated herbal in Scandinavia

PAULLI, Simon (1603–1680)

Flora Danica Det er: Dansk Urtebog: udi huilcken, . . . icke alleeniste Urternis Historiske Beskrifvelse, Krafter oc Virckninger, med zijrligste Figurer andragis: Men endocsaa Lægedomme til alle Siugdomme gafnlige, korteligen oc klarligen antegnis: Saa at den er baade en Urtebog oc Lægebog

Copenhagen, printed by Melchior Martzan for Joachim Moltke and Jørgen Holst, 1648.

Quarto – *leaf*: 190 x 145 *mm. Ff.* [18] *title & prelims,* [482], [48] *index.* Atlas: *pp.* 393, [3]. *Sign.*: A-4Z4, 5A-5E4, 5F2 a-m4; Atlas: A-3E4 3D2. *Last leaf with Plantin's device,* 'Labore et Constantia'. *Atlas with four separate titles with woodcut floral borders, one for each season, and* 384 *full-page woodcuts of plants. Engraved frontispiece, engraved portrait, and* 4 *engraved plates. The last leaf supplied from another copy. Contemporary calf.*

First edition of the first illustrated herbal in Scandinavia. The atlas part with 384 full-page woodcuts of plants was printed on better paper at the Plantin Press in Antwerp, who had a large stock of wood blocks. All the woodcuts had been used in other works published and printed by Plantin, e.g. in the herbals of Clusius, Dodonaeus and Lobelius, except for two, depicting *Cochlearia.* The Danish printers had neither the facilities nor experience for such an enterprise at that time.

The frontispiece and the four allegorical plates, representing the four seasons, are engraved by Albert Haelwegh. The plate of Spring probably depicts Princess Leonora Christina, daughter of Christian IV, to whom the book is dedicated. The plate of Autumn shows Paulli's wife and their son Holger. The frontispiece shows *Flora* with a view of Copenhagen in the background. The fine portrait of Paulli, which he inserted in most of his books, was engraved after a painting by Karel van Mander. Paulli's *Flora Danica* is one of the chief works within Danish botanical literature and one of the finest books printed in Denmark during the first half of the seventeenth century. It should not be confused with the later *Flora Danica*, published over a period of 122 years (1761–1883), whose 3060 plates makes it one of the most sumptuous copperplate works ever published, and which also enjoyed the honour of being transferred to a royal porcelain set.

Simon Paulli was born in Rostock, the son of a physician-in-ordinary at the Danish court. He studied at Rostock, Leiden and later in Paris under Jean Riolan. He then practised medicine at Rostock and was in 1639 professor of medicine at Rostock. In the same year as he published his *Flora Danica* he was appointed professor of anatomy, surgery and botany at Copenhagen and also became physician-in-ordinary to the Danish king, who granted him the revenue from the bishopric of Aarhus. Simon Paulli made notable contributions to the literature of anatomy and botany. He did not only compile from existing botanical knowledge but also compared it with information derived from his own experiments. He was the founder of the Anatomical Theatre in Copenhagen.

Paulli's *Flora Danica* is arranged according to the seasons and, besides descriptions of plants, includes information on their synonyms and medicinal properties. More a practitioner than a theoretician, he recommended the use of simple medications. There is a description of *Digitalis*, and two woodcuts of the tobacco plant (p. 103 and p. 211), the latter described on no less than twenty-one pages of text. Upon order of the king Paulli later wrote a separate treatise on tobacco and tea, which would dissuade the people from using these 'drugs'. The indices gives the names of the plants in Latin, German and Danish. The book was rare and sought-after already at the time of Linnaeus, who as a student at Lund used a copy in the library of professor Kilian Stobaeus, who had written the Swedish names beside the illustrations in his beautiful and legible hand. Linnaeus later found a copy of his own and quotes Paulli frequently in his writings. There exist a few copies with all the woodcuts hand-coloured.

A fascimile edition in three volumes was published in Copenhagen in 1971 with introduction and commentaries by Johan Lange and Vilhelm Møller Christensen.

Nissen BBI, 1497; Christensen, *Den Danske Botanikens Historie*, vol. II, p. 11; DSB, X, p. 426-7; Ballhausen & Johansen, 589; Waller 11703.

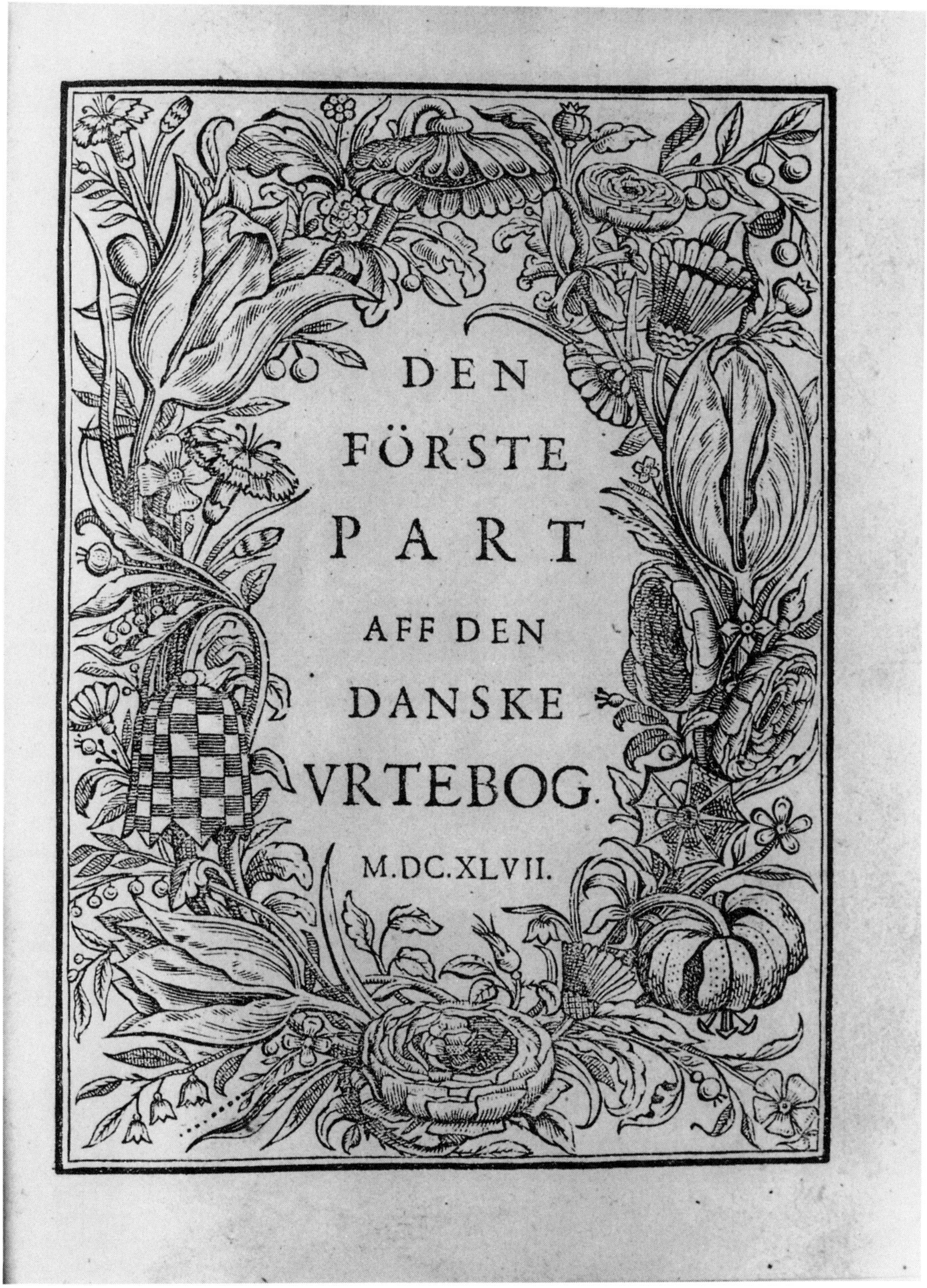
DEN
FÖRSTE
PART
AFF DEN
DANSKE
VRTEBOG.
M.DC.XLVII.

The first Danish Pharmacopoeia

BARTHOLIN, Thomas (1616–1680)

Dispensatorium Hafniense, Jussu Superiorum à Medicis Hafniensibus adornatum.

Copenhagen, Georg Lamprecht for Joachim Moltke, 1658.

Quarto – *leaf*: 185 *x* 150 *mm. Pp.* [8], 1-61, 62-283, [18]. *This copy lacks the engraved frontispiece, here replaced in facsimile. Contemporary vellum, new red morocco spine label.*

Bound with:

[TARIFF] Catalogus & Valor . . . / Apotecker Taxt paa alt hvis i Kiøbenhaffn hos de fire privilegerede Apotheckere til Kiøbs findis / Apothecker TAXA aller dehrer Medicamenten und Waaren . . .

Copenhagen, Georg Gøde for Peter Haubold, 1672.

Quarto – *Pp.* [8], 125, [3] *errata.*

Bound with:

[MEDICAL DECREE] Forordning om Medicis oc Apotecker . . . / Constitutiones Regiæ de Medicis & Pharmacopœeis . . . / Königliche Verordnung angehend die Medicos und Apothecker . . .

Copenhagen, Georg Gøde for Peter Haubold, 1672.

Quarto – *Pp.* 24.

The *Dispensatorium Hafniense* is the first Danish pharmacopoeia. It is also the first in Scandinavia, as it appeared twenty-eight years earlier than the *Pharmacopoeia Holmiensis* (1686). There is a later issue with the same date, in which the first sheet of four leaves has been replaced, with the title page reset, naming as printer and publisher Daniel Paulli, son of Simon Paulli, who after Joachim Moltke's death had taken over the bookshop.

In the *Dispensatorium Hafniense* Thomas Bartholin is named as author, even though two professors of medicine and eight physicians (but no pharmacist) are named in the preface as co-authors. After ten years of study abroad Bartholin had returned home to succeed Simon Paulli as professor of anatomy in Copenhagen and there he discovered the thoracic duct and, simultaneously with Olof Rudbeck, the lymphatic system. As the most distinguished physician in Denmark, and held high in esteem by the King, Bartholin was responsible for the Royal Decree of 1672 that settled the organization of Danish medicine for the next hundred years.

The main source for the Danish pharmacopoeia was the 1640 edition of *Pharmacopoeia Augustana*, which is known to have been in extensive use in Danish pharmacies. The *Dispensatorium Hafniense* was intended to be of assistance to the pharmacies in Copenhagen but by the Decree of 1672 it was stated that it was to be obligatory for all pharmacies in the Kingdom of Denmark, which at the time also included Norway and the duchies Schleswig, Holstein and Lauenburg. The total number of medicaments in the *Dispensatorium Hafniense* is about 800, while the tariff of 1672 mentions about 3000 drugs. The *Dispensatorium Hafniense* remained the valid pharmcopoeia until the first edition of the *Pharmacopoea Danica* was published in 1772.

The most important legal right given to the apothecaries in the 1672 Royal Decree was the monopoly of selling medicine and the exclusive right of preparing the physicians' prescriptions. The license gave the apothecary permission to deal also with those groceries and other articles, with which others than apothecaries dealt, and in many cases also permitted them to keep a wine cellar and to sell wine. This very soon led to the generation of real wine bars, where the citizens could meet. From here it was only a step further to innkeeping, a business which was more profitable for some apothecaries than the pharmacy itself.

Kurt Berentsen, 'Dispensatorium Hafniense in the light of history', in the Facsimile edition (1966); The History of Pharmacy in Denmark (*Theriaca*, VI, August 1960); Ballhausen & Johansen, 364; Waller 3134 (*Forordning*, 1672).

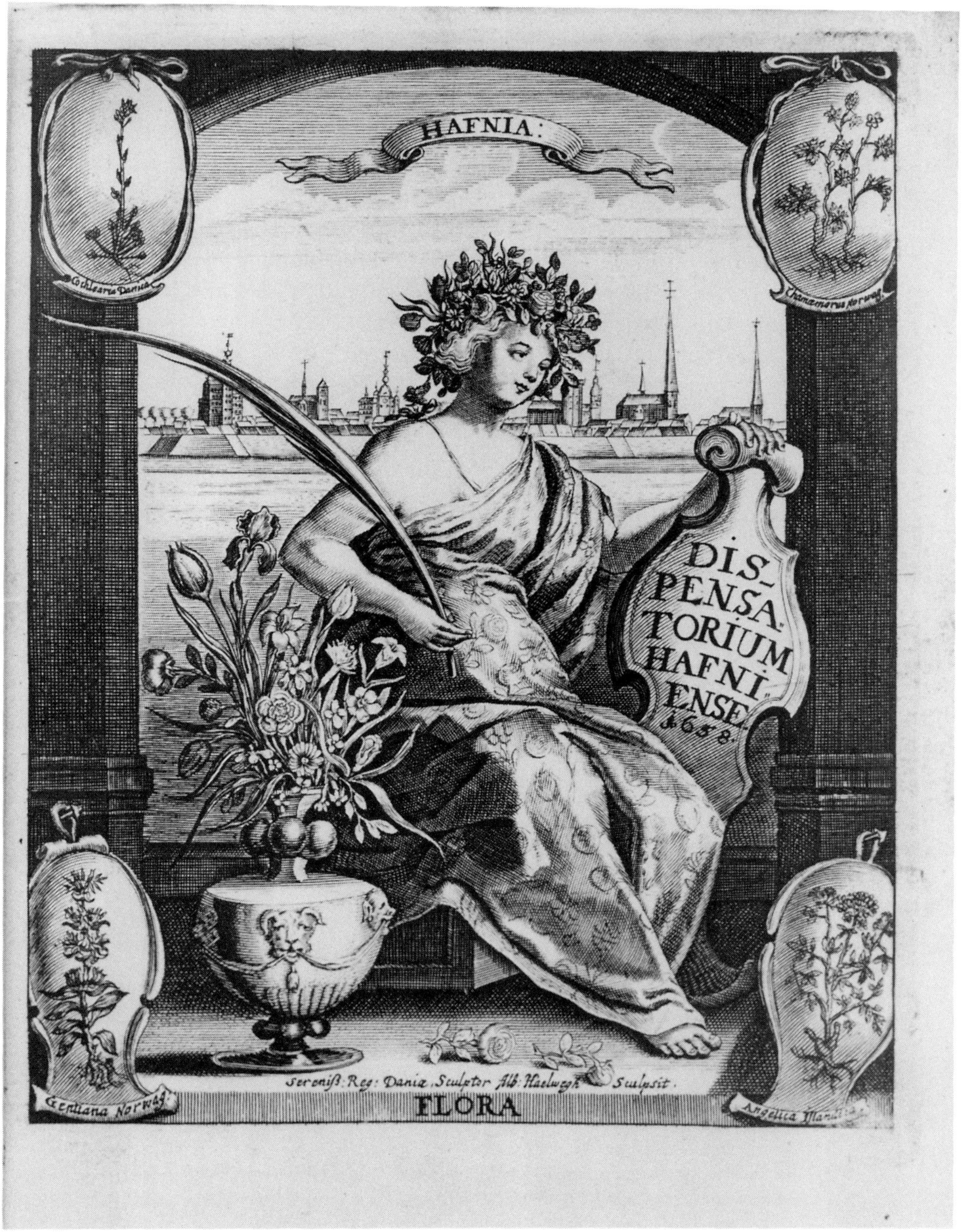

The fine frontispiece to *Dispensatorium Hafniense* with Flora sitting in front of the moats of Copenhagen is the same as the one Albert Haelwegh engraved for Simon Paulli's Danish herbal ten years earlier. The text in the shield, '*Dispensatorium Hafniense* 1658' has replaced '*Flora Danica*' and the banderole with *Hafnia* in the sky has been added and also the word *Flora* at the foot. The plants in the corners represent Denmark, Norway and Iceland.

The most used apothecaries' handbook of its time

SCHRÖDER, Johann Christian (1600–1664)

D. Johann Schröders trefflich-versehene Medicin-Chymische Apotheke, oder: höchstkostbarer Arzeney-Schatz, darinnen so wol einfache, als aus vielen Stücken bestehende, bewährteste Hülf-Mittel, welche nicht allein die dem Menschen zu kräftigster Gesundheit dienende Mineralien oder Bergsäffte, Pflantzen und Kräuter, sondern auch unterschiedliche Theile der Thiere betreffen, auf Medicinisch-Chymische Art kernreich erörtert werden, dabey ferner zu mehrerm Verständnis aller Materien, einzymahl höchst-dienlich-nöthig und nützlicher Schlüssel, in Herrn D. Friedrich Hoffmanns herrlichen Anmerckungen bestehend, befindlich, deme noch über das um mehrer Vollkommenheit willen eine nahmhaffte Anzahl Baconianisch-Cartesian- und Helmotianischer Vernunffts-Gründen, wie auch rarester Arzneymittel der fürtrefflichsten Herren Medicorum insoderheit des in gantz Sachsenland und andern Orthen höchstberühmten Herrn D. Johann Michaelis beygefüget, und dann endlich . . . Zum andernmahl gedruckt und an vielen Orthen verbessert. Von Johann Ulrich Müllern.

Nuremberg, Johann Hoffmann, 1686.

Quarto – *leaf*: 205 *x* 165 *mm. Pp.* [6], 1560, [8] Register der Bücher und Capitel, [14] Register über Fr. Hoffmanns Apoteker-Schatzes, [20] Verzeichnis Lateinischer Wörter, [18] Teutsches Register. *Engraved frontispiece. Title page printed in red and black. Contemporary vellum.*

From the C.D. Carlsson Collection.

Second edition of Müller's German translation, being a revised and enlarged version of the first edition printed in the previous year. At the end is Hoffmann's *Apotheker-Schatz* (pp.1409-1560), first published in Latin in 1675 as *Clavis Pharmaceutica Schroederiana.*

The pharmacopoeias of the seventeenth century were still tinged with the occult and magical, a fact that is illustrated in the work of Johann Schröder. His *Pharmacopoeia medico-chymica* was first printed in 1641. It became the universal textbook of the German apothecaries for at least one hundred years and went through a great many editions and translations. It was considered to be the best apothecaries' handbook and was the most commonly used. It gives a complete and exhaustive account of everything that concerns their trade in the seventeenth and early eighteenth century. After the author's death his book was edited, revised and supplied with extensive addendas by physicians like Johann Daniel Horst, Friedrich Hoffmann and Georg Daniel Koschwitz. Our library possesses the fourth Latin edition of 1655, the above German translation of 1686, Johann Jacob Manget's edition issued under the title of *Pharmacopoea Schrödero-Hoffmanniana* (Geneva, 1687) and Koschwitz's greatly enlarged version in its second edition (1709), a thick folio of over 1500 pages.

Schröder held the position as surgeon to the Swedish armies during the Thirty Years' War and was physician to the General Field Marshal Gustaf Horn. He later became municipal physician at Frankfurt-am-Main. His 'Pharmacopoeia' is divided into five Books: the first is introductory, the second is concerned with the apothecary shop and has 87 chapters on such topics as waters, cortices, flowers, fungi, clysters, confections, electuaries, pills, potions, tinctures and trochees. The third, fourth and fifth books deal with the mineral, vegetable and animal kingdoms respectively. Belief in sympathy and antipathy, the doctrine of signatures, and the employment of amulets, run through the book. The third book, *Bergwerck-Lehre,* contains considerable material on minerals and gemstones as used in medicine. Thorndike discusses some of the extraordinary recipes found in Schröder's book.

Thorndike, VIII, pp. 88-92; Schelenz, pp. 495-6; Ferchl, p. 487; Heilmann, *Kräuterbücher*, pp. 381-5; Sinkankas, *Gemology*, 5871. This German edition not in Ferguson, Duveen, Neu, Krivatsy, or Waller; Waller 8698 (Latin ed., 1649).

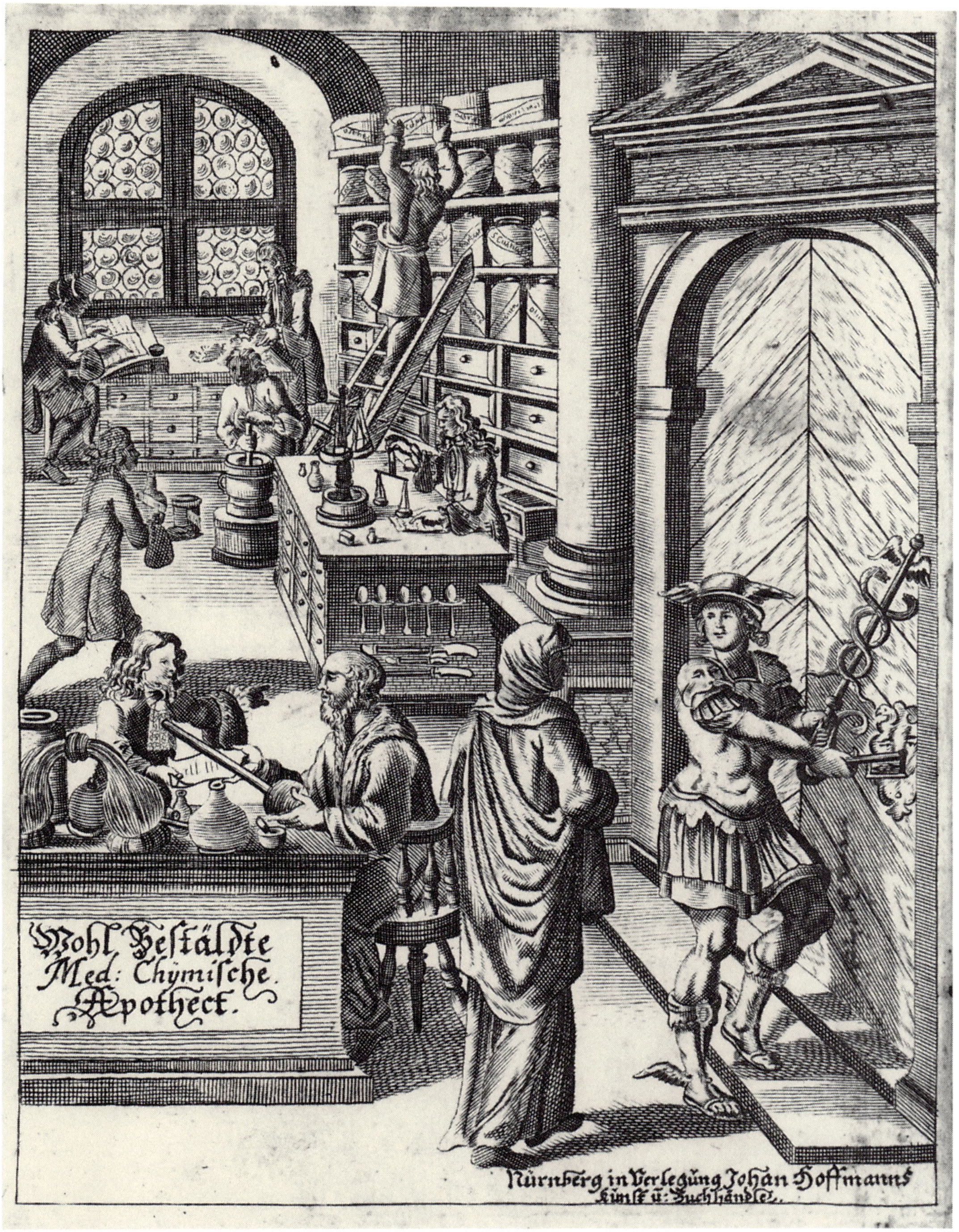

The engraved frontispiece to Johann Ulrich Müller's German edition of Schröder's famous handbook for apothecaries. It represents the interior of an apothecary shop. At the door is Hermes, holding the *caduceus* and a key with which he is about to unlock the door for Hygeia, the Greek goddess of health, and let her out.

An apothecary's advertising booklet

FLURER, Johann Georg (fl. 1660)

Eigentlicher und gründlicher Bericht, was ich Endesbenanter principaliter in meiner Reiss Apotheken führe, worzu eins und das andere dienet, und auff was mass und weise ein jedweders appliciret und gebraucht werden soll. Alles auffs treulichste, aus langwiriger (und zwar 36.jähriger) Experientz und Erfahrung zusammen getragen, jedermänniglichen zu Nutz und Diensten in offenen Druch übergeben, und verfertiget . . . Elixir Vitæ Majus. Hujus Elixiris . . .

Freyberg, Georg Beuthern, 1660.

Small quarto – *leaf*: 170 x 142 *mm. Pp.* [8]. *Title page within typographical floral border. Modern marbled boards, red morocco label on the upper cover, gilt. From the* C.D. Carlsson *Collection.*

This rare booklet cannot be traced in any of the standard bibliographies. The author, who on the title-page names himself 'Käyserlichen Privilegirten Medicum und Chirurgum', was at the time of publication a burgher of Rochlitz in Meissen. In this advertising booklet he describes the excellent drugs in his 'Travel Apoteck', that is to say medicine-chest, and offers complete sets of the chest together with current prices.

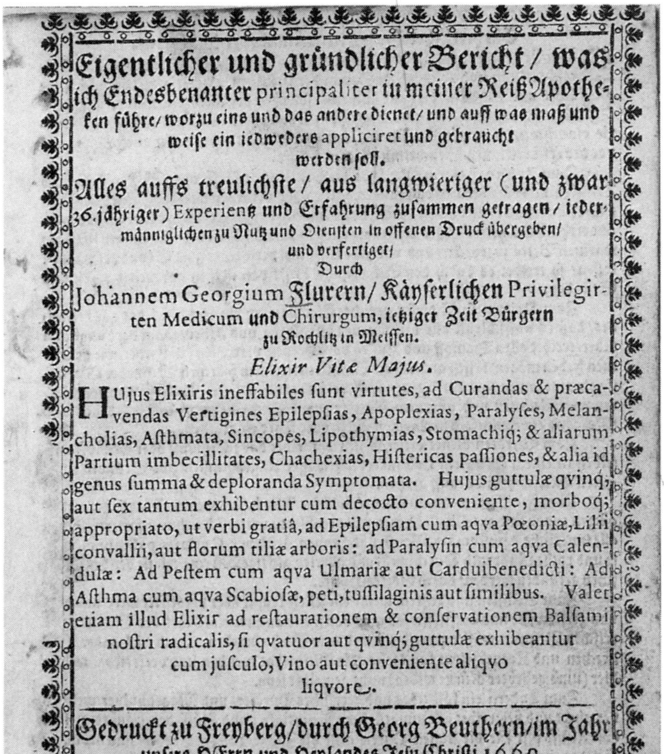

Eigentlicher und gründlicher Bericht / was ich Endesbenanter principaliter in meiner Reiß Apotheken führe / worzu eins und das andere dienet / und auff was maß und weise ein iedweders appliciret und gebraucht werden soll.

Alles auffs treulichste / aus langwieriger (und zwar 36. jähriger) Experientz und Erfahrung zusammen getragen / iedermänniglichen zu Nutz und Diensten in offenen Druck übergeben / und verfertiget / Durch

Johannem Georgium Flurern / Käyserlichen Privilegirten Medicum und Chirurgum, ietziger Zeit Bürgern zu Rochlitz in Meissen.

Elixir Vitæ Majus.

Hujus Elixiris ineffabiles sunt virtutes, ad Curandas & præcavendas Vertigines Epilepsias, Apoplexias, Paralyses, Melancholias, Asthmata, Sincopes, Lipothymias, Stomachiq; & aliarum Partium imbecillitates, Chachexias, Histericas passiones, & alia id genus summa & deploranda Symptomata. Hujus guttulæ qvinq; aut sex tantum exhibentur cum decocto conveniente, morboq; appropriato, ut verbi gratiâ, ad Epilepsiam cum aqva Pœoniæ, Lilii convallii, aut florum tiliæ arboris: ad Paralysin cum aqva Calendulæ: Ad Pestem cum aqva Ulmariæ aut Carduibenedicti: Ad Asthma cum aqva Scabiosæ, peti, tussilaginis aut similibus. Valet etiam illud Elixir ad restaurationem & conservationem Balsami nostri radicalis, si qvatuor aut qvinq; guttulæ exhibeantur cum jusculo, Vino aut conveniente aliqvo liqvore.

Gedruckt zu Freyberg / durch Georg Beuthern / im Jahr unsers HErrn und Heylandes Jesu Christi 1660.

He starts with an offer of a marvellous antidote or *Gifft Electuarium oder Mithridat,* useful during times of plague, *ein köstliches und herrliches Purgier- und Magenpulwer, ein gutes Edelhertzpulver, ein köstliche Rothe Bezoarpulver Pulvis Bezoardicus Rubeus* a splendid medicament for epilepsy, *ein herrliches Wurmpulver, ein gutes Zahnpulver, ein Haupt- und Hirnpulver*, which, used as a substitute for snuff tobacco, clears the brain and relieves dizziness and buzzing in the ears, etc. The listing of about twenty drugs for all conceivable ailments including toothache ends with the extraordinary *Tinctura Bezoardica Catholica*, a universal remedy for thirty-two specified ailments.

FRAUNDORFFER, Philipp (c.1650–1701)

Tabula Smaragdina Medico-Pharmaceutica; . . . Revidit emendavit, auxit JOH. ABRAHAM. MERCKLINUS . . .
Nuremberg, Leonhard Singer for Johann Friedrich Rüdiger, 1726.

A quite unusual format for a book

Tall narrow duodecimo – *leaf*: 165 x 65 *mm. Folding double-page title leaf printed in red and black, pp.* [20], 468, [48]. *Interleaved copy with Ms annotations. Contemporary blindstamped pigskin over wooden boards, two brass clasps, red edges.*

Provenance: 'ad Bibliothecam Christiani Josephi Udesheim, Coloniensis 1741; Ant. Balatka Bélensis, 1870; Carl Sommer. *From the* Ernst Matérn Collection.

This book, first published in 1699, is in an unusual tall and narrow format. A new enlarged edition, in the same 'catechismus' format, was edited by Johann Abraham, the son of the more famous Georg Abraham Mercklin, in 1714, of which this 1726 edition is a reprint. The original 600 recipes have now been increased to 800 and the pages from 408 to 536. Moreover this copy is interleaved with writing paper in the pharmacopoeia part, lending it an extraordinary physical shape, as it makes it thicker than it is deep. Both Fraundorffer, provincial physician in Brünn, and Mercklin were members of the illustrious *Academia Naturae Curiosorum* and often contributed to their transactions.

The book is a collection of 800 recipes taken from no less than 224 various authors. Fraundorffer has taken the title from the legendary Emerald Table (*Tabula Smaragdina*) of Hermes Trismegistus, the alleged father of the 'Hermetic Art' and the patron of its practitioners. According to legend, the original emerald slab, upon which the precepts of Hermes were written in Phoenician characters, was taken by Sarah, wife of Abraham, from the hands of the dead Hermes in a cave near Hebron some time after the Flood. This legend is a typical example of the extra flavour so often adopted in order to lend authority to alchemical assertions. The Emerald Table appears also to carry veiled directions for preparing the 'Philosopher's Stone', or the 'Elixir of Life', and thus served as an appropriate title for a book of medical recipes.

Waller 3236 (1713 ed.).

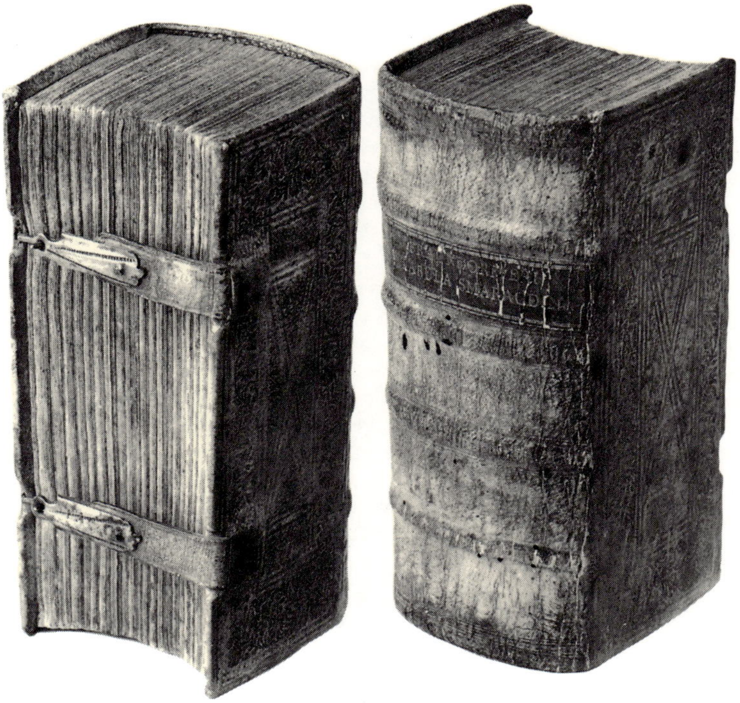

A well-equipped German pharmacy of the 17th century

OELLINGER, Georg Erasmus (fl. 1630–1663)

Designatio alphabetica medicamentorum omnium in Officina Pharmaceutica Öllingeriana Noribergæ prostantium . . . In tres partes divisa: quarum prior, Medicamenta Dogmatica, posterior, Chymica seu Spagyrica, ulterior, Simplicia trium Regnorum, . . . Nuremberg, Johannes Andreas Endter & Wolfgang Jr, heirs, 1663.

Duodecimo – *leaf: 130 x 75 mm. Pp.* [24] *incl. extra engraved title leaf,* 524, [1] *errata,* [3] *blanks. Contemporary boards covered with an old manuscript leaf with a red initial, blue-green edges.*

Provenance: Christoph Wenzel Graf von Nostitz (1643–1712), *with his signature on the title page. From the* C.D. Carlsson Collection.

Georg Erasmus Oellinger was a descendant of Georg [Jörg] Oellinger, the ancestor of the famous Nuremberg family of apothecaries. From 1633 he was the owner of the *Apotheke zur weissen Schwane* in Nuremberg with premises 'am Krebsstocke an der Fleischbrücke.' In the present book he lists in alphabetical order all the simple, composite and spagyric drugs that are to be found in the Oellinger apothecary shop in Nuremberg. Also German names are given. It throws a great deal of light on the contents of a well-equipped German pharmacy of the seventeenth century. 'Wichtiges Register einer wirklich bestandenen Arzneimittelsammlung'. (Ferchl, p. 387).

The ancestor, the apothecary Georg Oellinger the Elder (1487–1557), was a great collector of natural history specimens and the founder of a botanical garden near the city gate in Nuremberg. He is known as a skilled botanist and horticulturist and was a friend of Hieronymus Bock and Otto Brunfels, whom he provided with rare plants from his garden. Bock calls Oellinger 'seinen getrew lieb herr Jörg'. His remarkable collection of about 700 paintings of plants and animals, the Oellinger Herbarium, or *Magnarum medicinae partium herbariae et zoographiae imagines* [UB Erlangen, sign. Ms 2362], many drawn by Oellinger himself, was after his death acquired by Joachim Camerarius the Younger (1534–1598), and later by Dr. Trew. The existence of this magnificent manuscrtipt was unknown until 1936 when the catalogue of the illuminated manuscripts in the University of Erlangen Library was published. The Nuremberg gardens were renowned for their many rare plants, many of which were sent to Camerarius by friends in Italy and abroad, including Charles de l'Ecluse. In 1596 Camerarius was commissioned by the Prince Bishop Johann Conrad von Gemmingen to design and supervise the construction and planting in his garden at Eichstätt. Upon Camerarius' death two years later, the work was carried out by his colleague, the Nuremberg apothecary Basilius Besler, who arranged to have the remainder of Camerarius' plants transferred to Eichstätt. Like his colleague Oellinger, Besler had his own garden in Nuremberg, as well as a private museum of natural wonders. The garden at Eichstätt soon became the greatest German garden of its time, celebrated in Besler's *Hortus Eystettensis* (1613). Members of the apothecary family of Oellinger held gardens, 'Horti medicinales', in Nuremberg until 1674.

The engraved title page to the younger Georg Oellinger's book, listing the medicaments in the apothecary shop of 1663, is full of alchemical symbols. Above the title, displayed on a drapery, is a shield, within which is depicted a snake biting its own tail [a symbol for eternity], and the Hebrew sign for God [Jehova]. The title is surrounded by various equipment found in an apothecary's laboratory, such as alembics, retorts, phials and other distilling vessels, scales, a lamp-furnace, a coal-box, etc. The tree in the left corner symbolizes the origin of the substances from the alchemical elements sulphur, mercury and sal ammoniac. The fruits represent copper, lead, tin, gold, silver, iron, antimony, saltpetre, alum, vitriol, sal. ammoniac and rock salt. Even the bouquet in the lower right-hand corner has alchemical meaning, as the bird on the vase symbolizes mercury, which can appear in the black, white, yellow and red colours of the flowers.

Versuch einer Geschichte des Apothekenwesens in der freyen Reichstadt Nürnberg. 1792; Ferchl, (ed.) *Illustr. Apotheken Kalender* 1936; Wickert, Konrad, 'Süddeutsche Gartenkultur in der zweiten Hälfte des 16. Jahrhunderts und das "Camerarius-Florilegium",' in: Schnalke, *Natur im Bild* (1995), pp. 75-97.

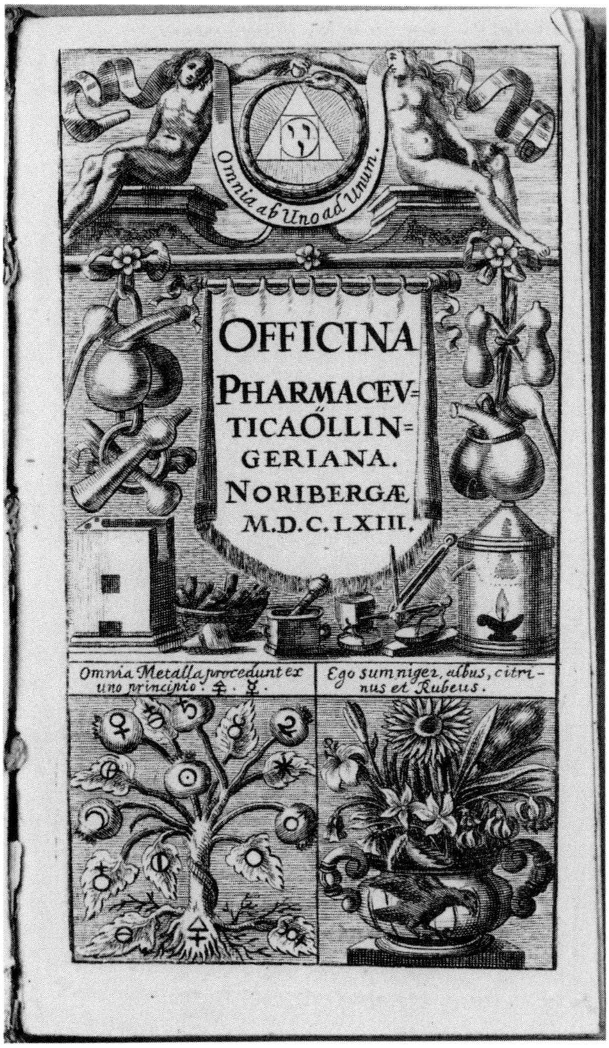
Omnia ab Uno ad Unum.
OFFICINA PHARMACEVTICA ÖLLINGERIANA.
NORIBERGÆ M.D.C.LXIII.
Omnia Metalla procedunt ex uno principio.
Ego sum niger, albus, citrinus et Rubeus.

An authority on viper bites

CHARAS, Moyse (1618–1698)

Nouvelles Experiences sur la Vipere, ou l'on verra une description exacte de toutes ses parties, la source de son venin, ses divers effets, et les remedes exquis que les Artistes peuvent tirer de la Vipere, tant pour la Guerison de ses Morsures, que pour celle de plusieurs autres Maladies.
Paris, printed for the author and Olivier de Varennes, 1669.

Octavo – *leaf*: 183 *x* 120 *mm. Pp.* [12], 1-58, 57-218, [6]. *Extra engraved title leaf and 3 folding engraved plates. Contemporary calf, gilt spine with five raised bands.*
Book-plate: C.D. Carlsson.

First edition, early issue, before the addition of the *'Suite des nouvelles experiences sur la vipere, avec une dissertation sur son venin, pour servir de replique à une lettre que Monsieur Francois Redi à écrite à Messieurs Bourdelot & Morus . . .'*. This letter, a reply to Francesco Redi's objections concerning the viper's venom, added to later issues, was first printed in 1671. It is paginated 201-78 and is found inserted after page 200 even in copies with the title page dated 1669 or 1670, followed by the *Echiosophium,* a description of the Viper in Latin verse, paginated 201-18. Not until the reissue of 1672 was it added to the text on the title page. A second edition, revised and augmented by the author, was published in 1694. There were also English and German editions. Charas' account of the viper's anatomy was also included in the important *Memoires pour servir à l'histoire des animaux* with anatomical descriptions of various animals conducted by a team of comparative anatomists, the 'Parisians', who, led by Claude Perrault, laid the foundations of our modern knowledge of comparative anatomy.

Moyse Charas, apothecary, physician, botanist, and for nine years demonstrator of chemistry at the Jardin de Roi in Paris, attained European celebrity in 1668, when the plague swept France, as the first French pharmacist to prepare the famous Theriac. This he did in the presence of a number of magistrates and physicians. It consisted of 65 ingredients and in his *Theriaque d'Andromacus* (1668) he gives a description of each of them. His chief work was the *Pharmacopée Royale galénique et chimique* (1676), which was in great vogue and went through several editions and translations into all principal languages, even into Chinese.

Charas was a Protestant, and in 1680, on account of the revocation of the Edict of Nantes, he left France and was cordially received by Charles II in London, who made him his pharmacist and doctor. He lived in England for five years and then went to Holland. There the Spanish ambassador persuaded Charas to go to Spain to see the king, who was in poor health. Here he got into trouble through his scientific habit of mind. Upon the canonization of an archbishop of Toledo, his successor announced that all snakes in that district should henceforth lose their venom. Charas was tempted to make an investigation of the facts, because he was an authority on vipers and had written a famous book on the subject. His investigation showed that the snakes were continuing to develop poison in the glands which nature had provided for that purpose, in evident ignorance of the archbishop's pronouncement. His investigation and his results were talked about with the effect that he was summoned by the Spanish Inquisition and imprisoned for some months. Charas' love for science was, however, greater than his adherence to Protestantism. He embraced the Catholic faith, was released and returned to France, where he was congratulated by Louis XIV on his change of views, and was elected to the Academy of Science.

In his work on vipers Charas alleged that he had shown by repeated experiments in the presence of numerous physicians that the yellowish liquor was merely a harmless saliva. He had wounded a number of animals with a detached viper-tooth and then poured the liquor into the wound with no ill effects. He therefore attributed the poisonous effect of the viper's bite rather to its vexed and enraged spirits. He was severely critizised by Redi, whom Charas answered in his *Suite* (pp. 201-78) added to later issues of his *Nouvelles experiences sur la Vipere.* His treatise is illustrated with three excellent anatomical plates.

Wellcome, p. 327; Krivatsy, 2366; *Biographie Médical,* III, pp. 219-20; Wootton, *Chronicles of Pharmacy,* I, pp. 279-80; Thorndike, VIII, pp. 24-5; Cole Library, 698; Cole, *History,* 406; Waller 11793 (2nd ed. 1694)

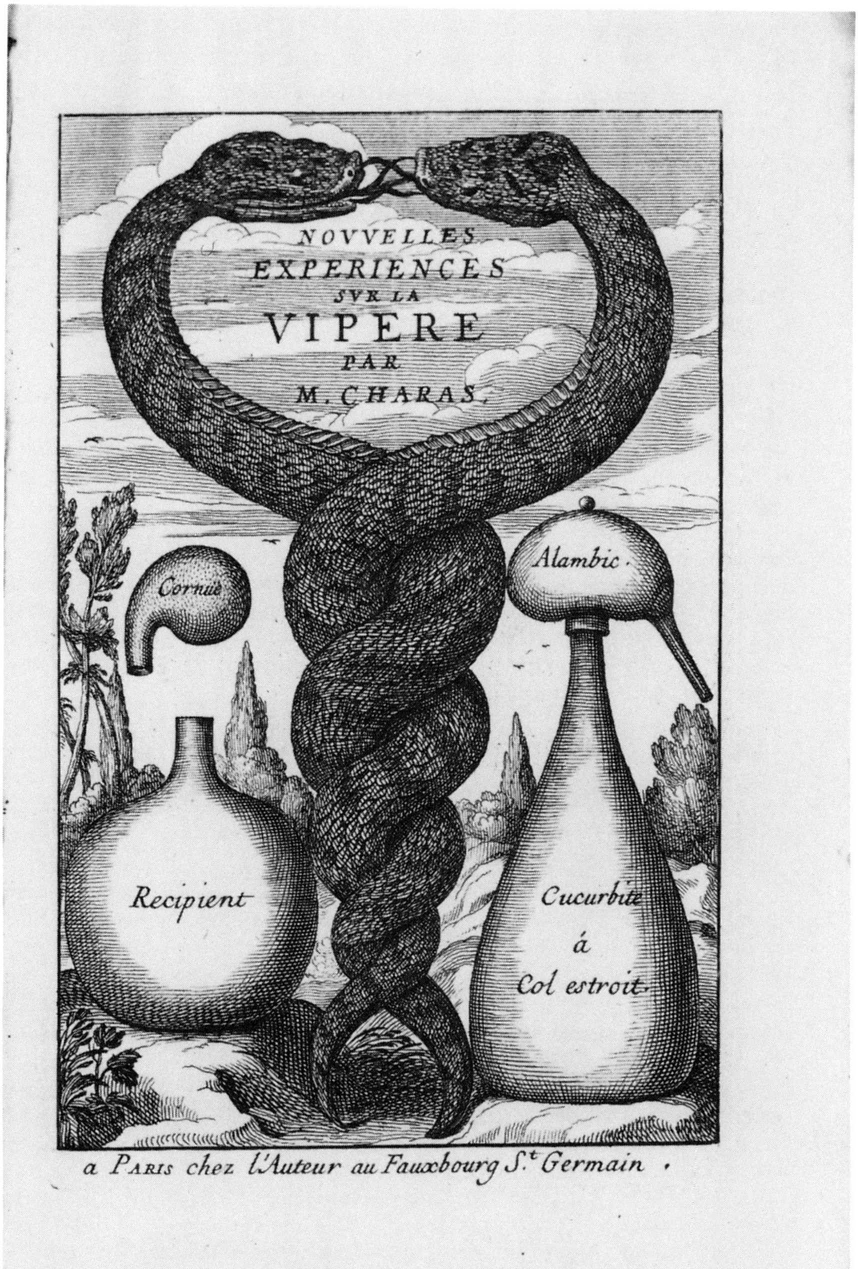

The engraved title, with two vipers entwined as in the *caduceus*, to Charas' '*New Experiments upon Vipers, Containing also an Exact Description of all the Parts of a Viper, the Seat of its Poyson, and the several Effects thereof, together with the Exquisite Remedies, that by the Skilful may be drawn from Vipers, as well for the Cure of their Bitings, as for that of other Maladies*' being the title of the English translation (1670).

A Carmelite monk's Persian pharmacopoeia

LABROSSE, Joseph (Père Ange de Sainct Joseph) b. 1636

Pharmacopoea Persica ex idiomate Persico in Latinum conversa. Opus Missionariis, Mercatoribus, caeterisque Regionum Orientalium Lustratoribus necessarium; nec non Europaeis Nationibus perutili. Accedunt in fine specimen notarum in Pharmacopoeam Persicam; . . .
Paris, Stephan Michallet, 1681.

Octavo – *leaf*: 186 *x* 120 *mm. Pp.* [6], 58, [6], 370, [28] = *Title* + [4] Epistola + [56] Missionariis Apostolicis + [4] Approbationes + [4] Discorso (*in Italian*) *&* Extraict de Privilege du Roy + 370 (*Pharmacopoeia*) + [26] *Index* + [2] *Errata, verso blank. Contemporary marbled boards.*

From the Ernst Matérn Collection *with his book-plate.*

The first European book on Persian medicine. Joseph Labrosse, or La Brosse, from Toulouse, was a Carmelite monk who took the name Père Ange de Sainct Joseph (Fr. Angelus of St. Joseph). After having studied Arabic in Rome for two years he went to Ispahan and began to study Persian. There he befriended a Carmelite father, Fr. Matthew, who having a considerable knowledge of medicine, used it as a means of propagating Christianity. Fr. Angelus envied his colleague his success, having seen him baptise both children and adults under the pretence of administering to them a medicine, and in addition to Persian began to study medicine. He tells that he visited the houses of the learned people of Ispahan and paid hundreds of visits to the shops of the druggists and pharmacists. Back in Paris he published his *Pharmacopoea Persica* in 1681, in which Persian types are also used. The translator's name appears in Persian on the title page (Wellcome).

According to Schelenz the book is a translation of a pharmacological treatise, *Tuhfat-ul-Mu'manín* or 'The Gift of the Two Mu'mans', father and son, completed in 1669, while Cyril Elgood in his *A Medical History of Persia,* as well as Wellcome, say that another pharmacopoiea, *Tibb-i-Shifá'i*, written in 1556 by Muzaffar bin Muhammad al-Husayní al-Shifá'i, formed the foundation of the *Pharmacopoea Persica* of Fr. Angelus.

Fr. Angelus himself says that he has read many Arabic and Persian books, above all the great medical encyclopaedia called 'Thesaurus of the Shah of Khwárazm', the *Zakhíra-i-Khwárazmsháhi*, written in the eleventh century by Ismail al-Jurj'aní, an important work that Elgood states did for Persian science what the Bible did for English prose.

However, it is generally agreed that many of the 1100 recipes in Fr. Angelus' very rare book, 'sehr seltene Werk' (Schelenz), go back to ancient Persian originals and primarily to the first pharmacological treatise to be written in Persian, composed in c. 975 A.D. by Abú Mansúr Muwaffaq, who flourished in Herat. A manuscript of his work copied by the poet Asudí in 1055 is preserved in the Austrian National Library, Vienna. It is not only the first pharmacological treatise to be written in Persian but the earliest known prose work in modern Persian as well as the oldest Persian manuscript in Europe. This work, called the *Kitáb-ul-Abniya 'an Haqá'iq-il-Adviya* or the 'Book of the Foundations of the True Properties of the Remedies', describes 585 drugs classified into four groups according to their action, about which the author had collected data from Greek, Syriac, Arabic, Persian and Indian sources.

About the same time as Fr. Angelus' book was published in Paris he was appointed visitor to the Carmelite Convent in Amsterdam, where he succeeded in buying the Oriental type which belonged to the heirs of the Elzevier press in Leiden and was thus able to publish the first Persian dictionary with the Persian words translated into Italian, Latin and French. The medically interested Carmelite monk paid far more attention to medical words than to others. His *Gazophyliacium linguae Persarum* appeared in Amsterdam in 1684. Fr. Angelus tells that he also translated the Aphorisms of Hippo-crates into Persian.

Cyril Elgood, *A Medical History of Persia and Eastern Caliphate from the Earliest Times until the Year* A.D. 1932, pp. 366-8; Schelenz, p. 69; M. Bouvet, 'La Pharmacopée Persane de 1681' in *Revue d'Histoire de la Pharmacie*, Sept., 1954, pp. 347-9; Wellcome, IV, p. 355; Parkinson/Lumb, 1893; Krivatsy, 8913; Waller 7403.

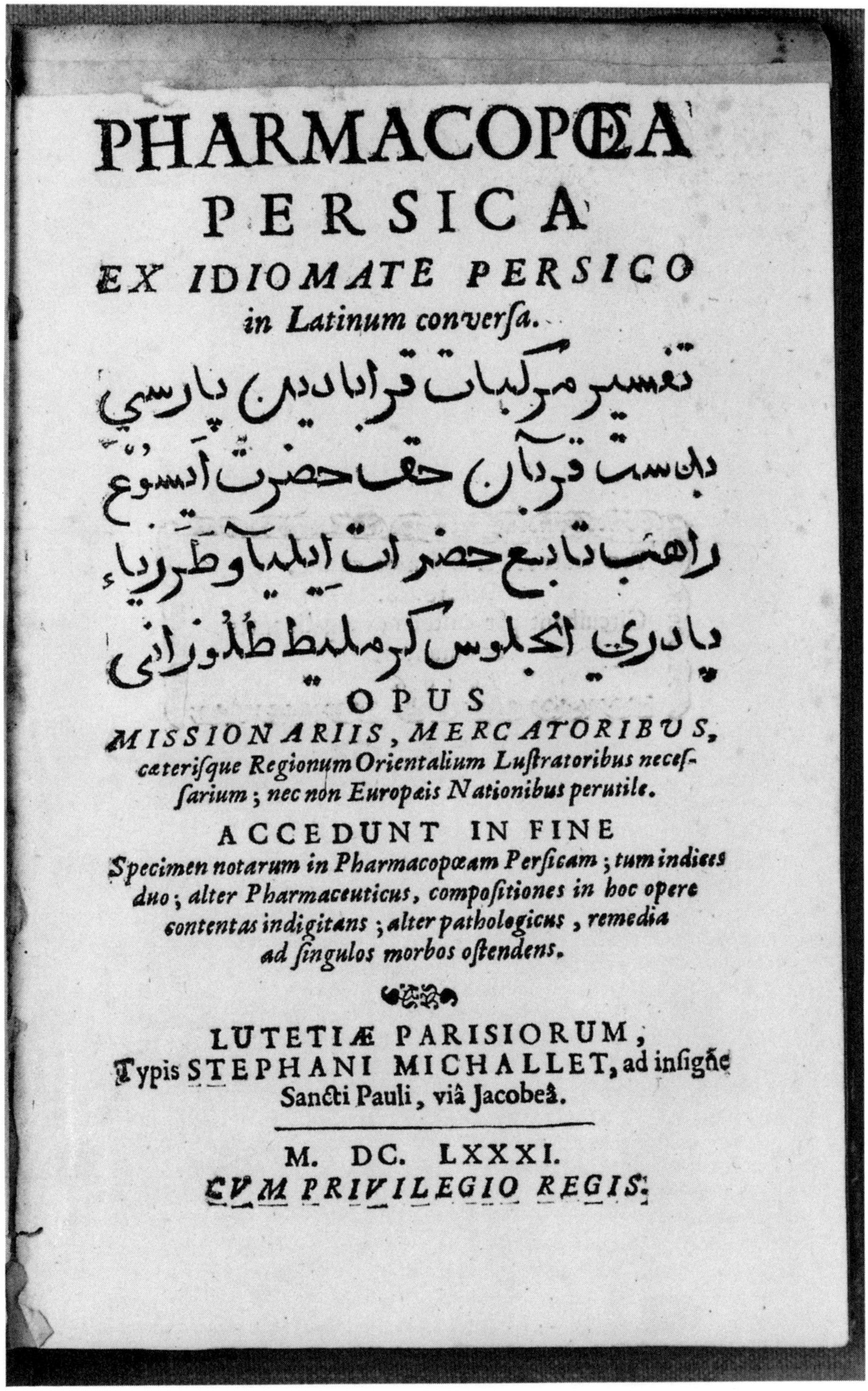

PHARMACOPŒA
PERSICA
EX IDIOMATE PERSICO
in Latinum conversa.

تفسير مركبات قرابادين پارسي
بدست قربان حقّ حضرت ايسوع
راهب تابع حضرات ايليا و طرزياء
پادري انجلوس كرمليط طُلوزاني

OPUS
MISSIONARIIS, MERCATORIBUS,
cæterisque Regionum Orientalium Lustratoribus necessarium; nec non Europæis Nationibus perutile.

ACCEDUNT IN FINE
Specimen notarum in Pharmacopœam Persicam; tum indices duo; alter Pharmaceuticus, compositiones in hoc opere contentas indigitans; alter pathologicus, remedia ad singulos morbos ostendens.

LUTETIÆ PARISIORUM,
Typis STEPHANI MICHALLET, ad insigne
Sancti Pauli, viâ Jacobeâ.

M. DC. LXXXI.
CUM PRIVILEGIO REGIS.

Scarce East India pharmacopoeia by a Swede

GRIM, Herman Nicolaus (1641–1711)

Compendium medico-chymicum, seu Accurata medendi Methodus, quæ excellentissimis Medicamentis, tam Europæ, quam Indiæ Orientali proficius, repleta, rariores Observationes, & curiosam optimorum Medicamentorum, in libelli hujus formulis contentorum, præparationem exhibet, . . .
Augsburg, Johann Jacob Schönigh for Theophil Göbel, 1684.

Octavo – *leaf*: 160 *x* 92 *mm. Pp.* [12], 475, [11] *index, one blank leaf. Engraved frontispiece* (Melchior Haffner sculp.) *and one woodcut in the text* (*p.* 414). *Contemporary vellum, manuscript spine title.*

This is the second edition of this scarce work that first appeared in 1679 printed at Batavia, Java, where the author was inspector of the barber-surgeons of the Dutch East India Company.

Of the numerous Swedish physicians who studied at foreign universities towards the end of the Swedish Great Power period, Herman Nicolaus Grim was surely one of the most remarkable. A native of Gotland, Grim left Sweden at an early age to learn the profession of his father, who was a barber-surgeon. He first studied for a short time in Copenhagen and then left for Holland, where he passed his examination. In 1663 he entered in the Dutch service as a ship's surgeon and probably took part in the war against the English. He sailed with a polar sea ship to Novaya Semlya and visited Greenland twice. He probably took his M.D. in Holland and may have served as a plague doctor in 1666. Two years later he returned to Denmark as a physician and took up further studies in chemistry for the famous Ole Borch and also made the acquaintance of the great professor Thomas Bartholin, to whose medical journal, *Acta Medica & Philosophica Hafniensia*, he contributed, amongst other things, with a paper concerning the cure for scurvy among the Eskimos.

In 1671 Grim was appointed physician to the Dutch East India Company and sailed for Ceylon, where he seems to have had his headquarters in Colombo, but he also stayed on the Coromandel and Malabar Coasts. About 1678 he served as chief surgeon at Batavia in Java. Due to his background in the field of chemistry and mineralogy he was also appointed inspector of the gold and silver mines in Sumatra, an experience on which he wrote papers published in Batavia.

During his stay in the East Indies, Grim's chief activities were in the field of medicine and pharmacy. His first pharmaceutical work, *Laboratorium Chymicum, gehouden op het voortreffelycke Eylandt Ceylon,* was on the *materia medica* of Ceylon dealing with drugs of the animal, vegetable and mineral kingdoms, how the native doctors prepared their drugs and for which diseases these drugs were used. The book was first published in Dutch, printed in Batavia in 1677. A pirated edition appeared in Amsterdam in 1679, translated into Latin by the French physician Bartholmaeus Pielat, who avoided any mention of the real author's name. In the same year Grim published his *Chirurgiæ & Medicinæ Practici Compendium Medico-Chimicum,* a more comprehensive work dealing with the medicinal plants of the Dutch East Indies, their pharmaceutical preparation for various afflictions, with the recipes extensively described. The first edition was printed at Batavia. The present copy is of the second edition printed in Augsburg. At the end is a *Pharmacopeia Indica* (pp. 387-474) with separate title page. It must be one of the earliest pharmacopoeias introducing colonial drugs to the European continent and is dedicated to Lucas Schröck, member and later president of the illustrious German *Academia Naturae Curiosorum.* Schröck was editor of the academy's journal, the *Ephemerides*, to which Grim contributed several articles on the natural history and medicinal plants of the East Indies.

After ten years Grim returned to Holland and in 1683 he turned up at Nyköping, Sweden, where he served as municipal physician for some years and then practised for a time in Stockholm. He then went to Germany, where he first served as town physician in Aurich and was physician-in-ordinary to the count of Ost-Friesland. He later became military surgeon in the garrison at Tönningen. After some ten years he returned to his native Visby and was in 1697 provincial physician of Gotland. In 1698 he settled in Stockholm and was for a time inspector of Urban Hiärne's chemical laboratory and was also received in the Collegium Medicum, to which he donated his exotic natural history collections. He made a respected name for himself during the plague of 1710, to which he himself succumbed, dying in the spring of 1711.

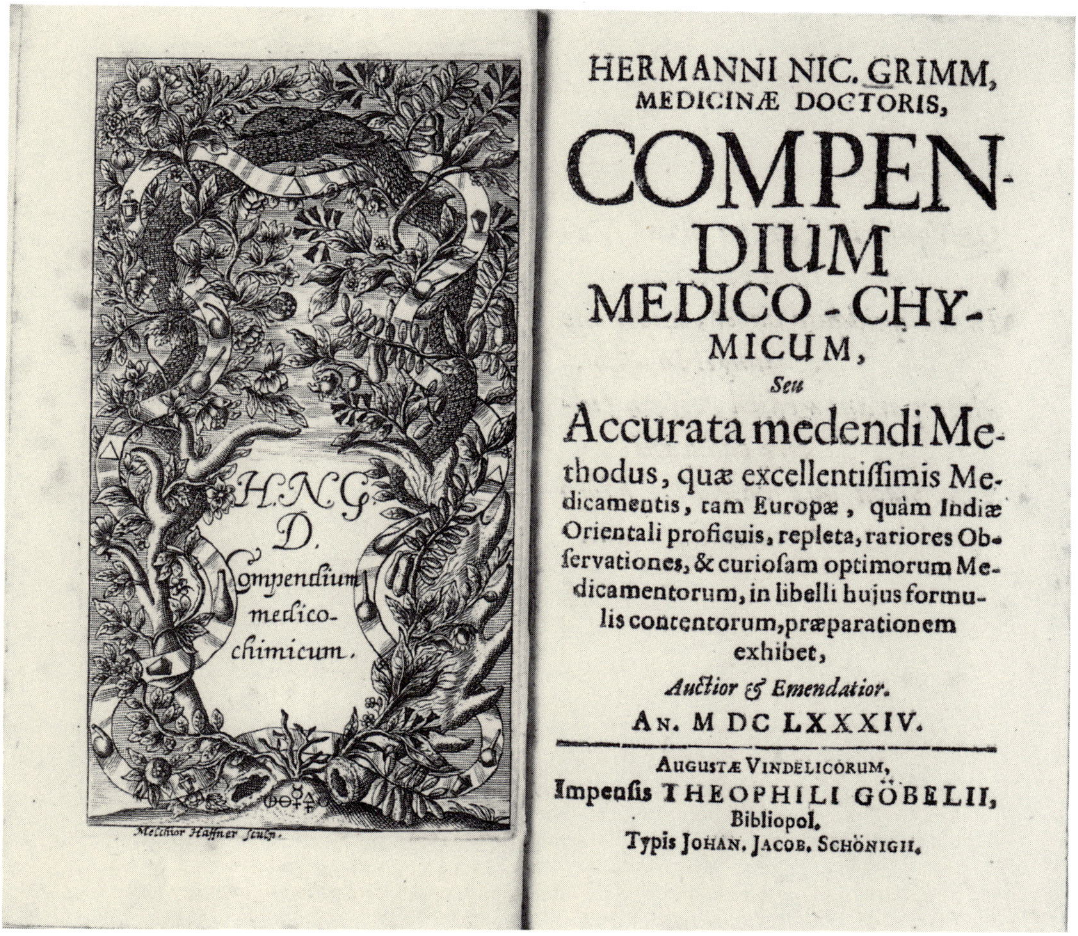
H.N.G. D. Compendium medico-chimicum.

Melchior Haffner sculp.

HERMANNI NIC. GRIMM,
MEDICINÆ DOCTORIS,
COMPENDIUM
MEDICO-CHYMICUM,
Seu
Accurata medendi Methodus, quæ excellentissimis Medicamentis, tam Europæ, quàm Indiæ Orientali proficuis, repleta, rariores Observationes, & curiosam optimorum Medicamentorum, in libelli hujus formulis contentorum, præparationem exhibet,
Auctior & Emendatior.
AN. M DC LXXXIV.
AUGUSTÆ VINDELICORUM,
Impensis THEOPHILI GÖBELII,
Bibliopol.
Typis JOHAN. JACOB. SCHÖNIGII.

Grim's very scarce publications on the pharmaceutical plants of the East Indies are pioneer works. The Dutch botanist, Johannes Burman, friend and patron of Linnaeus, names Grim's book in his *Thesaurus Zeylanicus* (1737) and calls the *Compendium* a 'golden book' (*aureus libellus*). Otherwise very little is found about Grim and his pharmaceutical books, certainly much because of their great rarity. There was no copy of the first edition in any Swedish library, not even in the *Bibliotheca Walleriana*, until 1992, when our National Library acquired a copy of the first edition of the above work, printed by the first printer at Batavia, Abraham van de Eede, in 1679.

Collijn, col. 327; Sten Lindroth in SBL, 17, pp. 292-4; T.J. Arne, 'Svenska läkare och fältskärer i holländska Ostindiska Kompaniets tjänt', in *Lychnos*, 1956, pp. 132-46; Sten Lindroth, 'Medicinen i Sverige under Stormaktstiden', in *Ciba-Journalen*, (1950), pp. 748-9; Sacklén, I, 73; IV, 11; Ferguson, I, 347 (Batavia, 1677); Ferchl, 200-01; Tjiang Beng Jap, 'Über die Wechselwirkungen europäischer und indonesischer Pharmazie im 17. Jahrhundert nach der Pharmacopoeia Indica', pp. 37-44 in *Veröffentl. d. Internationalen Gesellschaft f. Geschichte d. Pharmazie*, N.F., Band 21 (1963); Waller 3747.

PALMBERG, Johannes (d. 1691)

The first Swedish illustrated herbal

Serta Florea Svecana eller Swenske Örtekrantz.
Strängnäs, Zacharias Asp, 1684.

Octavo – *leaf:* 160 *x* 90 *mm. Pp* [16], 416, [44]. *This copy* 'A' *has only* 16 *of the* 44 *pages of indices at end. Those missing are to be found in copy* 'B' *lacking its title leaf. Floral border around the title page and with* 130 *woodcuts of plants in the text. Contemporary calf. Inner covers and endpapers filled with annotations by previous owners:* Christina Lars Dotter *and* Johannes Joh: Erenberg, *c.*1720. *Later owner was* Lars Svangren, *proprietor of the pharmacy at Alingsås in* 1862, *who opened the spa at Torpa, Lilla Edet.*

This small octavo, printed in the small medieval town of Strängnäs, is the first Swedish herbal with illustrations, if we exclude the second edition of Elias Til-Landz' *Catalogus Plantarum*, whose *Icones* (Åbo, 1683) has 158 woodcuts of plants growing in the neighbourhood of Åbo, Finland (at that time belonging to Sweden).

Johannes Palmberg, born in the 1640s, was the son of the vicar of the parish of Tuna in Södermanland. Having completed his collegiate studies at Strängnäs, he registered at the University of Åbo in Finland in 1663 to study medicine. At this time, medical education lay at a very low level in Åbo. There were hardly any medical books, and the professor, Erik Daniel Achrelius, was quite incompetent, having during his twenty-year tenure never issued a single dissertation and being seldom seen at the academy. A petition had been submitted to the king to have the decrepit professor pensioned off and replaced by a competent doctor, a post that Palmberg may have coveted. Among the sparse information extant on Achrelius' medical views is that he was accused of having poisoned the bishop's wife by prescribing a drug containing '*succus fimi equis*' (horse dung). After four years at Åbo, practising as a physician, Palmberg finished his medical dissertation, but never got to present it as Achrelius refused to preside. In 1669 Palmberg returned to his native Strängnäs without his titulary examination.

In Strängnäs there was at this time neither physician nor apothecary, and Palmberg had to share a practice with the town barber and surgeon. After several years of dispute, Palmberg was appointed schoolteacher of medicine and physics, which meant that he was to lecture on the medical effects of herbs. It is said that he founded a botanical garden in Strängnäs patterned on that of Rudbeck's at Uppsala. His first medical papers were published in the Strängnäs almanacks of 1670–1672 and he is thus the first Swedish physician to contribute to Swedish almanacks.

In 1672 Palmberg was given the Royal privilege to publish an illustrated herbal in Swedish ('at uppå wårt swenska Språk i Trycket låta uthgå een Örtebook medh sine Figurer och Örternes Affmålningar och färgor'), from which we may construe that the original intent was to have the figures coloured. Due to the death of the provincial printer, Brockenius, already in 1671, and in 1674 that of Bishop Emporagrius, who had granted the publication, the work was interrupted.

When printing finally started after a delay of twelve years there was friction between Palmberg and the successor of Brockenius, Zacharias Asp. Palmberg complained that Asp was too slow in printing the work, and Asp defended himself by saying that Palmberg had not provided him with money to buy candles. An edition appeared already in 1683 with only pictures and a separate title leaf. It contained 123 woodcuts with no other text than the plants' names in Latin and Swedish, with an index at the end. The woodcuts may have been completed already in 1672, as Bishop Emporagrius in a letter of recommendation declared that Palmberg had had a proof printed. Of this extremely rare edition only a handful of copies have survived. When the complete book was ready in 1684 it consisted of 476 pages with 130 woodcuts and a beautiful title page framed with a floral wreath in allusion to its title. It is supposed that no more than 500 copies were printed.

A new, enlarged, but unillustrated edition was published in 1733, reprinted in 1738, edited by the headmaster of the German School in Stockholm, J.B. Steinmeijer, who was keen on botany in his teaching.

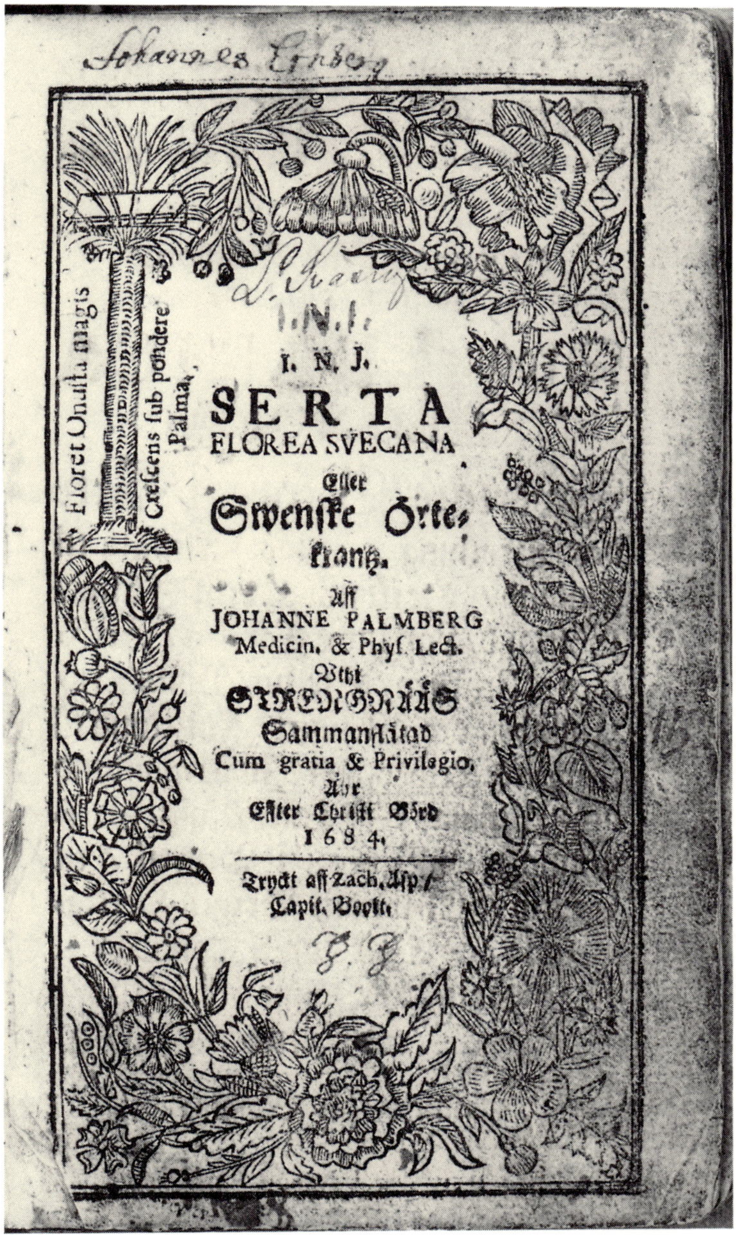
Floret Onusta magis
Crescens sub pondere Palma.
I. N. J.
SERTA
FLOREA SVECANA
Eller
Swenske Örte-
krantz.
Aff
JOHANNE PALMBERG
Medicin. & Phys. Lect.
Uthi
STRENGNÄS
Sammanfattad
Cum gratia & Privilegio.
Åhr
Effter Christi Börd
1684.
Tryckt aff Zach. Asp /
Capit. Boektr.

As most herbals, Palmberg's *Swenske Örtekrantz* is a compilation of old and foreign authors, to whom he admits his debt. Those who dared criticize these authorities were harshly compared by Palmberg to 'blowflies on an honest man's table'. Even if later botanists considered his herbal extremely poor, it remained the one and only Swedish floral handbook until Linnaeus' *Flora Svecica* (1745) appeared, and it was from Palmberg's 'wretched handbook' that the great master himself acquired his first botanical knowledge.

Krok, 570; Vilhelm Djurberg, 'En svensk medicinsk folkskriftförfattare på 1600-talet', in: *Hygiea*, 1900, pp. 357-405; 1906, pp. 145-59; Waller 11698.

PHARMACOPOEIA HOLMIENSIS

The first Swedish pharmacopoeia

Pharmacopoeja Holmiensis Galeno-Chymica complectens compositiones apprimé necessarias, usibus hodiernis destinatas; earumque conficiendi modos.
Stockholm, Johan G. Eberdt, 1686.

Quarto – *leaf:* 200 x 160 *mm. Pp.* [12], 173, [9]. *Interleaved copy with Ms annotations on the blank leaves. At the end is bound* Collegii Medicii Underrättelse (1757) *and* 48 *leaves with* Taxa *in manuscript. Old vellum, spine divided into four compartments with Ms title later added in the upper compartment and blind ornament stamps in the others. Double fillets around sides with a fleuron in each corner. Centrepiece with the initials* 'D.V.' *on upper and* 'D.L.' *on lower cover. Copy without the engraved frontispiece (see next item).*

The first Swedish pharmacopoeia. Before 1686 there was no official Swedish medical formulary. The first apothecaries in Sweden were brought from Germany. These immigrants used German pharmacopoeias, dispensatories or herbals with descriptions of the collecting of plants, their preparation and effects. The *Pharmacopoeia Augustana* was of special influence.

When the Swedish *Collegium Medicum* was founded in 1663, one of its foremost tasks was by Royal decree to ensure the compilation of an official pharmacopoeia. However, the work of this dispensatorium was not to commence until the autumn of 1680, when the main responsibility was entrusted to one of the youngest members of the *Collegium Medicum,* Johann Martin Ziervogel (1657–1701). He was the son of Samuel Ziervogel, the immigrated German court apothecary and founder of the renowned Ziervogel dynasty of pharmacists. Johann Martin began studying medicine at Uppsala under Hoffvenius and Rudbeck. As was customary at the time he went abroad to pass his M.D. at Leiden in 1679 on a dissertation on scurvy, *De scorbuto.* He then proceeded to Italy and returned home through France, Germany and Holland. Back in Stockholm, he was admitted to the *Collegium Medicum* in 1680. He ran a respected medical practice in Stockholm and in due course became court physician-in-ordinary. In 1698 he was ennobled Rothlöben.

By the time the *Pharmacopoeia Holmiensis* was finally completed, twenty-three years had elapsed since its commissioning. Legislation was now required to commit apothecaries and physicians to the use of the new pharmacopoeia. This was achieved by the new medical proclamation of 1688, which was not printed until 1699, and decreed that all apothecaries in the entire kingdom were required for their guidance to use the Stockholm pharmacopoeia. Now only a list of official tariffs remained to be determined. This *Apothekare Taxa* or *Catalogus et Valor*, printed in Latin, Swedish and German, appeared in 1698 (see next item).

The *Pharmacopeia Holmiensis* in Latin comprises over 800 preparations, divided into 22 classes. It contains both the old 'Galenic' and the new chemical or 'Spagyrical' pharmaceutics, the latter collected in the final class as a supplement, the '*Medicamentis chymicis*' with some fifty remedies (a full description is found in Ahlberg, p. 341 ff.) The main source for the Galenic part was Johann Zwelfer's revisions of *the Pharmacopoeia Augustana;* the chemical preparations were to a great extent derived from the *Collectanea Chymica Leydensia* (not published until 1684) by the three Leyden chemists De Maets, Marggraf and Le Mort, whose courses Ziervogel may have attended during his studies in Leyden.

Many of the Galenic preparations were of a most complicated composition, which resulted in complaints being voiced against the mandatory pharmacopoeia. Apothecaries even refused to take the prescribed oath largely because the dispensatory contained recipes almost impossible to prepare and which they claimed to be opposed to pharmaceutical practise. The 1756 Sumptuary Enactment, forbidding the importation of foreign luxury and superfluous goods, included many pharmaceutical articles. The *Collegium Medicum* was therefore forced to produce a provisional revision of the pharmacopoeia, which is why a supplement, the *Underrättelse*, appeared in 1757 (see next item).

Collijn, *Sveriges Bibliografi*, 1600-*talet,* col. 713 (without the frontispiece); Hjelt, III, p. 489 ff.; Ahlberg, pp. 392-5; Facsimile edition (*Suecica Rediviva*, 1979); Sten Lindroth, 'Pharmacopoeia Holmiensis 1686', in *Lychnos*, 1943, pp. 67-96. E. Louis Backmann 'Om den äldsta svenska farmakopén, dess medicinskt-historiska bakgrund och dess ställning till folkmedicinen', in *Upsala Läkareförenings Förhandl.* N.F., vol. 29 (1924) pp. 63-98; Waller 7393.

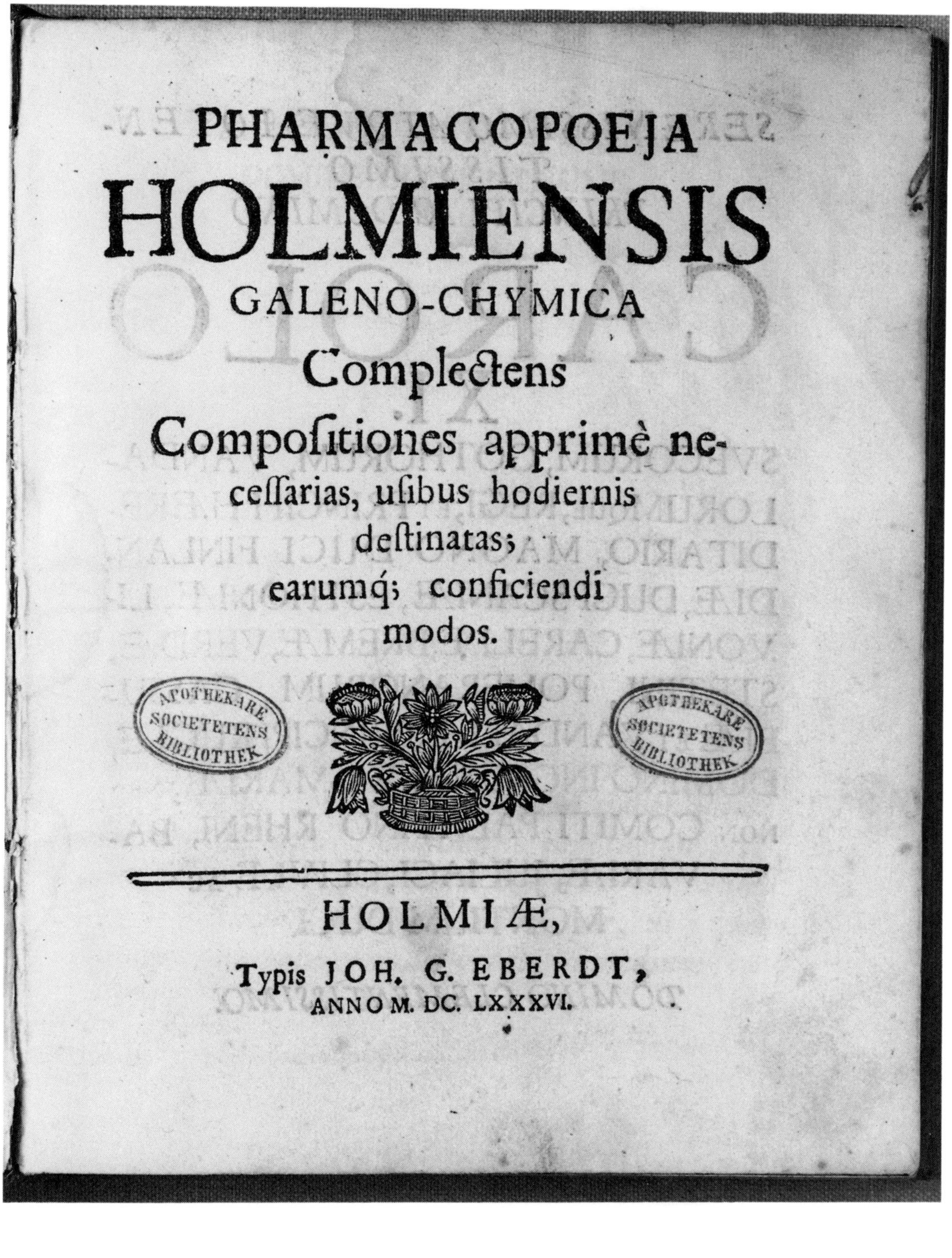

PHARMACOPOEJA
HOLMIENSIS
GALENO-CHYMICA
Complectens
Compositiones apprimè necessarias, usibus hodiernis destinatas; earumq; conficiendi modos.

HOLMIÆ,
Typis JOH. G. EBERDT,
ANNO M. DC. LXXXVI.

In its original binding with the rare frontispiece

[MEDICINAL-ORDNINGAR 1699]

Kongl. May:tz i Nåder Utgifne sidste Medicinal-Ordningar af Trycket utgångne Åhr 1699. / Sac:æ Reg:æ Maj:tis Clementis-simæ Constitutiones Medicæ, Publicatæ Anno M.DC.XCIX. / Ihro Königl. May:tz Allergnädigste Medicinal-Ordnungen. Durch den druck herausgegeben Anno 1699.
Stockholm, (1699).

Bound and issued with:

Kongl. May:tz Nådige Resolution, och Förklaring angående några Måhl, beträffande Collegium Medicum, Apothekare Societeten och Barberare Embetet, gifwen Stockholm den 1 Augusti 1698. (12 *pages*)

and:

[TAXA] Catalogus et Valor Medicamentorum in Officinis Pharma-ceüticis Stockholmiensibus prostantium. / Apothekare-TAXA, uppå alla de Medicamenter och Wahror, som på Apotheken i Stockholm finnes til Sahlu. / Apotheker-TAXT, Aller Medicamenten undt Wahren, welche in denen Stockholmischen Apotheken zu finden seyn.
No imprint (Stockholm, 1698).

Quarto – *leaf*: 187 x 150 *mm*. Medicinal-Ordningar: 66 *pages;* Resolution: 12 *pages;* Taxa: *pp.* [4], 1-96, [28]. *Sign.*: (a)[1] (*title*), A-H4; (*Resolution*): I4 K2; (*Taxa*): A4, A-L4 M2 N2 O-Q4 R2. *This copy, in its original binding, is bound with the rare engraved frontispiece (see reproduction on the opposite page). Contemporary brown calf over thick boards, sides with floral border within double fillet and the lettering*: 'MEDICINAL ORDNING' *on upper cover. The blind stamps may have been gilt, but if so, they are now faded.*

The first edition of the important medical decree of 1699 issued together with the tariff and preserved in its original binding. The text is printed in Swedish, Latin and German. The *Taxa* of 1687 was to be made a general ordinance in 1688, but the printing was delayed until 1698. The *Medicinal-Ordning* of 1699 was reprinted in 1742 and issued together with the the *Taxa* of 1739 (Stockholm, 1741).

[UNDERRÄTTELSE] – Kongl. Collegii Medici Underrättelse om Några ändringar i Stockholmska Pharmacopéen til underdånigst följe af Hans Kongl. Majts Nådiga Bref af den 19. Januarii 1757; samtelige Rikets Apothekare till efterlefnad, til thess nya Pharma-copéen af trycket utkommer.

Stockholm, Kongl. Tryckeriet, 1757.

Quarto – *leaf*: 200 *x* 160 *mm*. *Pp.* (8). *This quarto sheet, here bound with our copy* 'A' *of the* Pharmacopoeia Holmiensis (*see preceding item*), *is in fact a type facsimile printed on old paper.*

With our copy of the *Pharmacopoeia Holmiensis* is bound the *Underrättelse* of 1757, according to which no less than 44 compounds were to be expunged from the *Pharmaopoeia Holmiensis* and the preparation of several others was to be modified. About the same time, preparatory efforts began for a new official Swedish pharma-copoeia. Up to the first edition of the new *Pharmacopoea Svecica*, which appeared in 1775, the above regulations constitute what was officially applicable for the apothecaries in Sweden.

Medicinal Ordning 1699: Collijn, col. 598; Taxa: col. 913; Waller 5376 (Med. ord. 1699), 1823 (Taxa), 5372 (Underrättelse, also a reprint).

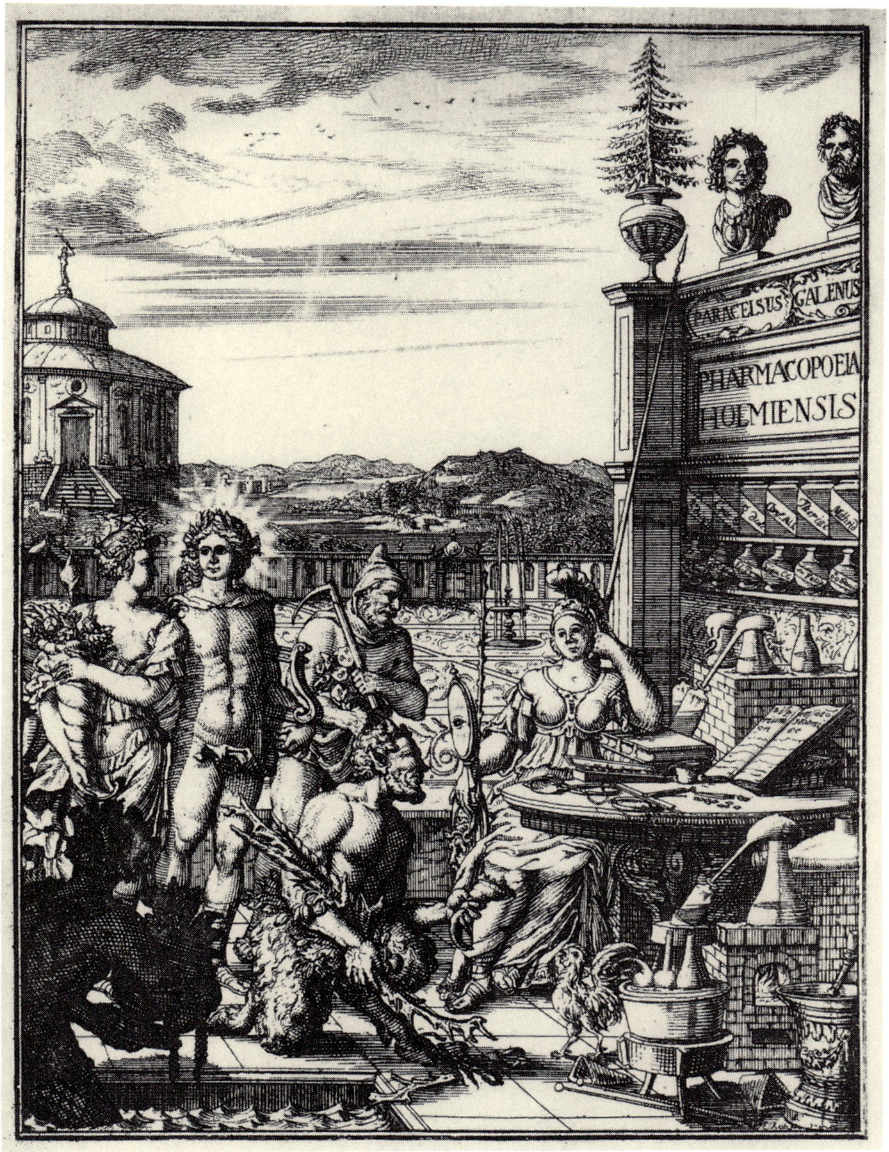

The rare frontispiece that was intended to adorn the *Pharmacopoeia Holmiensis* is found in a very few copies only. Ernst Matérn had not seen the frontispiece in any of the about ten copies that had passed through his hands. It is, however, more often found in copies of the Medical Proclamation with the *Taxa* of 1698-99.

The plate was engraved by Erik Reitz, who also made a number of plates for the renowned topographical work *Suecia Antiqua et Hodierna*. Drawing inspiration from frontispieces of foreign pharmacopoeias, it sets mythical figures in an allegorical scene. Minerva, the goddess of wisdom, is sitting at a table surrounded by furnaces and chemical apparatus and instruments. Pan kneels by her side, holding some animal horns, including that of a unicorn, in his arms. Beside him is Vulcan with a miner's pickaxe and minerals. Standing behind Vulcan we see Apollo, god of the healing art, with Ceres holding a cornucopia filled with flowers. These figures represent the *materia medica* from the animal, vegetable and mineral kingdoms. In the left corner an Indian emerges from a tub of water, holding gifts in a jar, presumably representing drugs from the New World. Representing the Galenic and Spagyrical compounds, the busts of Galen and Paracelsus are set atop a simplicia cabinet, its shelves laden with drug jars.

The drugs displayed are: *Antimonium diaphoreticum, Crocus metallorum, Mercurius dulcis, Confect. alkermes, Theriaca Mithridates, Tinctura cordialis, Essentia ambrae, Elixir proprietatis, Liquor cornu cervi, Spiritus fuliginis,* and *Oleum succinis.*

One of the filthiest books in world literature

PAULLINI, Kristian Frantz (1643–1712)

Heilsame Dreck-Apotheke; wie nehmlich mit Koth und Urin fast Alle, ja auch die schwerste, gifftige Kranckheiten, und bezuberte Schaden, vom Haupt biss zum Füssen, inn- und äusserlich. glücklich curirt worden; Durch und durch mit allerhand curieusen, so nutz- als ergetzlichen Historien, und anderen feinen Denckwürdigkeiten, bewährt und erläutert, . . .
Frankfurt am Main, Friedrich Knoch, 1696.

Octavo – *leaf*: 165 x 100 *mm. Pp.* 32, 268, [4]. *With extra engraved title leaf. Vellum-backed marbled boards, new endpapers.*

From the C.D. Carlsson Collection.

First edition. – In a world history of pharmacy, faeces and urine are listed among the oldest remedies still in use, and occupy a place in popular medicine even in the history of pharmacy in the Western world. Both human and animal excrement were common already in the times of Dioscorides and Galen, and are to be found in official pharmacopoeias and tariffs well up to the eighteenth century. The *Pharmacopoea Wirtenbergica* of 1741 lists *Album Graecum:* white dog dung, the white and odourless excrements, dried and cleaned, of a dog fed with bones, especially useful in the treatment of colic and dysentery. Also listed is *Pavonis stercus*: peacock droppings, useful for epilepsy and vertigo. It is prescribed as a powder, but in the treatment of epilepsy is to be rectally injected. Antidotaries often had special chapters devoted to urine and dung. This fashion reached its climax with the publication of a work compiled by Kristian Frantz Paullini, ducal physician and imperial poet laureate. His *Heilsame Dreck-Apoteke*, a work more notorious than famous, is described by Faber du Faur in his *German Baroque Literature* as 'one of the filthiest books in world literature', the purpose of which, according to the title page, was to cure successfully almost all ailments, even the most serious diseases and curses, from head to toe, internally and externally, with excrements and urine.

The first edition of this singularly scatophagous work appeared in 1696, a book of 304 pages. It went through several enlarged editions. The 1714 edition, (also in our library) totalling no less than 756 pages, having received the addition of a second volume. The book is not exclusively devoted to faeces but to all kinds of secretions such as urine, menstruation blood, ear-wax, sweat, mucus, etc. Paullini describes with hundreds of examples from medical literature and also from his own practice, the outstanding virtues of man's stools and urine, both inwardly given, and outwardly applied – but also excrements from domestic and wild animals and birds, e.g. squirrels, elephants, camels, wolves, bears, cuckoos, peacocks, owls, crocodiles, lizards, spiders and bees. The book was apparently very popular and a lucrative business for the publishers as it went through seven editions, the last (?) published as late as 1847. A facsimile of the 1734 edition was published in Munich, 1969.

The book is full of nasty prescriptions and relates hundreds of curious cases: Regina Hubaldin of Vissbeck drank her urine every morning with a raw egg, which cured her pulmonary consumption; Zacharias Medard used butter-fried crows' droppings against diarrhoea; the white dung from foxes was of outstanding value and used in many drugs. Paullini recommends distilled water from human excrements as a cosmetic: it gives a nice colour to the face. Other noteworthy cosmetics were excrements from crocodiles or lizards, making the skin both smooth and soft, recommended for finer ladies. A less nasty case was that of a patient who went to the doctor, who wrote down his prescription on a piece of paper and then strew sand on the ink, folded the paper and gave it to the patient with the ordination to take it every day. After a few days there was no 'medicine' (=sand) left on the paper, and the poor man, becoming desperate, swallowed the entire prescription form – and was cured!

Paullini was born in Eisenach and studied at various German universities and also in Copenhagen, where he even acted as interpretor for the Italian adventurer and conspirator Giuseppo Francesco Borri. On his return from a visit to England he graduated M.D. in Leyden. He travelled extensively, visited Sweden and Norway and is said to have visited Lapland and Iceland as well. He then practised in Hamburg up to 1675, which year he spent in France, after having been created Count Palatine. On his return to Germany he was engaged by the Bishop of Münster as premier physician and historiographer, but in 1689 he removed to Eisenach where he died in 1712, having been paralysed on his right side for seven years.

Paullini possessed a thoroughly facile pen and is the author of *Zeit-kürzende Lust*, a sort of encyclopedia of curiosities and anomalies, which was exceedingly popular, as were his numerous monographs on the dog, the wolf, the mole, the eel, the hare, the ass, and on different herbs, written according to the norm of the illustrious *Academia Naturae Curiosorum,* of which he was a member. Two of these, *De Theriaca* (1701) and *Jalapa* (1700) are in the Scheele-room, Biomedical Library, Faculty of Pharmacy, University of Uppsala.

Ferguson, II, p. 76; Kremers & Urdang, p. 79; Faber du Faur, *German Baroque Literature* pp. 205-06; Wolfgang Schneider, 'Über Paullini's Dreckapotheke' in *Veröffentl. d. Intern. Gesellschaft f. Geschichte d. Pharmazie*, N.F. Band 26 (1965), pp. 131-8; Waller 7240 (1697 ed.).

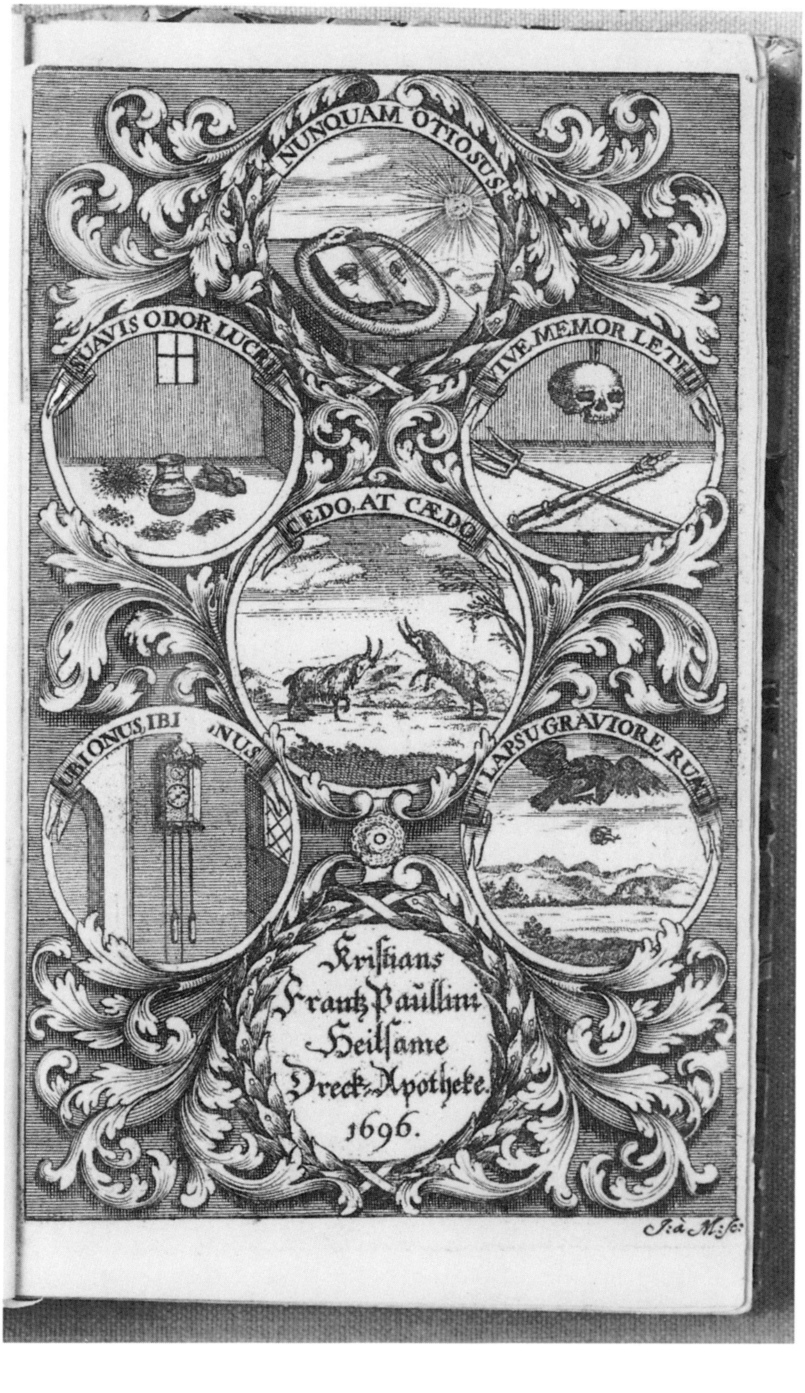

Merian's copperplates coloured by hand

VALENTINI, Michael Bernhard (1657–1729)

Viridarium Reformatum, . . . Das ist: Neu-eingerichtetes und Vollständiges Kräuter-Buch, worinnen auff noch nicht geschehene Weise derer Vegetabilien, als Kräutern, Sträuchen, Bäumen, Bluhmen und anderer Erd-Gewächsen Art, Krafft und Würckung dergestalt beschrieben werden, . . . jedes Kraut zu seiner rechten Haupt-Art bringen, auch dessen Nutzen in der Artzney deutlich und umständlich finden: Über dem einige besondere, aber bewährte Arcana zur Dämpffung des Podagras und Vertreibung des Steins, nebst vielen Praeparationen unterschiedlicher zur Medicin dienlichen Dingen antreffen kan; Denen, so kein Latein können, zu Lieb, auch zum Besten derer Aertzten, Apotheckern, Materialisten, Laboranten, Barbierern, Hebammen, Gärtnern, Mahlern und Andern Künstlern, sonderlich aber allen Hauss-Vätern und Hauss-Müttern zum Vorteil Teutsch verfasset; . . [*the comprehensive title comprises no less than 42 lines*]

Frankfurt am Main, Anton Heinscheidt, 1719.

Folio – *leaf*: 346 x 205 *mm. Pp.* [18], 584, [24];. Icones: *title leaf with instructions for the bookbinder on verso and* 387 *engraved plates (mostly with several figures on each plate), numbered* I-CCCLXXXIII, *with a supplement plate* CCCLXXXIII b, *one unnumbered double-page plate between p.*215 *and p.*216 *depicting the* Aloe, *and two unnumbered plates at the end of the preface representing a floral system* (A-Z). *Moreover there are* 223 *fine engravings in the text, those on p.*47 *and p.*241 *being cancels pasted over misplaced engravings. Complete except for one leaf in the prelims. The* Appendix: *Georg Welling's* Opus Mago-Cabalisticum, *a curious work on the origin of salt, is missing as in most copies. Contemporary calf.*

Provenance: Axel Kockum, 1927.

First and sole edition of this magnificently illustrated work on medicinal, economic and decorative plants and flowers. The present copy has nearly all of the engravings neatly coloured by hand. In 1704 the author had published another gigantic and fascinating work in three folio volumes entitled *Museum Museorum* (also in our library), the single most valuable contribution to the history of natural history collections or *Wunderkammers*, as it reprints many early collection catalogues and lists the c. 160 museums known to exist at the time. That book forms an inexhaustible repertory of all overseas products, including medicinal plants, of the late seventeenth century, sumptuously illustrated with nearly 400 engravings copied from other works and depicting thousands of exotic plants, animals, and minerals, as well as scientific apparatus. This costly enterprise apparently met with success, as Valentini subsequently carried out another herculean task: the present work on medicinal and other useful plants, exquisitely illustrated with engravings and plates derived from earlier works.

Of particular beauty are the superb emblematic engravings in the text with charming representations of flowering plants against scenic backgrounds of landscapes, gardens, farmhouses, castles, etc. They are printed from the copperplates made some 75 years earlier by Matthäus Merian (1593–1650) in Frankfurt am Main to illustrate the catalogue of the members of the *Fruchtbringende Gesellschaft,* a society founded in 1617, its intention being the fostering of an elegant language which, serving as a model and extending over the entire German-speaking world, would produce results by example and stimulation. Its president was Prince Ludwig of Anhalt-Köthen, who initiated the members, gave them the insignia of the society in the shape of a medallion hung around the neck, assigned to them a characteristic name, and immortalized each new member with a picture of a plant and a stanza in the society's manual, engraved by Merian. A collection of 400 such engravings was published in 1646 under the title of *Der Fruchtbringenden Gesellschaft Nahmen, Vorhaben, Gemählde und Wörter: nach jedes Einnahme ordentlich in Kupfer gestochen, und in achtzeilige Reimgesetze verfasst.* These copperplates were taken over by the new Frankfurt publisher, who after replacing the member's symbolic name with the German and Latin names of the plant, used them to illustrate Valentini's *Viridarium Reformatum.* The separate plates in the

VIRIDARIUM REFORMATUM,

SEU

REGNUM VEGETABILE,

Das ist:

Neu-eingerichtetes und Vollständiges

Kräuter-Buch,

Worinnen auff noch nicht geschehene Weise
Derer Vegetabilien / als Kräutern / Sträuchen /
Bäumen, Bluhmen und anderer Erd-Gewächsen Art,
Krafft und Würckung dergestalt beschrieben werden,
daß man dieses Werck statt einer

BOTANIschen BIBLIOTHEC

haben / jedes Kraut zu seiner rechten Haupt-Art
bringen, auch dessen Nutzen in der Artzney deutlich und umständlich
finden: Uber dem einige besondere, aber bewährte Arcana zur Dämpffung
des Podagras und Vertreibung des Steins, nebst vielen Præparationen
unterschiedlicher zur Medicin dienlichen Dingen antreffen kan;
Denen / so kein Latein können / zu Lieb / auch zum
Besten derer Aertzten, Apotheckern, Materialisten, Laboranten,
Barbierern, Hebammen, Gärtnern, Mahlern
und andern Künstlern,
sonderlich aber allen

Hauß-Vätern und Hauß-Müttern

zum Vortheil Teutsch verfasset;
Denen zu Lieb auch vortreffliche, und durch die Experienz
bewährte Recepte für allerley Kranckheiten, als eine kurtzgefaste
Hauß-Apotheck, beygefüget.
Und endlich denen Liebhabern Göttlicher Wunder
in der Natur ein OPUS MAGO-CABALISTICUM
eines wahrhafften ADEPTI beygefüget und communiciret,
alles übrige aber
Aus denen berühmtesten Botanischen und Medicinischen Schrifften
Alter und Neuer Zeiten, auch selbst-eigener viertzigjähriger Erfahrung
zusammen gebracht, und mit etlich tausend saubern Kupffer-Figuren vorgestellet wird
Von

D. MICH. BERNH. VALENTINI,

Hochfürstl. Hessen-Darmstädtischen Leib-Medico, der Artzney-Kunst ordentlichen Professore zu Giessen, auch Mitglied verschiedener Kayserlichen und Königlichen Societäten der Wissenschafften in Teutschland / Italien / Engelland und Preussen.

Franckfurth am Mayn, gedruckt bey Anton Heinscheidt, 1719.

atlas part were the same used to illustrate Merian's *Florilegium Renovatum* (1641), being an enlarged edition of Johann Theodor de Bry's *Florilegium Novum* (1612), with the plates copied from Pierre Vallet's *Le Jardin de Roy* (1608), Basilius Besler's *Hortus Eystettensis* (1612) and Chrispin van de Passe's *Hortus Floridus* (1614). Other illustrations were copied from woodcuts in Bauhin's German edition of Mattioli's herbal. The Frankfurt publishers apparently had access to a large stock of old copperplates, which came to be of great use in collaboration with the copious writer and compiler Valentini, and resulted in such richly illustrated works.

The artist and engraver of the emblems, Matthäus Merian (1593–1650), was married to the eldest daughter of Johannes de Bry, the famous engraver, publisher and book- and print-seller in Frankfurt am Main. After the death of his father-in-law he took over the business, which remained in the family till 1726, when it came to an end as a result of a fire destroying most of the stock. It was Merian's long series of topographical views that inspired Erik Dahlberg for his *Suecia Antiqua*. Another of De Bry's daughters married William Fitzer, the printer of Harvey's *De motu cordis*. Maria Sibylla Merian, the famous artist of hand-coloured copperplate works on Surinam insects and plants, was a daughter of Matthäus Merian.

Michael Bernhard Valentini was a man of broad interests in natural history and experimental sciences. He was born at Giessen and studied at the university there, obtaining his licence in 1680. In addition to his medical practice he gave private courses in which he tried to imbue others with a love of natural phenomena. In 1683 he was admitted a member of the illustrious *Academia Naturae Curiosorum* and later became editor of their *Ephemerides*. During the 1680s he visisted many German cities and also studied in Holland, England and France, before his appointment to the medical chair at Giessen. Valentini received many honours and distinctions during his life and was a member of many foreign scientific societies. In 1728, the year before his death, he was appointed Imperial Physician, Count of the Holy Roman Empire and Count Palatine. He was the author of numerous papers and academical dissertations and a great compiler, who abstracted or reprinted important texts of others into comprehensive works illustrated with a tremendous amount of engravings, of which his *Museum Museorum* and the above *Viridarium Reformata* are telling examples, with their thousands of illustrations. His celebrated treatise, *Amphitheatrum zootomicum* (1720) is the first extensive work on the comparative anatomy of vertebrates – and his *Corpus juris medico-legale* (1722), a huge storehouse of well-arranged facts, is the first systematic work on forensic medicine. He wrote on the Ipecacuanha (1698), St Ignatius' Bean (1701) and was one of the first in Germany to use the Cinchona Bark (*De China-China*, 1697) as a therapeutical agent.

It was to Valentini that Rudolph Jacob Camerarius in 1694 addressed his *De Sexu Plantarum Epistola* (Letter on the Sex of Plants) containing the first experimental proof that in flowering plants, the anthers are male organs, the ovaries and styles female organs, and that viable seeds cannot be formed without the addition of pollen, an important discovery that was entirely adopted by Linnaeus, who early in life had access to a copy of Valentini's *Polychresta exotica* (1701), in which Camerarius' letter was reprinted.

Ferguson, II, pp. 494-5; Hirsch, V, pp. 693-4; Hunt, 447.

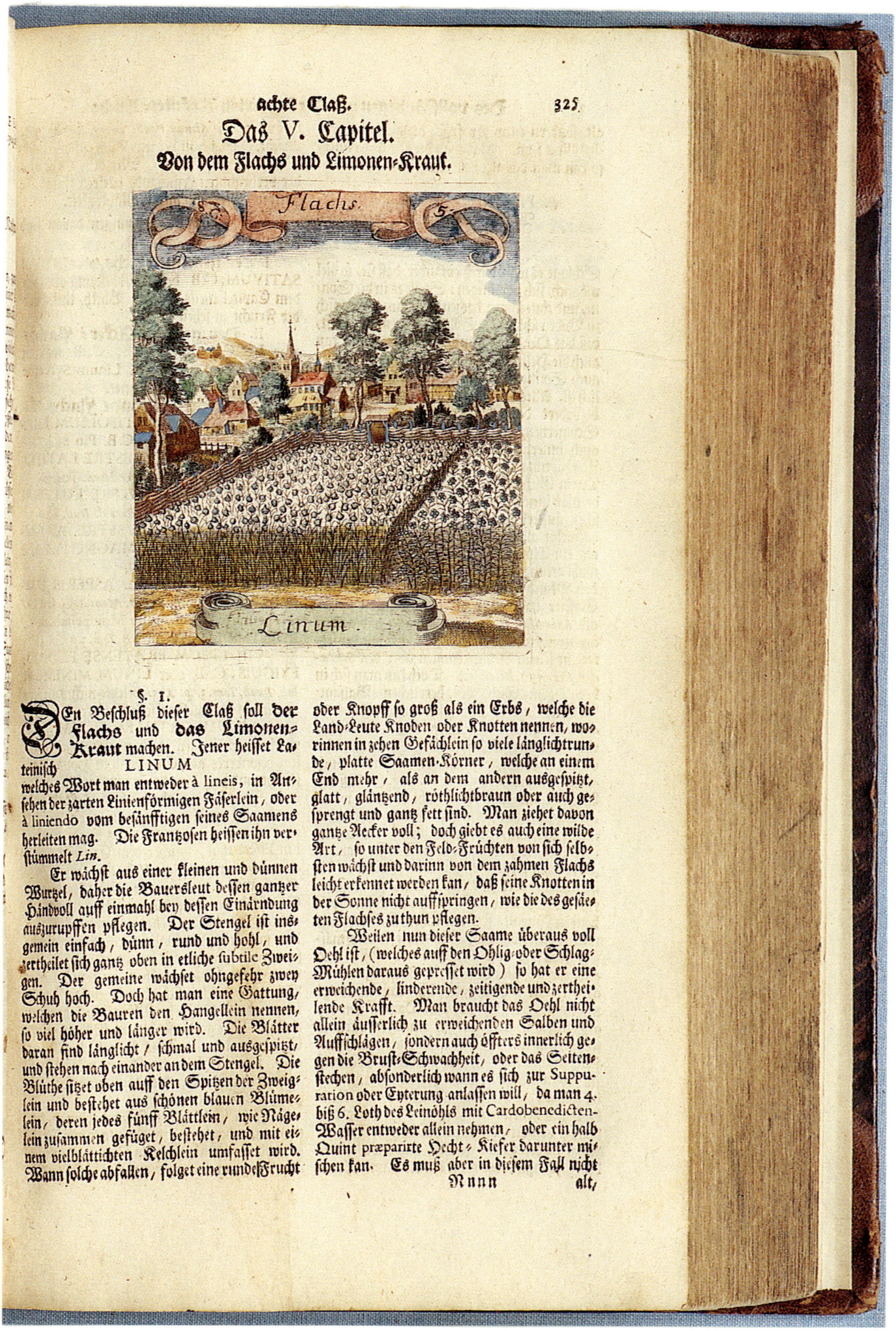
achte Claß. 325

Das V. Capitel.

Von dem Flachs und Limonen-Kraut.

§. 1.

DEn Beschluß dieser Claß soll **der Flachs** und **das Limonen-Kraut** machen. Jener heisset Lateinisch LINUM welches Wort man entweder à lineis, in Ansehen der zarten Linienförmigen Fäserlein, oder à liniendo vom besänfftigen seines Saamens herleiten mag. Die Frantzosen heissen ihn verstümmelt *Lin*.

Er wächst aus einer kleinen und dünnen Wurtzel, daher die Bauersleut dessen gantzer Händvoll auff einmahl bey dessen Einärndung auszurupffen pflegen. Der Stengel ist insgemein einfach, dünn, rund und hohl, und zertheilet sich gantz oben in etliche subtile Zweigen. Der gemeine wächset ohngefehr zwey Schuh hoch. Doch hat man eine Gattung, welchen die Bauren den Hangellein nennen, so viel höher und länger wird. Die Blätter daran sind länglicht / schmal und ausgespitzt, und stehen nach einander an dem Stengel. Die Blüthe sitzet oben auff den Spitzen der Zweiglein und bestehet aus schönen blauen Blümelein, deren jedes fünff Blättlein, wie Nägelein zusammen gefüget, bestehet, und mit einem vielblättichten Kelchlein umfasset wird. Wann solche abfallen, folget eine rundeß Frucht oder Knopff so groß als ein Erbs, welche die Land-Leute Knoden oder Knotten nennen, worinnen in zehen Gefächlein so viele länglichtrunde, platte Saamen-Körner, welche an einem End mehr, als an dem andern ausgespitzt, glatt, gläntzend, röthlichtbraun oder auch gesprengt und gantz fett sind. Man ziehet davon gantze Aecker voll; doch giebt es auch eine wilde Art, so unter den Feld-Früchten von sich selbsten wächst und darinn von dem zahmen Flachs leicht erkennet werden kan, daß seine Knotten in der Sonne nicht auffspringen, wie die des gesäeten Flachses zu thun pflegen.

Weilen nun dieser Saame überaus voll Oehl ist, (welches auff den Ohlig- oder Schlag-Mühlen daraus gepresset wird) so hat er eine erweichende, linderende, zeitigende und zertheilende Krafft. Man braucht das Oehl nicht allein äusserlich zu erweichenden Salben und Auffschlägen, sondern auch öffters innerlich gegen die Brust-Schwachheit, oder das Seitenstechen, absonderlich wann es sich zur Suppuration oder Eyterung anlassen will, da man 4. biß 6. Loth des Leinöhls mit Cardobenedicten-Wasser entweder allein nehmen, oder ein halb Quint præparirte Hecht-Kiefer darunter mischen kan. Es muß aber in diesem Fall nicht

Nnnn alt,

One of Merian's emblematic engravings originally made to illustrate the catalogue of the members of the *Fruchtbringende Gesellschaft* (1646).

FERBER, Johan Eberhard (1678–1761)

One of the rarest works by Linnaeus

Hortus Agerumensis, exhibens Plantas saltem Rariores, Exoticas & Officinales, quas Horto Proprio intulit, secundum Methodum Linnæi Sexualem digestus.
Stockholm, Peter G. Nyström, 1739.

Octavo – *leaf*: 187 *x* 122 *mm. Pp.* [4], 76, [4]. *Original blue paper wrappers.*

Provenance: Johan Arvid Afzelius (1753–1837), *professor of chemistry, metallurgy and pharmacy at the University of Uppsala, and teacher of Berzelius;* Isidor Nordin (1846–1906), *owner of the Lion pharmacy in Stockholm and director of the Royal Pharmacy at Drottningholm (now at Skansen open air museum). Besides books, Nordin had an important collection of matchbox labels.*

First and only edition of this rare catalogue listing the plants in the pharmaceutical garden of J.E. Ferber at Agerum in the south of Sweden, with an appendix listing the specimens in his natural history museum. The book is in fact written by Linnaeus, even though he does not appear as author on the title page. In this work he introduces for the first time his new sexual system of classification in Sweden. This little book is one of the greatest rarities to grace any Linnaeus collection.

In 1711, Johan Eberhard Ferber, apothecary to the Admiralty and to the city of Karlskrona, established a large pharmaceutical garden on his country estate at Agerum, some miles outside Karlskrona. By the time the catalogue was published, this garden had become one of the greatest in Sweden, comparable 'to the Edens of Kings and Princes'. Besides the customary orangeries with exotic fruit trees and ornamental plants and flowers, Ferber had gone to great lengths and great expense to introduce medicinal plants from remote corners of the earth, the whole of which was tended to by the most accomplished gardeners available (two of which were taken over by King Fredrik I after his visit at Agerum). Ferber had also collected specimens from the animal, vegetable and mineral kingdoms in a museum, which Drake calls the first pharmaceutical museum in Sweden. Ferber was renowned among collectors far and wide and made many purchases from his famous colleague Albertus Seba in Amsterdam. At the end of the book is a list with a selection of the museum's contents: seeds, shells, corals, fishes, amphibians, snakes, insects, minerals, fossils, birds of paradise, humming birds, birds' eggs including that of the cassowary, unicorn's horns, bezoar stones, penises from deer and walrus, elephant's tusks, human foetuses, etc. In addition to this listing the museum contained another 600 items.

The book was written in the context of Linnaeus' return from his four-year stay in Holland, where he had been appointed manager of the botanical garden at Hartecamp owned by the wealthy banker George Clifford, for whom Linnaeus compiled the *Hortus Cliffortianus*, the famous catalogue of the exotic plants found there. Linnaeus, who by now had made a name for himself on the Continent, had a wish to publish a similar catalogue of a Swedish garden. He had never seen Ferber's garden, but his old teacher at Växjö, Johan Rothman, had made a first draft of a list of the plants, and now passed the task on to his former pupil in order to accommodate his wishes. The *Hortus Agerumensis* can be said to be a collaboration of Ferber, Rothman and Linnaeus, to which a fourth hand may be added, that of Olof Rudbeck the Younger, who re-read and revised Linnaeus' manuscript before it went to print.

The book opens with a dedication to nine notable persons including Olof Rubeck [*sic*], Rothman and Linnaeus, signed by Ferber, who had paid for the printing. It is followed by a 14-page preface by Rothman with a description of the wonderful garden. The catalogue lists nearly 400 species divided into the 24 classes. At the end is the *Rariora Musei Ferberiani.*

When the book appeared, the garden was at its finest, but when Ferber retired and passed the pharmacy to his son, he grew tired of the large grounds and sold the lot for a mere pittance. In the early 1750s the garden is said to have fallen into decline, hedges and alleys were chopped down and the soil cultivated with tobacco and grain instead of medicinal plants.

Soulsby, 340; Junk Rara, p. 92; Fries, *Linné*, I, pp. 273-4; G. Eriksson, *Botanikens historia i Sverige*, p. 97; Y. Löwegren, *Naturaliekabinett i Sverige under 1700-talet,* pp. 71, 87; Pehr Johnsson, 'Apotekare Ferber i Karlskrona och hans stora trädgård å Agerum', in *Sv. Farm. Tidskr.* 25 (1921), pp. 353-7; Gustaf Drake, 'Medicinalväxterna i Agerums trädgård', in *Sv. Farm. Tidskr.* 25 (1921), pp. 337-42, 358-62,506; Gustaf Drake, 'Apotekare Ferbers museum', in *Sv. Farm. Tidskr.* 26 (1922) pp. 187-8, 198-200, 261-5; Waller 11506.

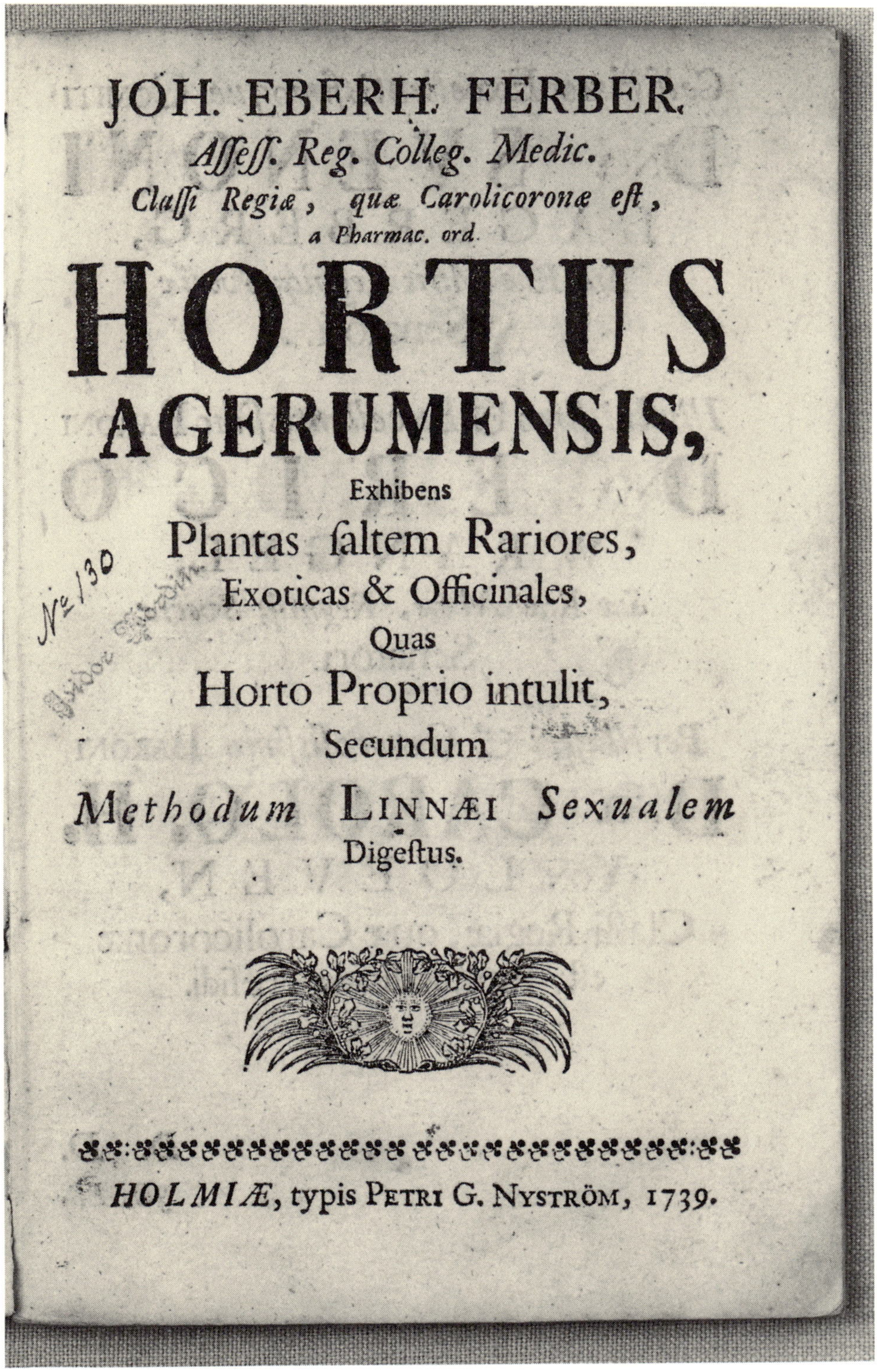
JOH. EBERH. FERBER.

Assess. Reg. Colleg. Medic.

Classi Regiæ, quæ Carolicoronæ est,

a Pharmac. ord.

HORTUS AGERUMENSIS,

Exhibens

Plantas saltem Rariores,

Exoticas & Officinales,

Quas

Horto Proprio intulit,

Secundum

Methodum LINNÆI *Sexualem*

Digestus.

N° 130

HOLMIÆ, typis PETRI G. NYSTRÖM, 1739.

The whole art of the apothecary

ERNSTING, Arthur Conrad (1709–1768)

Nucleus totius medicinae quinque partitus. Pars I. continent Lexicon & Dispensatorium Pharmaceuticum. Oder: Der Volnkommene und allezeit Fertige Apothecker. Darinnen alle und jede Stücke so würcklich in den Apothecken zu finden, ihre Gestalt und Gehalt, Herkunfft, etc. auch was daraus zu machen ist, und wie die Composita auf das beste daraus zu bereiten, erkläret worden sind . . . Pars II. [- V.] . . . Alle diese Theile so wohl aus denen alten als neuern Autoribus (auch Theils aus selbst eigener Erfahrung) mit Mühe und Fleiss colligiret und in solche Ordnung gebracht, . . .
Helmstädt, for Meissner in Braunschweig & Leipzig, 1741.

Quarto – *leaf:* 207 *x* 160 *mm. Pars* I: *pp* [2] *title in red and black,* [8] *dedication to Frederick* II, *King of Prussia, with engraved headpiece,* [32] *preface,* 872, [54] *index*; *Pars* II: *pp.* [8], 314, [14]; Appendix chymica: *pp.* [44], *with one large* [355 *x* 900 *mm*] *folding engraved table*; *Pars* III: *pp.* [8], 320, [24]; *Pars* IV: *pp.* 86, [8]; *Pars* V: [8], 127, [15]. *Engraved portrait of the author in volume* I. *Complete in five parts, bound in two volumes, contemporary calf, richly gilt spine with red title labels.*

Old owner's signature on the title: Peter Nystedt. *Gift from* Mr and Mrs Axel Kockum.

First edition of Ernsting's major and most extensive work. In the absence of a real comprehensive handbook written in the German language, Ernsting compiled his *Nucleus* to serve all those who wanted to learn the whole art of the apothecary, 'aller in der Apothecken vorkommenden Sachen'. The five volumes of nearly 2000 pages must have taken him several years to compile, and are today of the greatest value for the student of the history of pharmacy.

The first part, the *Lexicon Pharmaceuticum*, is separately bound, while the succeeding four parts are bound together in one volume: Part II. *Lexicon Practico-chemicum,* III. *Lexicon Theoretico-Medicum,* IV. *Lexicon Chirurgicum,* and V. *Lexicon Theoretico-Anatomicum.* In his comprehensive preface Ernsting writes that the apprentice will not only find 'ein vollnkommenes *Dispensatorium*, welches bey weiten von keinem andern Buche zu rühmen ist, darinnen auch die allergeheimesten *Compositiones* mit ihren *processen* oder Bereitungen zu finden sind; welche öffters von den Herren Apotheckern so geheim gehalten werden, dass man solche mit ihren *modum præparandi* nur verstohlner weise erhaschen muss, oder es stehet öffters in einem kostbahren Buche, so sie sich nicht anschaffen können, und auch bisweilen nicht verstehen, weil es nehmlich in Lateinischer oder Frantzösichen Sprache etc. geschrieben ist . . .'

At the age of fourteen Arthur Conrad began, like his elder brother, as an apprentice at his father's pharmacy in the small town of Sachsenhagen in Schaumburg. In 1734 he entered the University of Helmstädt to study medicine. After having obtained his M.D. on a dissertation on *Materia perlata* (1737), 'ein zartes, weisses Pulver, durch Aceto aus dem Elixir antimoniale gefällt, das . . . in seinem Glanze den Perlen gleichkommt', [named in various pharmacopoeias as *Magisterium antimoniale diaphoreticum*] he settled in Braunschweig where he practised as physician for fifteen years. In 1739 his *Phellandrologia* appeared, in which the Water Fennel was introduced as a remedy. It had earlier been used only for horses and was popularly called 'Peer-Saat'.

Ernsting's father had died in 1742 and the pharmacy in Sachsenburg was taken over by his elder brother, upon whose death in 1751 Arthur Conrad moved back to his native town and took over the business. In the meantime his brother's widow married an apothecary who received the privilege for the Sachsenburg pharmacy, resulting in Ernsting losing the family business and receiving instead the privilege for the apothecary shop in Hagenburg, where he then moved, bringing his younger brother Johann Conrad to manage the shop while he devoted himself to medical practice and writing. In 1762 he published a botanical work in two volumes with copperplates, *Historische und physikalische Beschreibung der Geschlechter der Pflanzen, welcher Hrn. Linnäus systematisches Verzeichnis von den Geschlechtern der Pflanzen beigefüget worden.* (Lemgo, 1762). Ernsting died at Hagenburg in 1768.

Paul Haarbeck, *Arthur Conrad Ernsting. Ein Apotheker und Arzt des Barock.* (Veröffentlichungen der Internationalen Gesellschaft für Geschichte der Pharmazie, Neue Folge, Band 3, 1953.)

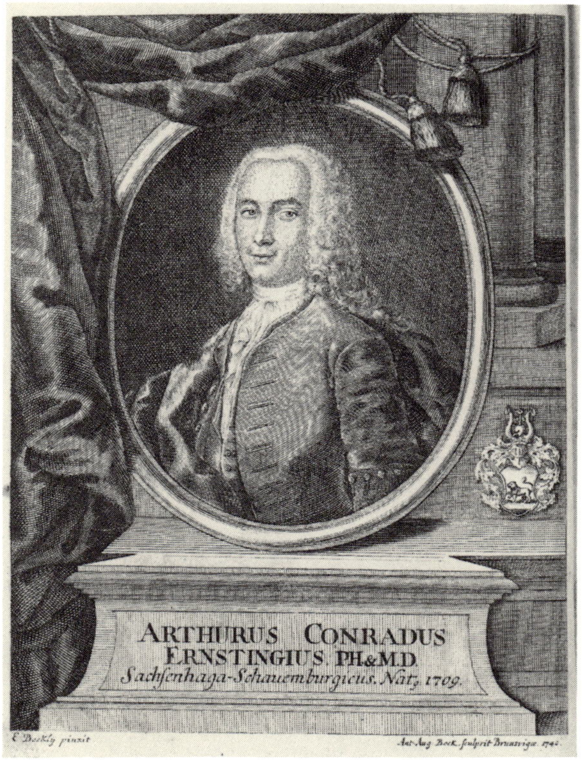

NVCLEVS TOTIVS MEDICINAE
QVINQVE PARTITVS.
PARS I. CONTINET
LEXICON & DISPENSATORIVM
PHARMACEVTICVM.
Oder: Der
Volnkommene und allezeit Fertige
Apothecker.

Darinnen alle und jede Stücke so würcklich in den Apothecken zu finden/ ihre Gestalt und Gehalt/ Herkunfft ꝛc. auch was daraus zu machen ist/ und wie die Composita auf das beste daraus zu bereiten, erkläret worden sind. Dabey auch nach dem Alphabeth die Kunst-Wörter und vielen andern Beynahmen mehr folgen. ꝛc.

PARS II. CONTINET
Lexicon Practico-Chymicum, oder der richtig führende Chymiste. Cum Appendice Brevi loquus Chymicus, oder der kurze Chymische Redner genannt, darinnen alles so zur Chymie gehöret, zu finden ist.

PARS III. CONTINET
Lexicon Theoretico-Medicum, oder der zur Heilungs Gelahrheit leitende Artzt ꝛc. welcher die Medicinischen Kunst-Wörter und was sonsten dazu gehöret, erkläret.

PARS IV. EST
Lexicon Chyrurgicum, ein Chyrurgisches Wörter-Buch.

PARS V. SISTIT
Lexicon Theoretico-Anatomicum, oder der sich selbst erkennende Mensche.

Alle diese Theile so wohl aus denen alten als neuern Autoribus (auch Theils aus selbst eigener Erfahrung/) mit Mühe und Fleiß colligiret und in solche Ordnung gebracht,
Auch jedweden Theil mit einem Deutschen Register versehen;
Damit jedweder die Nahmens, auch was sonsten in der gantzen Medicin vorfällt, gleich darinnen finden und nützlich gebrauchen kan.
Herausgegeben durch
ARTHVRVM CONRADVM ERNSTINGIVM
Ph. & Med. D. & Pr. Brunsvic.

Gedruckt Helmstädt 1741.
Zu finden Braunschweig und Leipzig in Meißnerischen Buchladen.

A famous Swedish provincial apothecary

AKEN, Frantz Michael (d. 1760)

Hus- och Rese-Apotheque, huru man sin hälsa rätt skjöta, och the rätta approberade medel, uti ett hushåll, bruka skal, . . .
Skara, Herman Arnold Möller, 1746.

Octavo – *leaf:* 165 *x* 100 *mm. Pp.* [14], 15-368, [24]. *Title printed in red and black. Copies exist with an extra inserted errata leaf at the end, which is missing here. Contemporary calf, gilt spine, gilt edges.*

From the C.D. Carlsson Collection.

First edition of a popular 'House- and Travel Apotheque' divided into six parts. The first gives some infallible household remedies, the third deals with coffee, tea, chocolate, beer, spirits, tobacco and spas. The fourth part has dietary rules for the sick, the fifth deals with child care.

The second part is of special interest as it is a Swedish translation by L[ars] B[ælter] of Rosén von Rosenstein's dissertation *De compositione medicamentorum Hallensium* (1739), for which Peter Lundberg was respondent. There was much discussion on the balsamic purgatives of Halle, especially the pills prepared there by the famous professor of medicine Johannes Juncker. Halle was the main centre of the Stahlian school and the Stahlians considered that nature itself cured all diseases and doubted the efficacy of strong drugs like opium and quinine, but favoured copious blood-letting and mild purgatives. In this paper, *Academiskt Prof, om the Halliska Läkedomars Tilredelse samt Theras Sanna och Inskränkta Nytto*, Rosén agrees that these medicines of Halle can be of certain value but is critical of their extreme cost. These medicaments of Halle which, in spite of being forbidden to import, were offered for sale in many Swedish towns, and were so highly commended in an accompanying booklet by Christian Friedrich Richter of Halle 'that anyone inexperienced in the Art of Medicine could easily believe that they were endowed with a hidden Divine power, and a panacea for all diseases'. – 'med så öfwerflödande beröm alt in til himmelen upphöijer sina Läkemedel, hwilka han i så högt prijs til salu utropar, at en uti Läkare-Konsten oförfaren skulle lätteligen komma på the tankar, at uti them låge en aldeles Gudomelig kraft förborgad, til at fördrifwa allahanda krankheter. Thesse wahror lemnades, såsom och nu för tiden skier, icke allenast åt Apothekare at försäljas, utan och åt Kiöpmän, som togo dubbelt werde af them'. This Swedish translation of Rosén's dissertation on the pills from Halle was first published in 1744 but is here reprinted by the business-minded apothecary in his 'House and Travel Apotheque'.

The sixth and concluding part concerns the extermination of vermin and pests, including crickets and finches, who occasionally stole grains of wheat. This part, which also deals with wolf-pits and how to catch ravens, moles, hawks, owls, eagles, etc, appeared separately in 1747 with the title *Hus- och Land-Apotheque.*

Frantz Michael von Aken was born in Rostock in Swedish Pomeriana and arrived in 1723 to Sweden, where he purchased the famous apothecary shop *Hjorten* (The Deer) in Örebro and soon acquired the title of both court apothecary and court physician. He also received the special privilege of having the monopoly on all pharmacies in all the towns in the provinces of Närke and Värmland.

Aken was said to be knowledgeable and his shop was always well stocked. Besides his ordinary profession he dedicated himself to inventions. In his domestic travel books Linnaeus claims to have seen designs of von Akens hawk- and sparrow-traps.

Von Aken was succeeded by his son, Frantz Joachim von Aken, who made himself famous for several inventions, on which he published numerous pamphlets which caused him to be involved in polemics with competitors. Especially famous were his fireworks and the so-called Aken's 'Fire Extinguishing Substance', demonstrated for the king, an event immortalized in a large copper engraving in one of his advertisements.

Hebbe, I, 1724; Schreber, 5; Anna-Lena Pehrsson, 'Nils Rosén von Rosenstein and iatromechanics', in: *Acta Pædiatrica, Supplement,* 156; Ingrid Odelstierna, 'Curant exspectando' in *Svenska Linné-Sällskapets Årsskrift,* XLIII, 1960, pp. 45 ff. The reprint of Rosén's dissertation in Aken's book has escaped the notice of Dintler in his bibliography of Rosén von Rosenstein; Waller 252.

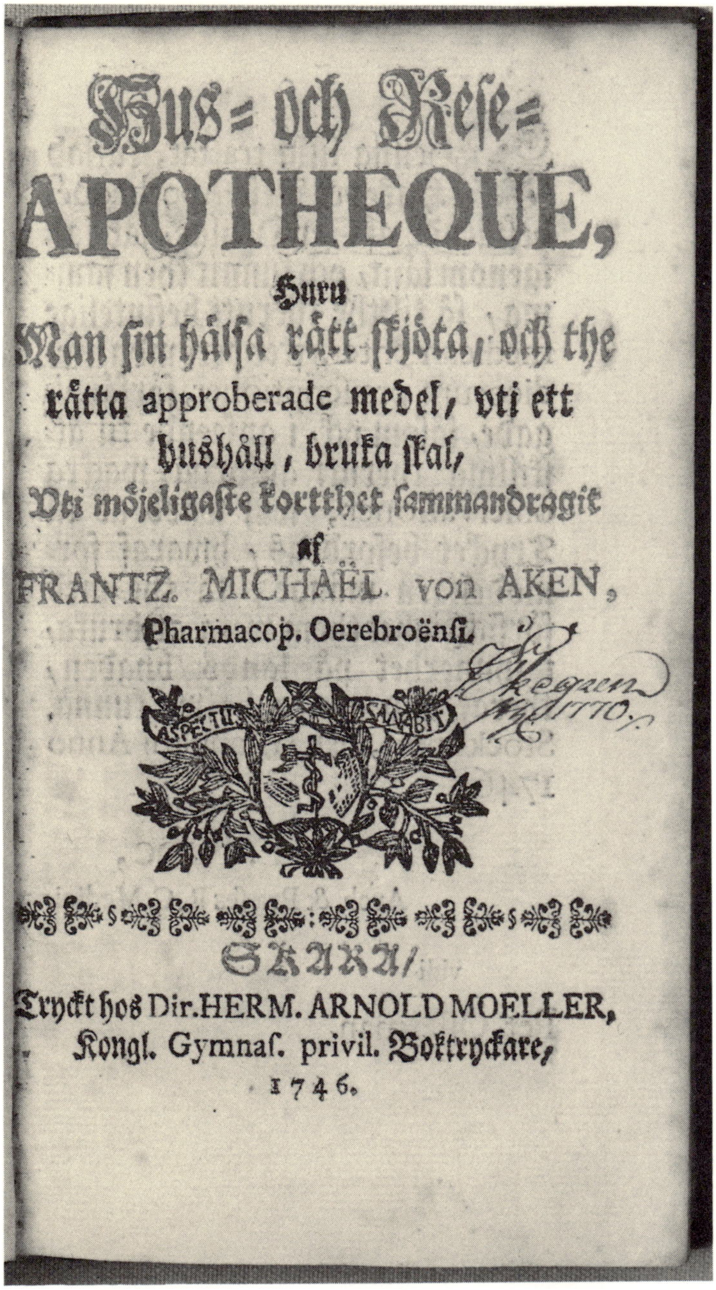
Hus= och Rese=
APOTHEQUE,
Huru
Man sin hälsa rätt skiöta, och the
rätta approberade medel, uti ett
hushåll, bruka skal,
Uti möjeligaste kortthet sammandragit
af
FRANTZ. MICHAËL von AKEN,
Pharmacop. Oerebroënsi.

SKARA/
Tryckt hos Dir. HERM. ARNOLD MOELLER,
Kongl. Gymnas. privil. Boktryckare,
1746.

A classic of pharmacological work in world literature

LINNAEUS, Carl (1707–1778)

Materia Medica, Liber I. De Plantis.
Stockholm, Lars Salvius, 1749.

Octavo – *leaf*: 200 x 123 *mm. Pp.* [32], 252. *Frontispiece and one folding plate.* (Serpentum Radix), *engraved by Carl Bergqvist after Johan Gustaf Hallman. Contemporary half calf, worn.*

The first edition of this classic work within pharmacological literature. It covers the vegetable kingdom only, Liber I. *De Plantis*, the animal and mineral kingdoms appearing as academic dissertations: *Materia Medica in Regno Animalium,* resp. Jonas Sidrén (1750) and *Materia Medico in Regno Lapideo*, resp. Johan Lindhult (1752). That was all published by Linnaeus himself. Pulteney says 'it is only to be lamented that he did not republish it, with all the improvements which many subsequent years of observation enabled him to make, and which are actually shown to have been numerous and important by the many notes inserted with his own hand in the printed copy that belonged to his own library'. The *Materia Medica* was in its day an invaluable reference work for pharmacists and doctors. The great Albrecht von Haller held it to be one of the best works of Linnaeus.

In 1772 a second edition (editio altera) appeared, including also animals and minerals but now edited and published in Leipzig & Erlangen by Johann Christian Daniel Schreber (1739–1810). He was one of Linnaeus' German pupils who in 1760 had received his M.D. at Uppsala and upon his return to Germany was appointed professor of medicine and natural history. Schreber's edition had, however, been preceded by a small twelvemo edition edited by Ludovici Tessari, published in Venice in 1762 (Soulsby, *Addenda*, 968a). Schreber published two more editions, the last one, *editio quinta*, of 1787, was dedicated to Carl Peter Thunberg. It was increased to 384 pages with many additions by Schreber from notes made after Linnaeus' lectures on *materia medica,* and was the one on which the works on *materia medica* by Peter Jonas Bergius, William Cullen, Johan Anders Murray and several others were mainly based.

The *Materia Medica* of 1749 contains the Linnaean names of 535 medicinal plants, several of which are for the first time reduced to their proper genera and species, followed by the synonym in Bauhin's *Pinax*, or if the plant was unknown to Bauhin, the synonym of the first discoverer. This is followed by LOC., the country of origin, if it is a herb, shrub or tree, whether it be annual, biennal, or perennial, and also whether it be indigenous, or, if not, whether it may thrive well by common cultivation in gardens, or require defense from the cold of the winter in Sweden; PHARM., the Swedish officinal name, what parts are used, and the doses adminstered; OUAL., the taste and smell of the plant, whether bitter, aromatic, acid, etc. whether uncertain, well known, and approved, or whether to be cautiously used; VIS., its reputed effects on the human body; USUS., the diseases for which it is most frequently prescribed; COMP., the composed medicines into which it enters in the Swedish pharmacopeia.

Linnaeus also gives instructions as to the proper time and mode of collecting simples. He recommended the choice, as far as possible, of native plants, not only as they were cheaper but also because they were more likely to be fresh and unadulterated. At the end are several indices including an *index morborum,* with the simples appropriate to each disease, and an *index virium* adapted to Linnaeus' classification of medicines, founded on their reputed effects and divided into six classes, and indices of the officinal and of the botanical names. An English translation of Linnaeus' vegetable *Materia Medica* (1749) appeared as volume 2 of Charles Whitlaw's *New Medical Discoveries* (London, 1829).

Hjelt states that it is the merit of Linnaeus to have laid the foundation of the independent development and arrangement of pharmacodynamics, the branch of pharmacology concerned with the action of drugs on the physiology of the body, a favourite subject for Linnaeus during his entire life.

Soulsby, 968; Krok, 98; *Tax. Lit.*, 4751; Pulteney, 2nd ed., (1805), pp. 94-101; Otto E.A.Hjelt, *Carl von Linné som läkare och medicinsk författare* (1907), pp. 98-115; Waller 5907.

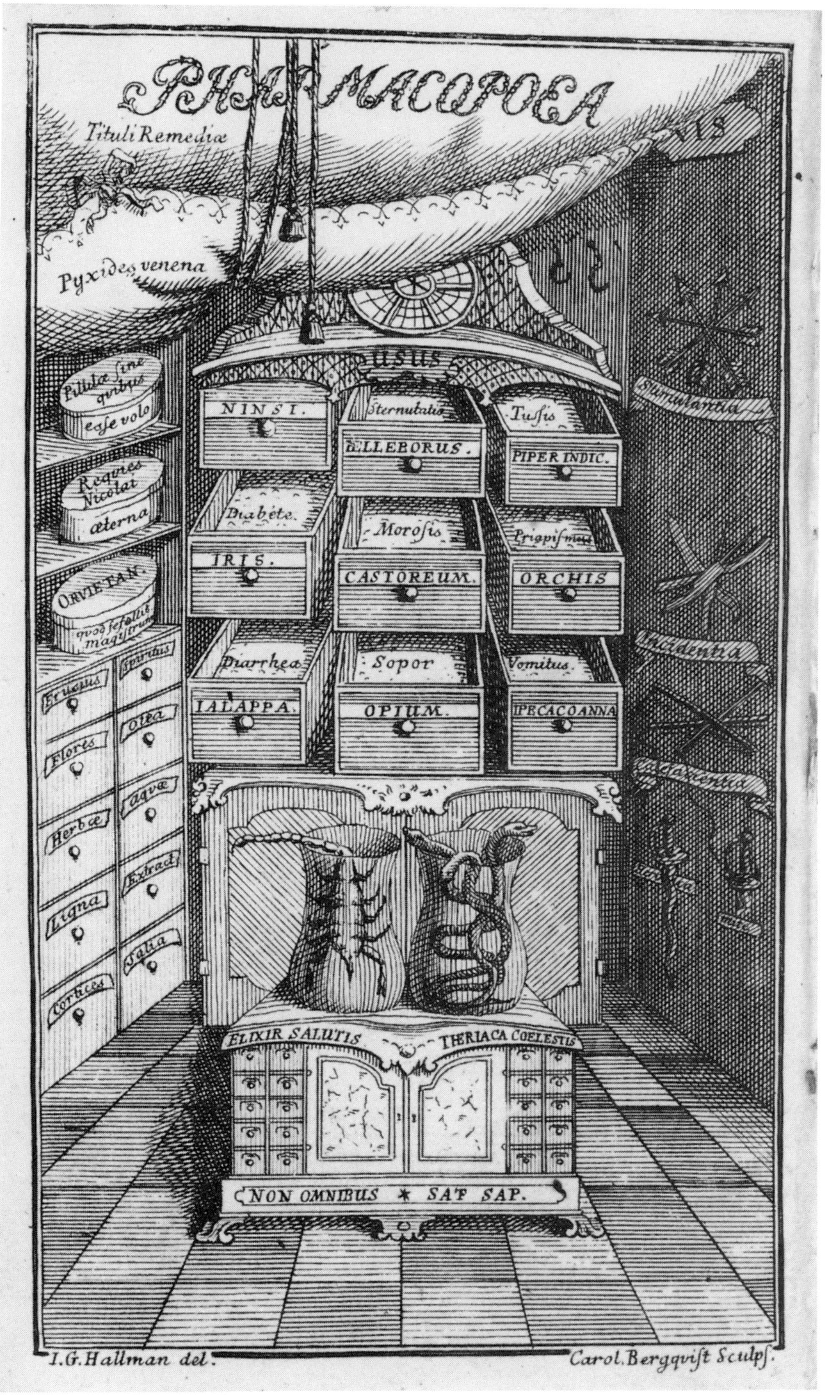

The engraved frontispiece, showing the equipment in a pharmacy with cabinet and medicine chests, two glass vases, one with a giant scorpion, the other with snakes, is drawn by Johan Gustaf Hallman, a pupil of Linnaeus, who in the same year as the book appeared was sent to study abroad. He stayed away for five years and visited Vienna, Paris and the main medical centres in Italy. During the course of his travels, he met many famous men such as Voltaire. In his youth he was a most talented draughtsman often engaged by Linnaeus and the Academy of Sciences to draw natural history objects.

Dr. Trew's edition of Mrs Blackwell's Curious Herbal

BLACKWELL, Elizabeth (c.1700–1758)

Herbarium Blackwellianum . . . / Vermehrtes und verbessertes Blackwellisches Kräuter-Buch das ist Elisabeth Blackwell Sammlung der Gewächse die zum Artzney-Gebrauch in den Apothecken aufbehalten werden, deren Beschreibung und Kräfften aus dem Englischen übersetzt angezeiget die Abbildungen grossen Theils nach der Natur verbessert mit Beyfügung der Theile der Blume und Frucht vermehret wie auch mit bewährten Namen der Kräuter-Lehrer erläutert werden. Mit einer Vorrede Christoph Jacob Trews [*and Christian Gottlieb Ludwig, in vol.* VI]. Verlegt gemahlet und in Kupfer gestochen von Nicolaus Friedrich Eisenberger. *In Six Volumes.*

Nürnberg, Christian de Launoy [vols. I-IV], the heirs of C. de Launoy [vol. V] and Johann Joseph Fleischmann [vol. VI], 1757 [1747]–1773.

Folio – *leaf*: 370 x 240 *mm. Text*: *vol.* I [1757]: *pp.*[4] *titles,* [14] *preface,* [54] Catalogus Auctorum, [64] *expl. of the plates*; *vol.* II [1754]: *pp.* [4] *titles, pp.* 54-80 (Catalogus Auctorum), [84] *expl. of the plates,* [4] *index*; *vol.* III [1757] *pp.* [4] *titles,* [4] *preface,* [82] *expl. of the plates,* [6] *index*; *vol.* IV [1760]: *pp* [4] *titles,* [4] *preface,* [84] *expl. of the plates,* [4] *index*; *vol.* V [1765]: *pp.* [4] *titles,* [4] *preface,* [70] *expl. of the plates,* [6] *index*; *vol.* VI [1773]: *pp.* [4], *titles,* [4] *preface,* [64] *expl. of the plates,* [14] *index.* Atlas: *Engraved title to vols.* I-II, *plates* 1-200; *engraved title to vols.* III-IV, *plates* 201-400; *engraved title to vols.* V-VI, *plates* 401-600. *There are two plates* (a *and* b) *issued for Nos.* 269, 322, 341, 497, 498, 522, 523, 533, 536, 539, 547, 573 *and* 600; *three plates* (a, b *and* c) *are issued for No.* 574. *This makes a total of* 615 *plates. The engraved title pages and all the plates are hand-coloured. Six volumes bound in four, modern cloth, gilt spine with green morocco spine lables, red edges.*

This comprehensive German work on pharmaceutical plants, illustrated with 615 hand-coloured plates, is a greatly superior version of Mrs Blackwell's *A Curious Herbal*, originally published in London, 1737-39. The *Herbarium Blackwellianum* was published on the initiative of the famous physician Christoph Jacob Trew (1695–1769), whose versatility as a scholar, promotor of natural history iconography, and collector of natural objects was outstanding in the Germany of his time. His library of 35 000 volumes was donated to the University of Altdorf (later Erlangen). By giving support, scientific instruction and financial aid to a fine team of local artists and engravers, he made Nürnberg one of the most important centres of botanical art. One of his discoveries was Georg Dionysius Ehret, flower painter extraordinary, who inaugurated 'The Golden Age of Botanical Art'.

The publication of the *Herbarium Blackwellianum* started in 1747 by the painter N.F. Eisenberger on a subscription basis, the work being issued in instalments up to 1773. The above copy is one of the sets sold complete, with the title page of the first 'century' reprinted with the date 1757, as distinct from subscription copies. Trew wrote the lengthy text for the first 90 plates, a text provided in addition to a translation of the brief notes in Blackwell's *A Curious Herbal.* Thereafter the text was written mainly by Georg Rudolph Böhmer and Ernst Gottlob Bose under the supervision of the botanist Christian Gottlieb Ludwig, whose *Ectypa vegetabilium* is described on pp.182-5 in the present catalogue. The plates are drawn and engraved by Nicolaus Friedrich Eisenberger. The first 500 are copied from Blackwell's plates, but are much more carefully drawn, engraved and coloured, and have alterations and additional details of flower parts, fruits, etc. The last 100 plates are entirely original. All the plants depicted are those used in pharmacy, except for some poisonous and ornamental plants in the last 'century'.

The story of Elizabeth Blackwell and her *Curious Herbal* is 'a drama of heroism, intrigue and torture which seems strangely out of place in the sober chronicles of botanical illustration' (Blunt/Stearn). Her husband, Alexander Blackwell, a native of Aberdeen, was an adventurer, whose career is enveloped in mystery and contradiction. Some sources say he studied medicine and even was apprentice to an apothecary, and that he travelled extensively in Europe. He seems, however, never to have taken any degree. According to one biographer, Alexander secretly married his second cousin

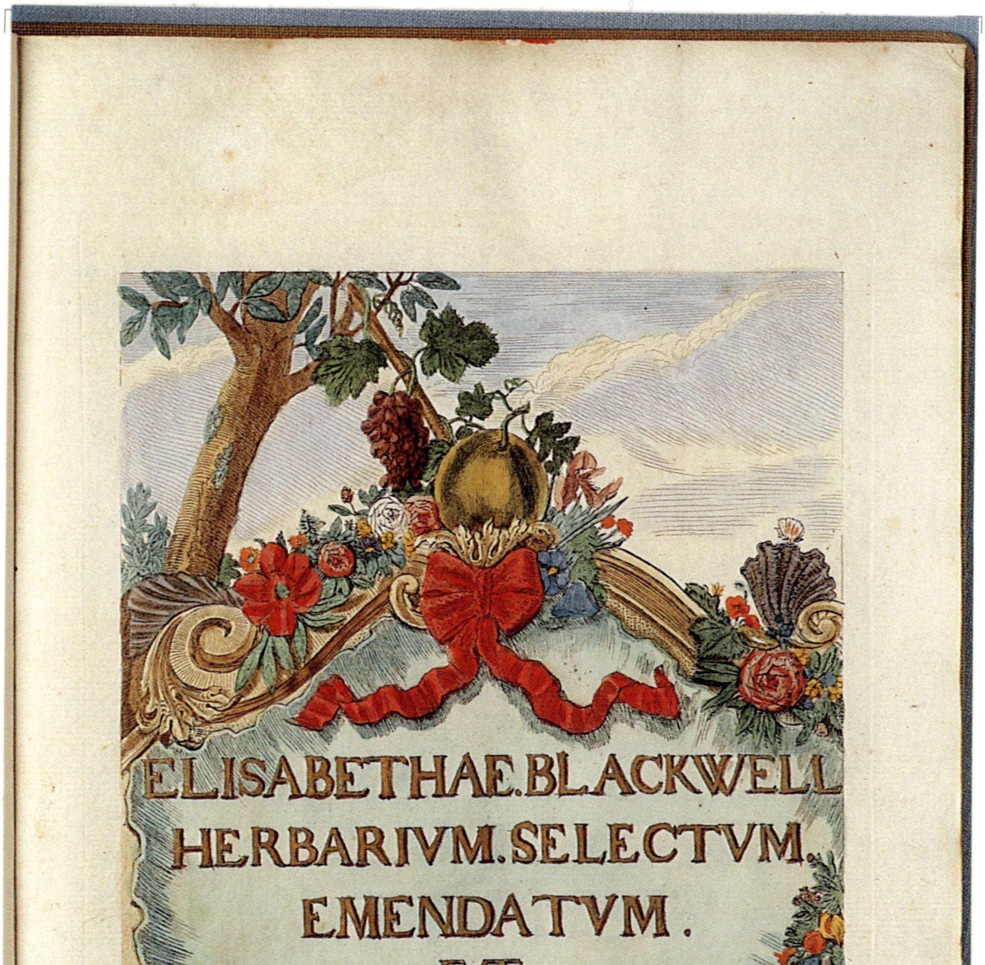
ELISABETHAE. BLACKWELL
HERBARIVM. SELECTVM.
EMENDATVM.
ET.
AVCTVM.
CENTVRIÆ.
III·IV

Elisabeth Blachrie, the daughter of a wealthy stocking merchant, before completing his studies. The young couple went to the metropolis of London to seek their fortune, where Alexander was employed as a corrector of the press of a London printer. In 1730 he set up as a printer on his own account.

He had not been long in business before action was brought against him for not having received an apprenticeship to the trade. The jury found him guilty. Blackwell was caught up in debt, became bankrupt in 1734 and condemned to a debtor's prison, where he might have languished indefinitely had his talented wife not come to his rescue. Learning that a herbal of medicinal plates was much needed, Elizabeth Blackwell started a grand enterprise in an attempt to free her ruined husband from financial embarrassment. She received great encouragement from various members of the Society of Apothecaries, and on the advice of Isaac Rand took a house opposite the Botanical Garden at Chelsea, 'whereby she had the opportunity of receiving the plants and flowers fresh out of the garden' to have them delineated. After finishing the drawings, Elizabeth engraved them herself on copper and coloured all the prints herself by hand. The complete work, illustrated with 500 plates, was published in two volumes in 1737 and 1739 respectively. Alexander Blackwell had assisted his wife in the compilation of the text from his prison cell.

As a monument of marital devotion, the *Curious Herbal* is a most touching and admirable work. It was reissued several times, the last time as late as in 1782. A much inferior pirated edition of the work was also begun, but only the first fascicule was issued before legal action stopped further publication. Its practical value was apparently great and its merits received the most substantial recognition from the fine, enlarged and superior republication undertaken by Doctor Trew in Nürnberg.

The *Curious Herbal* was issued to subscribers in weekly parts, each consisting of four engraved plates and an engraved page of text. The plates were available either plain or coloured and on large paper if required. On September 28, 1737, by which date 320 copperplates with figures of plants and 80 with descriptive text had been engraved, Alexander Blackwell, with the consent of his wife Elizabeth, sold a third share of the herbal to the publisher, John Nourse, for a sum of £150. Later on, in 1740, the Blackwells sold a further sixth share of the copyright to Nourse, and in 1745, Alexander Blackwell, then residing in Sweden, granted his wife, who lived in a parish in Middlesex, power of attorney to act for him in his business dealings with Nourse.

After Alexander Blackwell was released from prison, he obtained employment as director of improvements in the service of the Duke of Chandos, who at the time was planning the grounds of his splendid mansion. But in 1742 Blackwell turned up in Sweden. Here he represented himself as a physician, prescribed successfully to the king, and was actually appointed one of the physicians-in-ordinary to King Fredrik I, but was soon suspected to be a quack. In 1745 he published *Försök til Landtbrukets bättring i Sverige* ('An Essay on the Improvement of Swedish Agriculture'), which in fact is a translation, almost word for word, of J. Tull's *The Horse-hoeing Husbandry* (London, 1733). He had been entrusted with the direction of a model farm at the Royal manor of Ållestad in Västergötland, where he was well-received by Jonas Alströmer. Linnaeus visited Blackwell at Ållestad in July, 1746, but was only modestly impressed. Soon Blackwell's methods were severely criticized and the precariousness of his appointment may perhaps have driven him to engage in political intrigue. He eventually became involved in a conspiracy to alter the Swedish succession, and tried to bribe the king with 100 000 pound sterling, a sum said to be guaranteed by the Danish queen. Alexander Blackwell was arrested, charged with high treason, and condemned to be variously tortured, broken alive on the wheel, and finally decapitated in Stockholm on the 27th of July, 1747.

The fate of Elizabeth Blackwell, who did not accompany her husband to Sweden, is unknown. She died in 1758 and was buried in the churchyard of Chelsea Old church.

Henrey II, pp.228-36; *Tax. Lit.* 546; Blunt & Stearn, pp. 151-3; Johnston, *Cleveland Herbals*, 444; *Great Flower Books*, p. 50; Dunthorne, 43; Nissen, BBI, 169; Lisney, pp. 114-15; Birger Strandell, 'Alexander Blackwell, Fredrik I:s livmedikus, Ett läkaröde', in *Svenska Läkaretidningen*, 48 (1940); Erik Naumann in SBL, IV, pp. 730-4; DNB, II pp. 604-06; Schnalke, Thomas, *Natur im Bild.* (1995), No. 141, pp. 117-21.

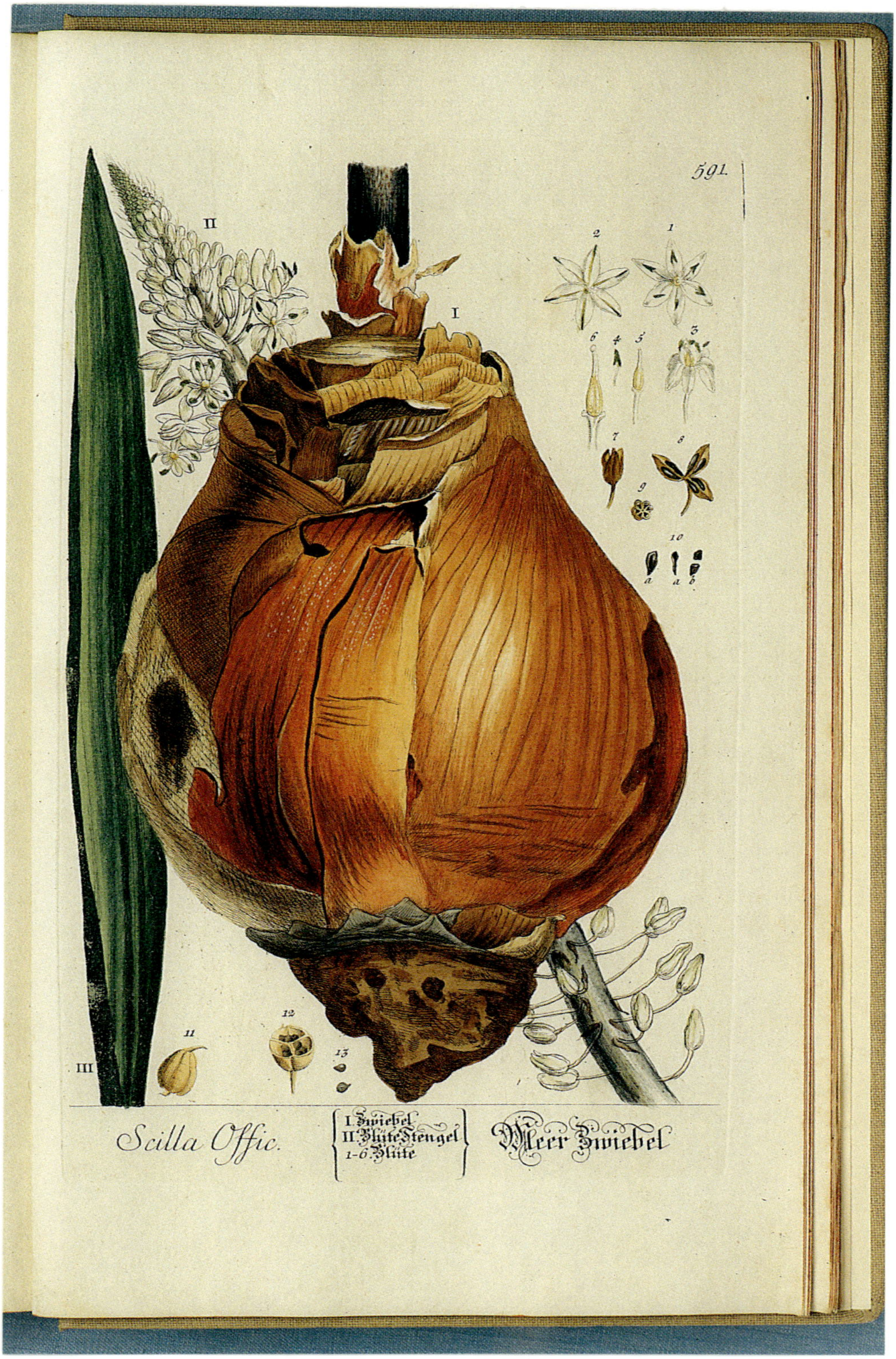

Radix Scillae (Swedish: *Sjölök*) is one of the most ancient of medicines. In Egypt a temple was built for the bulb, which was given the name of the 'eye of Typhon' (the god of Evil). Pythagoras' chief contribution to pharmacy was the invention of *acetum scillae*. It was well known to the ancient Greek physicians and Pliny wrote a treatise on squills, which he believed possessed magic virtues. Dioscorides describes how to make vinegar of squills, and the ancient Arabian physicians administered compounds of squill with honey.

A classic manual for pharmacists

BAUMÉ, Antoine (1728–1804)

Élémens de Pharmacie theorique et pratique: contenant toutes les Opérations fondamentales de cet Art, avec leur définition, & une Explication deces Opérations, par les Principes de la Chymie; La maniere de bien choisir, de prépater, & de mêler les Médicamens, avec des Remarques & des Réflexions sur chaque procédé; Les Moyens de reconnoîtres les Médicamens falsifiés ou altérés; Les Recettes des Médicamens nouvellement mis en usage; Les Principes fondamentaux plusieurs Arts dépendans de la Pharmacie: tels que l'Art du Confiseur, & ceux de la préparation des Eaux de Senteur & des Liqueurs de Table. Avec une Table des Vertus & Doses des Médicamens.

Paris, P. F. Didot, le jeune, (and others), 1762.

Octavo – *leaf:* 196 *x* 124 *mm. Pp.* XVI, 853, [3] *addenda & errata, pp.*1-4 *(publisher's catalogue of P.F. Didot). Two engraved plates, one facing p.*80 *(furnace and distillation apparatus) and one facing p.* 560 *(pill-making device). Fine contemporary half calf, richly gilt spine with raised bands, red spine label, sprinkled boards.*

Antoine Baumé is one of the important French apothecary-chemists of the eighteenth century who simultaneoulsy enriched pharmacy and chemistry. At the age of fifteen he was apprenticed to a pharmacist in Compiègne, and by 1745 he was a pupil of C. J. Geoffroy in his dispensary in Paris, soon becoming master apothecary and demonstrator in chemistry. At the age of twenty-five he was appointed to the Chair of Chemistry at the College of Pharmacy and opened his own shop in 1753.

Baumé established a manufacturing laboratory, making sal ammoniac, red precipitate, tin and mercury chlorides, sugar of lead, and many other chemicals and galenicals on a large scale. He was an authority on perfumes and liquors. In 1777 he won the first prize for an essay on the furnaces, alembics, and other apparatus to be used in the distillation of wine. He also invented processes for gilding clocks, dyeing in two colours, bleaching silk, and removing the bitter principle from horse chestnut starch. His name is still familiar in connection with his aerometer or hydrometer, with which it became possible to make an easy and fairly exact determination of the density (specific gravity) of liquids. Baumé's scale is till used in technology. In his large-scale drug manufacturing Baumé offered some 2000 preparations, of which about 400 were chemicals, produced in his laboratories.

In 1757, Baumé together with Macquer began a series of courses in chemistry and pharmacy that continued for sixteen years. During that time they are said to have given sixteen complete courses, each of which was illustrated with more than two thousand experiments. These lectures were attended by hundreds of students, some of whom later became famous in chemistry. During the Revolution Baumé lost his fortune, including his pension as a member of the Academy, but in 1795, as a result of an appeal to the Committee of Public Instructions, he received a sum of money that enabled him to open another dispensary in 1796.

Baumé's *Élémens de Pharmacie* is a classic textbook in the history of pharmacy. It was first published in 1762 and became very popular and went through at least nine French editions plus several pirated reprints, as well as translations into Spanish and Italian. It is a well-ordered, complete and useful manual for the pharmacist. It gives a clear exposition of all related processes, details as to gathering and preparing plant materials and describes pharmaceutical apparatus and procedures, and it also includes a review of the work that had been done to date in pharmaceutical chemistry. Our library has, besides the first edition, also the eighth edition of 1797 (*An* V). The preface to the 1797 edition says: 'La premiére édition de ces Élémens a essuyé des censures trés-vives. C'est le sort de tous les écrits sur les Sciences'. In consequence Baumé had removed polemical matter.

René Davy, *L'apothicaire Antoine Baumé* (1955); E. McDonald in DSB, I, p. 527; Cole, *Chemical Literature* 1700–1820, No. 52; Kremer & Urdang, pp. 344, 398; Partington, III, pp. 90-5; Cowan & Helfand, pp. 112-13, 161; Schelenz, p. 563; LaWall, pp. 365-6.

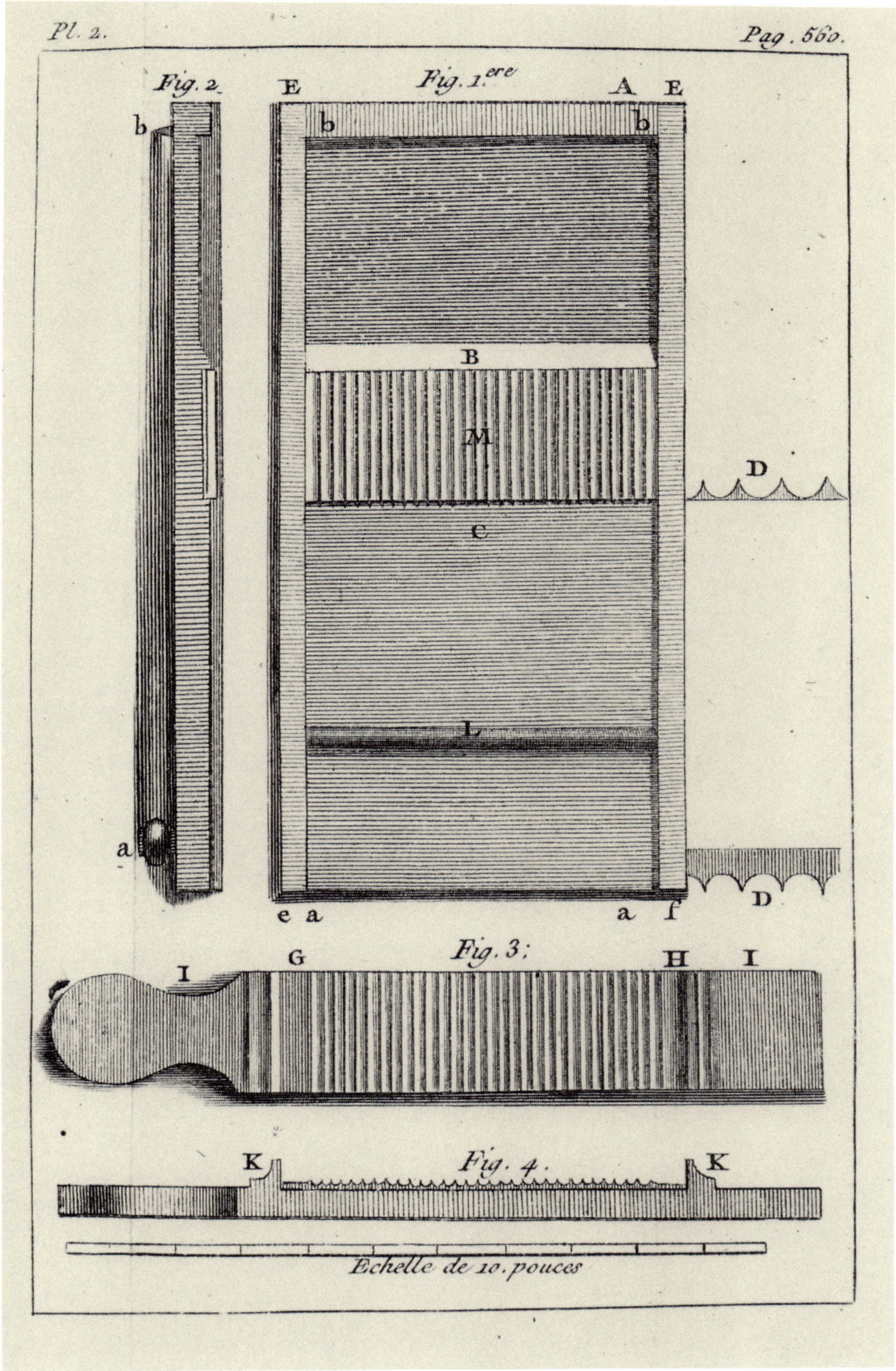

One of the two engraved plates in the first edition of Baumé's *Élémens de Pharmacie*.
It is the first plate in a book to show pill-making equipment.

Scheele's brother's recipe book from the Unicorn apothecary shop

SCHEELE, Johann Martin (1734–1754)

Laboratio Medicamentorum quae sunt usuales in Pharmacopoea Civitatis Gotaburgensi scripsi Anno 1748. – Catalogus medicamentorum & aliarum rerum quae Indiae Orientalis cistae sunt. Gothenburg, c. 1748–1754.

Quarto – *leaf*: 210 x 170 *mm. Manuscript of* 105 *leaves. First leaf with J.M. Scheele's name and date:* Johann Martien [*sic*] Scheele Gothenburg 1 Martio 1748, *verso blank.* Laboratio Medicamentorum: *pp.* 1-38, 41-194 (*lacks one leaf, pp.* 39-40); Catalogus medicamentorum . . . Indiae Orientalis: *pp.* 195-8; *Index*: *pp.* [199-210] *lacking the final leaf* (*or leaves*); *in the alphabetical index the text ends in the middle of the listing of syrups.*

Original leather-backed boards. Sides covered with decorative paper block-printed in blue and black on white paper in a design with interlinked hexagons (honeycomb), each containing an oak-leaf set in a triangular shape.

This interesting manuscript is of particular value for the Scheele researcher. It not only gives an accurate and complete picture of pharmaceutical practise in the mid-18th century, but also illustrates what Johann Martin's younger brother, Carl Wilhelm, the budding chemical genius, had to learn in his beginnings as an apprentice in the apothecary shop of the Unicorn in Gothenburg.

Johann Martin was the eldest brother of Carl Wilhelm Scheele. He was born at Stralsund, Swedish Pomeriana, on the 14th of February, 1734. As a young boy of about 14 he went to Gothenburg as an apprentice to the apothecary Martin Bausch in his shop under the sign of the Unicorn. Shortly after the completion of his apprenticeship he died of spotted fever (*typhus exanthemicus*) on the 15th of January, 1754, at the early age of 19. From his activities as apprentice all that remains is the above laboratory journal with prescriptions by his hand, in which we find all the medicaments in alphabetical order on the first 194 pages, followed by an extremely interesting listing of the number of medicaments, surgical instruments and other medical equpiment that a Swedish East India ship should bring along. The latter lists some 200 medicaments with even the correct dosage indicated. It is of interest to note that the Unicorn apothecary shop equipped the fleet of the East India Company with medicine chests.

Like his elder brother, Carl Wilhelm became interested in pharmacy at an early age. After his brother's premature death he presumably inherited the manuscript book of prescriptions, which he may have studied prior to his own decision to become an apothecary. It is said that while still a boy he was taught how to read prescriptions and to write chemical symbols by two friends of the family in Stralsund. Three years later the 15-year old Carl Wilhelm followed in his brother's footsteps and arrived in Gothenburg, also to be trained by Martin Bauch, who had a general reputation for competence among his contemporaries and came to have great influence on Scheele's development. Carl Wilhelm remained for eight years at the Unicorn apothecary shop, and the book stayed with him also when he left for Malmö and then followed him to Stockholm, Uppsala and finally to his own apothecary shop at Köping.

The meticulously written laboratory journal with hundreds of prescriptions thus followed Carl Wilhelm throughout his entire life and was after his death apparently left in his apothecary shop at Köping. In later times it was donated by one of his successors to the *Farmaceutiska Föreningen*, whose library stamp is found on the title page.

The Swedish pharmacist Axel Kockum, part of whose collection of old pharmacological books was donated to our library, informed Otto Zekert of the existence of this manuscript. Zekert's description of the formulary book, with a detailed list of its contents, form a separate 84-page part in his great Scheele biography (Otto Zekert, *Carl Wilhelm Scheele, Sein Leben und seine Werke,* Volume III, 1933).

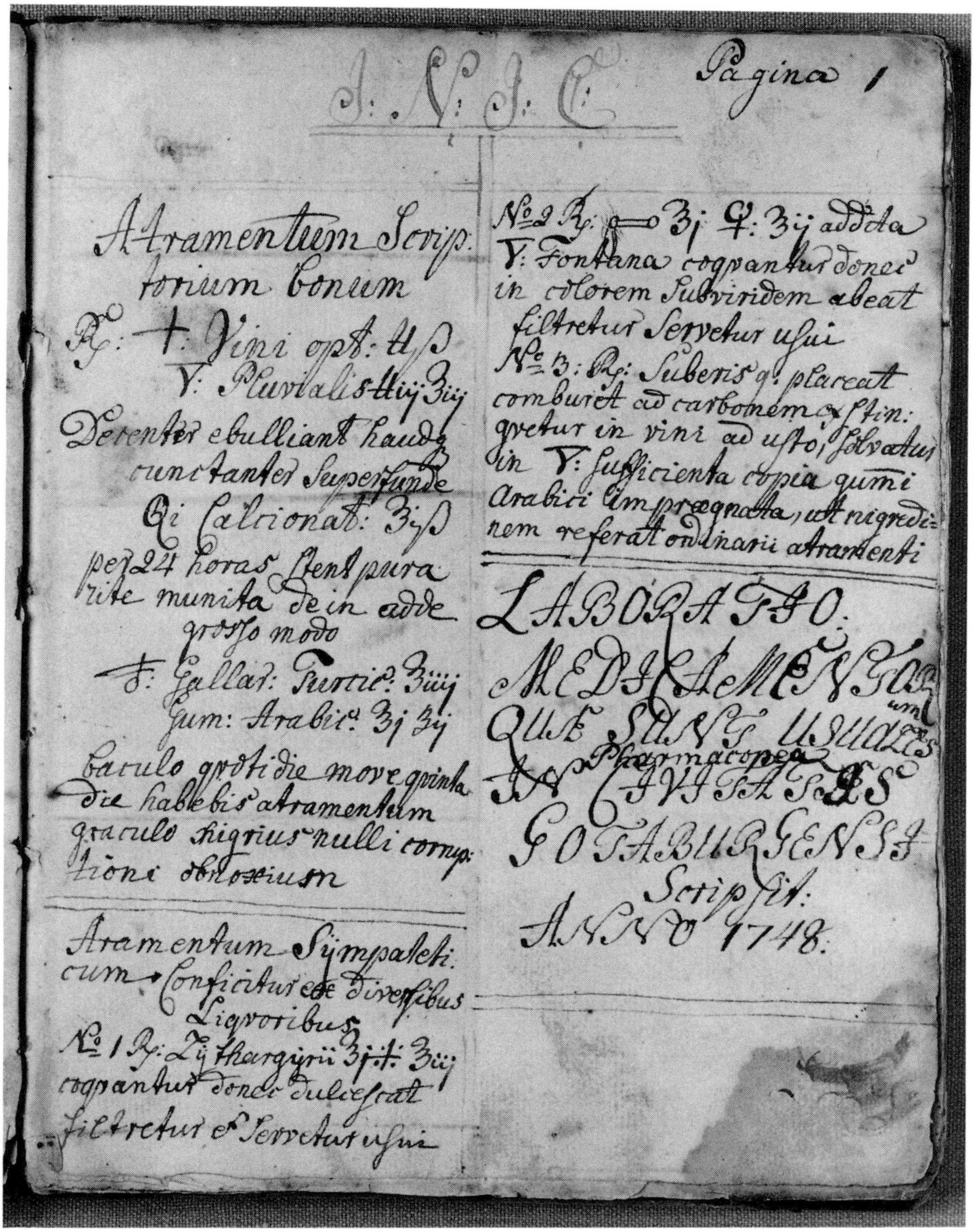

J: N: J: C: Pagina 1

Atramentum Scrip:
torium bonum
Rc: ♁: Vini opt: ℔ß
V: Pluvialis ℔ij ℥ij
Decenter ebulliant haud
cunctanter superfunde
Qi Calcionat: ℥jß
per 24 horas stent pura
rite munita dein adde
grosso modo
♁: Gallar: Turcic: ℥iij
Gum: Arabic: ℥j ʒij
baculo quotidie move quinta
die habebis atramentum
graculo nigrius nulli corrup:
tioni obnoxium

Atramentum Sympateti:
cum Conficitur ex diversibus
Liqvoribus
No 1 Rc: ʒij Lithargyrii ℥j ♁: ℥iij
coquantur donec dulcescat
filtretur et servetur usui

No 2 Rc: … ℥j … ℥ij addita
V: Fontana coquantur donec
in colorem subviridem abeat
filtretur servetur usui
No 3: Rc: Suberis q: placeat
comburet ad carbonem exstin:
guetur in vini ad usto, solvatur
in V: sufficienta copia gumi
Arabici impraegnata, ut nigredi:
nem referat ordinarii atramenti

LABORATIO
MEDICAMENTORUM
QUAE SUNT USUALES
In Pharmacopea
CIVITATIS
GOTABURGENSIS
Scripsit:
ANNO 1748.

LUDWIG, Christian Gottlieb (1709–1773)

Nature-printed coloured plates

Ectypa Vegetabilium . . . / Nach der Natur verfertigte Abdrucke der Gewächse, welche besonders zu dem medicinischen Gebrauche bestimmt sind, und im Apotheken aufbehalten auch auf verschiedene Art zubereitet werden. Nebst einer kurzen Beschreibung deren Wartung, Eigenschaften und Wirkungen, . . .
Halle, printed by Johann Gottfried Trampe for Bernard Christoph Breitkopf in Leipzig, 1760 (–1764).

Folio – *leaf*: 390 *x* 235 *mm. Pp.* [4], 96. *With* 200 *plates* (Tabula I-CC) *of flowering plants, nature-printed and partly hand-coloured; with names printed in Latin (generic names) and German Fraktur. Text in German and Latin in parallel columns.The last page has the catchword* 'CCI', *but no more was published. Two leaves inserted at the end with manuscript index of Latin names in alphabetical order. Recently bound in light brown half calf with all edges entirely uncut.*

Provenance: Wibyholm Library, *stamped* 'VIBYHOLM' *on the title. On a slip inserted at the end is a note that the book was read* 1 *of March,* 1779, *by Wiveka Trolle at Trolleholm* (1721–1806), *second wife* (1740) *to Count Gustaf Bonde* (1682–1764) *and owner of the Wibyholm Library. Her books from Wibyholm were transferred to Trolleholm Castle. Wiveka Trolle was interested in* materia medica *and collected Ms recipes of all kinds.*

This is a very rare and uncommon book. 'Along with J.H. *Kniphof's Botanica in Originali,* [it] was one of the eighteenth century's most valiant attempts at nature-printing' (Hunt). The number of copies printed must have been quite limited due to the processes involved, and no two copies are alike. This copy belonged to Wiveka Trolle, whose notes on the plant's various uses in medicine and in the household are written opposite many of the plates, that is on the verso of the preceding plate. Another copy of this rarity is in the Library of the Swedish Academy of Science.

It is unknown when the technique of taking direct prints from natural objects was originally invented. Bengt Danielsson, in his *Gauguin in the South Seas,* records that at one time the Tahitians decorated their tapa-cloth 'by dipping fern and hibiscus leaves in red sap and pressing them on the material by hand'. The earliest description and the oldest extant nature print (a leaf of *Salvia officinalis*) is found in Leonardo da Vinci's manuscript *Codex Atlanticus,* which he probably began to write in 1490. The dried leaf or plant was covered with a mixture of lampblack and oil, placed between sheets of soft paper, and rubbed hard with a smoothing tool to transfer the image of the leaf to the paper. The first description of nature printing to appear in print is found in Alexis Pedemontanus' *De secreti* or 'Book of Secrets', which first appeared in the mid-1560s and went through several editions and translations. The most widely spread being the German one by the town physician of Colmar, Hans Jacob Wecker, which edition, printed at Basel in 1576, is in our library. In Alexis' work these products of nature printing were described under the name of 'Ectypa plantarum'. Many similar descriptions are to be found in the seventeenth century.

[Many recent writers, Bradbury, Blunt, Cave & Wakeman, Hunt, all refer to a certain Mr Hessel who made leaf prints in America around 1707, quoting Linnaeus' *Philosophia Botanica* (1751) and even Kniphof (1733), adding that no nature prints by him are known. 'Mr Hessel' was in fact the Swede Samuel Hesselius (1692–1753), minister in the New Sweden Mission in Christina (Wilmington), Delaware, 1723–1731. He was the brother of Andreas and Gustaf, who spent many years in America and who both had a keen interest in natural history. Andreas was Samuel's predecessor and the author of a book on the Swedish Church in America (1725), Gustaf was a painter, who is sometimes known as 'The Father of Painting in North America' besides being probably the first builder of organs and spinets in America. When Samuel went back to Sweden in 1731 he brought with him a collection of natural history specimens, mostly snakes and amphibians in spiritus, which were taken care of by a fourth brother, Johan Hesselius, provincial physician, who presented the collection to Count Gyllenborg (described in Linnaeus dissertation *Amphibia Gyllenborgiana*), who in turn presented the collection to the University of Lund. That collection also included a volume of nature prints of American plants made by, or at least brought home by Samuel Hesselius. In 1750 Hesselius had sent a paper to the Swedish Academy of Science with a description of a method to print leaves on paper and linen, entitled 'Berättelse om et besynnerligt sätt at aftrycka löf och blader på papper och Linneväf, som til Tapeter och annat kunde brukas', which, however, was never published. From a letter from Olof Celsius the Elder to Linnaeus in 1739 we can learn that his son, Olof Celsius the Younger (he of the thermometer), also experimented with nature printing, and had a large number of prints made. They were considerably better than the American ones by Hesselius, which Celsius had had an opportunity to study. Some of Celsius' nature prints may be found in the Linnean Society. The volume with Hesselius' *Ectypa plantarum* with American plants has been missing from Lund for many years.]

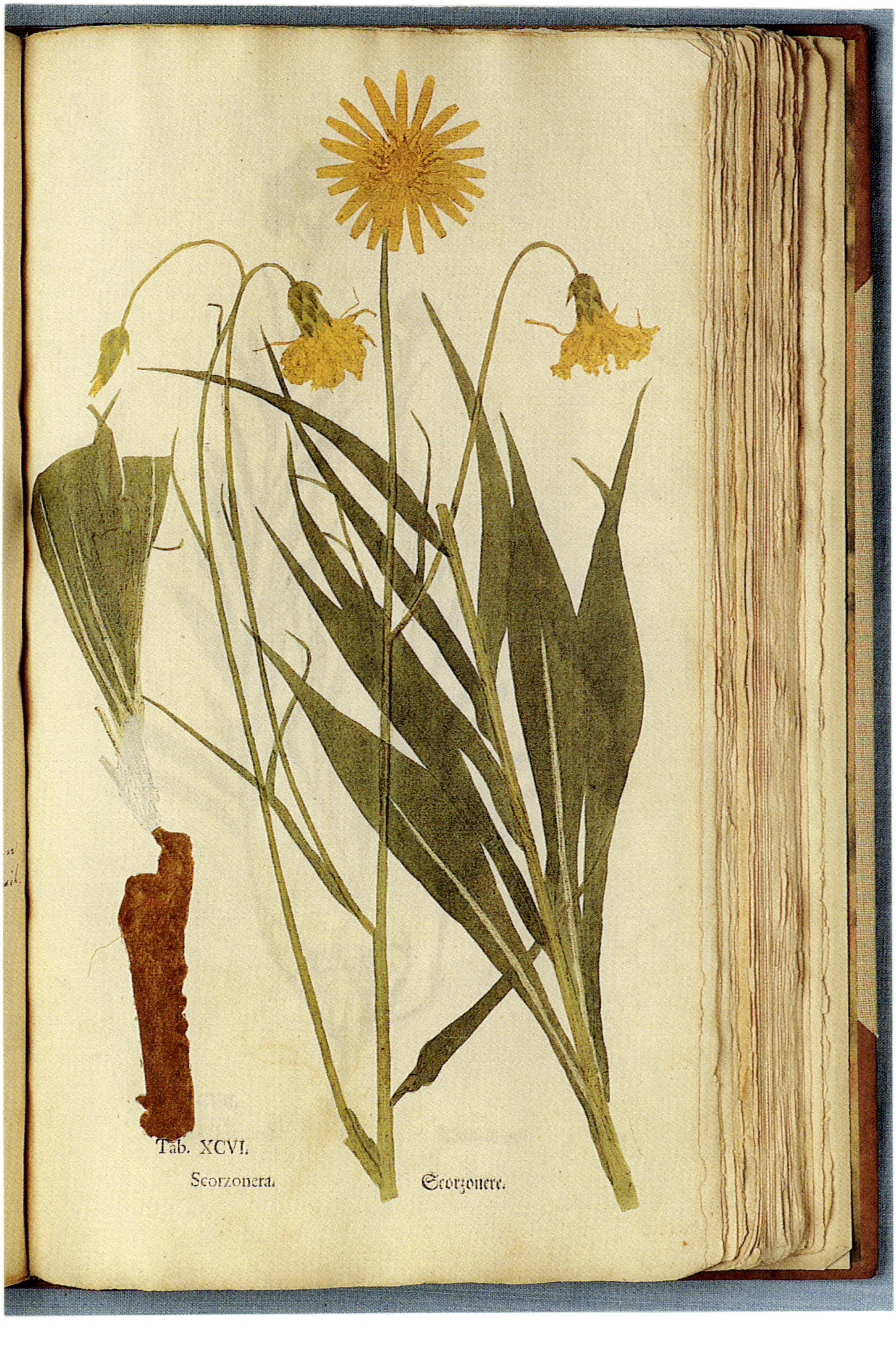
Tab. XCVI.
Scorzonera.
Scorzonere.

There does not appear to have been any considerable improvement in the technique of taking nature prints until 1733, when Johann Hieronymus Kniphof, professor of medicine and botany at Erfurt, published a small folio, *Botanica in Originali Pharmaceutica*, with two hundred nature-printed plates made by his improved method in which printers' ink was substituted for lampblack and the flat press was used for printing instead of the smoothing bone. Kniphof had in 1728 formed a working partnership with the printer Johann Michael Funcke in Erfurt for the experimental preparation of nature-printed plates. 'The book was issued in "centuries" or parts of one hundred plates each, but as issued by the Funcke-Kniphof partnership it progressed very slowly indeed and never got beyond a third century. The standard of production was, however, very high: indeed the skill with which satisfactory prints of fleshy plants such as radishes, cacti, etc. were obtained has never been surpassed. It is quite clear that the same plant did not serve to provide the total number of prints required by the size of the edition (though that was admittedly small); the action of re-inking and re-printing took its toll, and individual plants, as they became damaged beyond use or else too saturated with ink to be convenient to handle, would be replaced by other examples of the same species, sometimes as a considerably different stage of growth from the original' (Cave & Wakeman). Büchner in a review of Kniphof's *Nachricht von einer sehr bequemen und nützlichen Art, die Kräuter abzudrucken und nach ihrer natürlichen Gestalt abgebildet vorzustellen* (1729), tells that he had observed that from copperplates some 12-15000, and from woodblocks some 70-80000 impressions can be made, but from a dried plant no more than 4 to 6 impressions. Kniphof says that printing could proceed rather quickly, with 200 to 300 impressions a day. The *Botanica in Originali* was continued after Funcke's death by the printer-publisher Johann Gottfried Trampe at Halle, who persevered until twelve centuries had been completed. The definitive edition appeared between 1757 and 1764 with 1200 plates. It was obviously intended for hand-colouring, the impresssions in black being printed very much more lightly than those in the Funcke issue.

Trampe was also the printer of the *Ectypa Vegetabilium* by Ludwig. It is nature printed in the same manner as Kniphof's *Botanica in Originali*, 'but on a larger and more ambitious scale' (Dunthorne). The plates are not, as in Kniphof, printed in black, but in green, with flowers and other details coloured by hand, some seemingly applied by stencil or by stamps. The prints show evidence of great care in inking the very delicate plants uniformly. It was issued in eight fascicles from 1760, the title evidently issued with the first fascicle. 'Artistically and botanically the plates show both the advantages and disadvantages of coloured *Naturselbstdruck* . . . Although the object of the method was to obtain greater fidelity to nature, the effect produced is primitive, highly stylized, at times even coarse and childlike . . . The aesthetic value of the series varies greatly with the individual plants. Some, like that of the Iris [*germanica*], have the crude flashy vigour of a child's drawing book: others, like the *Gratiola* and the *Cynoglossum*, display an exquiste linear grace worthy of Chinese or Japanese drawings' (Hunt). [In the present copy these latter two prints are not especially delicate, maybe because they are printed from other specimens].

The book is an early publication of the Breitkopf firm. Bernard Christoph Breitkopf was the founder of the Leipzig business which in 1795 became Breitkopf & Härtel, who developed the printing of music with movable types. Surely Ludwig's *Ectypa Vegetablium* was one of their unusual ventures in printing.

Christian Gottlieb Ludwig, botanist and physician, was almost an exact contemporary of Linnaeus. His doctor's thesis was on *De sexu plantarum* (1737). In 1740 he was extraordinary professor of medicine at Leipzig. He was engaged as a botanist to accompany the Hebenstreit expedition to North Africa, one of the first purely scientific journeys of exploration. He wrote several botanical works and was a friend of Christoph Jacob Trew, the distinguished physician, under whose patronage so many talented artists, engravers and printers produced some of the finest natural history books ever published in Germany. Trew contributed the scientific text to another fine nature-printed book published in Nuremberg, 1748: Johann Michael Seligmann's *Die Nahrungs' Gefäse* [sic] *in den Blättern der Bäume*. Ludwig wrote the preface to Trew's Latin edition of Elizabeth Blackwell's *A Curious Herbal* [the *Herbarium Blackwellianum*. See pp. 174-7]. He is memorialized in the genus *Ludwigia*, Linn., belonging to the evening primrose family.

Hunt II, 569 [pp. 276-80]; Fischer, Ernst, 'Zweihundert Jahre Naturselbstdruck', in *Gutenberg Jahrbuch* 1933, pp. 186-213, No. 8; Roderick Cave & Geoffrey Wakeman, *Typographia Naturalis* (1967); *Tax.Lit.* III, p. 182; Nissen, BBI, 1252; Dunthorne, pp. 43-4. No. 188; Kampmann, Karl, 'Der Naturselbstdruck', in Eder (ed.) *Jahrbuch für Photographie*, 1899.

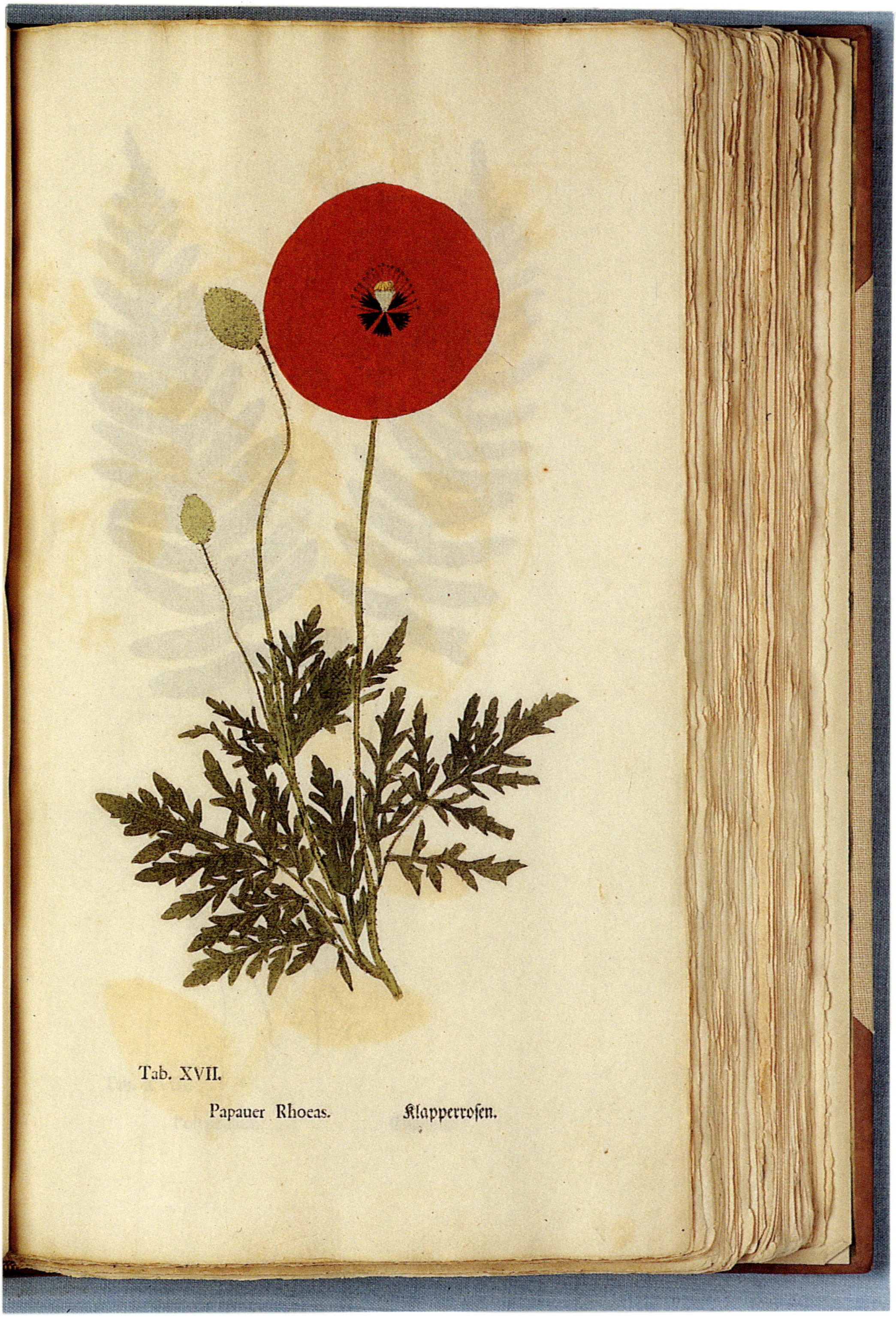
Tab. XVII.
Papauer Rhoeas.
Klapperrosen.

The final death of all quack's publications

ROSEN VON ROSENSTEIN, Nils (1706–1773)

Hus- och Rese-Apoteque.
Stockholm, Carl Gottlieb Ullf, 1765.

Octavo – *leaf*: 165 *x* 110 *mm. Pp.* 112. *Engraved title page with landscape vignette. Inner covers and endpapers filled with handwritten recipes. Contemporary half calf.*
Book-plate: C.D. Carlsson.

First edition. At the request of Her Majesty the Queen, Rosén published his 'House- and Travel-Apotheque' in 1765. The aim of the book was to enlighten people regarding scientific medicine and thus to diminish the influence of quacks. Ancient tradition in matters of health and hygiene, belief in medical charlatans who were much in demand, and the use of folk remedies was common and caused much suffering. In his oration to the memory of his colleague, held at the Academy of Science, Schultz von Schulzenheim says 'this book has given all quacks' publications their final death', an opinion that was certainly a little too optimistic. Nonetheless, the very popular book was of great value for the advancement of better knowledge of scientific medicine. No less than three editions appeared during the eighteenth century (1765, 1772, 1784) and the fourth and last edition in 1803. It was also translated into Danish (1768) and into German (1781).

Rosén, ennobled Rosén von Rosenstein, was professor of medicine at Uppsala and physician-in-ordinary to the royal family in Stockholm. He has been labelled 'The Father of Pediactrics' as the author of the first modern textbook of pediatrics, *Underrättelser om Barn-Sjukdomar,* which was first published in instalments in the Swedish almanacks 1753-71 and in book form in 1764 . That book is by far the most influential work published by a Swedish physician and went through twenty-five editions in eight different languages.

Bo Vahlquist & Arvid Wallgren, eds., 'Nils Rosén von Rosenstein' (*Acta Pediactrica*, Supplement 156, 1964); Waller 8191.

Pulvis Rhabarbari
Rhabarber - Pulver.

Dosis är 20 a 30 gran. Den drifwer något på watnet, gör det ljusrödt. Den öpnar ock Lifwet; men stoppar efteråt. God Rhabarber är tung, marmorerad inuti, och bör ej wara maskstungen. Den brukas

1) Enär man känner ref och buller inuti lifwet; hwilket betyder at något är i tarmarne, som med sitt aggande kan förorsaka Diarrhée eller Colique, eller, om det får tid at draga sig i blodet, göra Feber. Tager man straxt en dosis deraf, så förekommes sådant. Blott härmed förekoms i ganska många år siukdomar hos Högst-Salig Hennes Maj:t Drottning ULRICA ELEONORA.

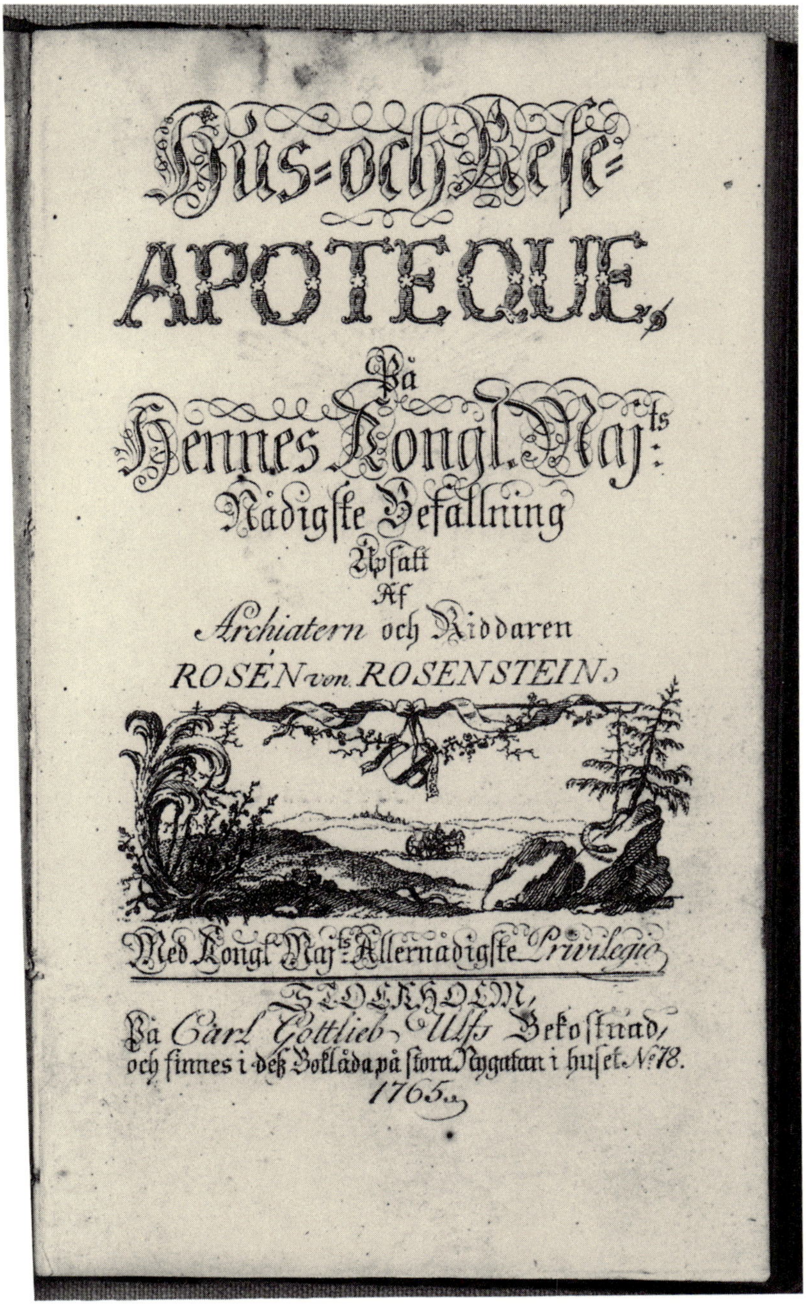

Hus- och Rese-

APOTEQUE,

På

Hennes Kongl. Maj:ts

Nådigste Befallning

Upsatt

Af

Archiatern och Riddaren

ROSÉN von ROSENSTEIN.

Med Kongl. Maj:ts Allernådigste Privilegio.

STOCKHOLM,

På Carl Gottlieb Ulfs Bekostnad,

och finnes i dess Boklåda på stora Nygatan i huset N:o 78.

1765.

The King's Travelling Apotheque

PETERSEN, Peter, ennobled von Heidenstam (1709–1783)

Beskrifning af Kongl. Rese-Apotheque jämte en kort underwisning huru de Sjukdomar, som wanligast påkomme resande, igenkiännas och botas.
Stockholm, Kongl. Finska Boktryckeriet, 1766.

Octavo – *leaf*: 170 *x* 110 *mm. Pp.* [16], 1-96, 96-102, [1] *blank. Contemporary half calf, pastepaper over wooden boards.*
Book-plate: C.D. Carlsson.

First edition of Petersen's 'Royal Travel Apotheque' dedicated to Crown Prince Gustav and Crown Princess Sofia Magdalena by Petersen's son, Johan Christian, who himself was a physician and had translated the work into Swedish. A German edition appeared in Lübeck in 1769.

Peter Peters was born at Heide in Dithmarschen. After studies at the universities of Kiel and Copenhagen he travelled extensively in England, Spain and the African coast. In 1737, when appointed town and garrison physician in Neustadt, he went by his new name, Petersen. He accompanied Adolf Fredrik, the successor to the Swedish throne, to Stockholm in 1743, later became the king's personal physician, and was also nominated *Archiater* from 1752.

Petersen's 'Travel Apotheque' was published at the request of the king one year after the appearance of Rosén's 'House- and Travel Apoteque', which was published at the request of the queen. She had been much impressed by Rosén's skill, while the king's physician, Petersen, was an antagonist of his. Rosén had recommended a cure for the king at Loka spa for a persistent headache, which Petersen, who accompanied the king to Loka, claimed was ill-advised. When Rosén in 1769 ordered variolation to protect the royal children from small-pox, the king was not too enthusiastic, as he was under the influence of Petersen, who was even suspected of placing anti-variolation pamphlets on the king's table. However, the inoculation was carried out by Schultz von Schulzenheim in the presence of Rosén, and all went well. The Swedish Court and Parliament were so pleased that Rosén was granted a national reward of 100 000 thalers, and Petersen was enobled von Heidenstam.

Peter von Heidenstam died in 1783 and was buried in the German church in Stockholm. His engraved portrait is to be found in Hedin's *Vetenskaps-Handlingar för Läkare och Fältskärer*, vol.2 (1795). Besides Johan Christian, who edited his father's book, he had two more sons, who deserve attention: Ernst Joachim Magnus von Heidenstam (1745–1803), who was a pupil of Linnaeus, later physician-in-ordinary to Gustav III and preses of the Collegium Medicum, and Gerhard Johan Baltazar von Heidenstam, famous Swedish ambassador in Constantinople, whose son, Gustaf Daniel, became fencing master at Uppsala, and wrote the first Swedish book on gymnastics (1821). Their half-brother, Werther Verner, was the grandfather of Verner von Heidenstam, Nobel Prize winner for literature in 1916.

Sacklén I, 375-7; SBL, XVIII, 522; Waller, 4203.

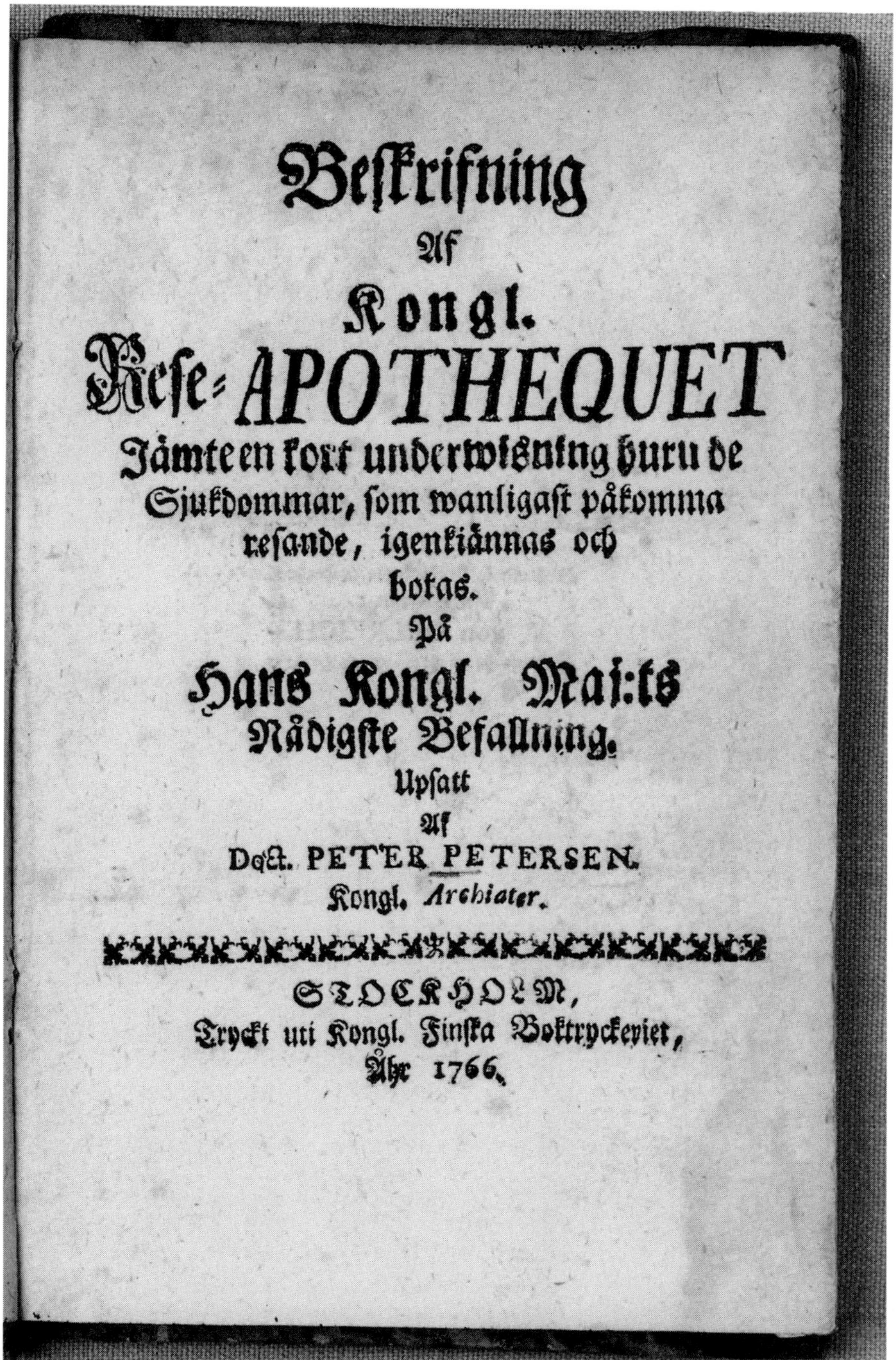

Beskrifning
Af
Kongl.
Rese-APOTHEQUET
Jämte en kort underwisning huru de
Sjukdommar, som wanligast påkomma
resande, igenkiännas och
botas.
På
Hans Kongl. Maj:ts
Nådigste Befallning.
Upsatt
Af
Doct. PETER PETERSEN.
Kongl. *Archiater*.

STOCKHOLM,
Tryckt uti Kongl. Finska Boktryckeriet,
Åhr 1766.

PHARMACOPOEA SVECICA.

A heavily annotated copy of the Editio Prima

Pharmacopoea Svecica.
Stockholm, Henrik Fougt, 1775.

Octavo – *leaf*: 190 *x* 115 *mm*. *Pp*. [10], 237, [3]. *Engraved title vignette. Contemporary half calf, paste paper boards.*

First edition of the *Pharmacopoea Svecica* edited by Abraham Bäck, assisted by several members of the Collegium Medicum and also by Linnaeus and Scheele. It was modelled after the London and Edinburgh pharmacopoeias and was simple and clear in its composition. The *Vegetabilia* in the *Materia Medica* section, written by Linnaeus, includes about 380 simples, and the *Praeparata et Composita* some 400 chemical and Galenic preparations. The second and third editions appeared in quick succession in 1779 and 1784, followed by the fourth edition in 1790 and the fifth in 1817. The Swedish pharmacopoeia, enjoying the cooperation of great names as Linnaeus and Scheele and in the early nineteenth century of Berzelius, has at all times shown the most progressive pharmaceutical standards.

In Sweden the art of pharmacy improved slowly. Even towards the middle of the eighteenth century a well-stocked apothecary shop was expected to supply approved remedies such as snake fat, pike jaws, earthworm oil and genuine Egyptian *mumia*. The old *Pharmacopoeia Holmiensis* of 1686 was still the guiding line for Swedish pharmacists, even if many superfluous medicaments had begun to be expunged.

In a letter to the President of the Collegium Medicum, Abraham Bäck, dated 23 Oct. 1749, Linnaeus proposes that his friend revise the pharmacopoeia, and to another letter he encloses a list with medicaments of animal origin available in apothecary shops and of which he wanted two thirds excluded. In 1752 the Collegium was instructed by the king to prepare for a new pharmacopoeia: 'en ny Apothecare boks eller dispensatorii inrättande, såsom i alla andra wäl bestälde Riken och samhälden skiedt är, sedan wettenskaperna kommit ur deras förra mörker'. The work progressed slowly, hindered by much discussion, and not until 1768 did Bäck have a first draft ready for further examination by experts, among whom we find Anders Jahan Retzius, Peter Jonas Bergius, Nils Dahlberg and many more. After many revisions, exclusions and additions, a definitive examination before printing was made by David Schulz von Schulzenheim, who in turn used expert assistance from Henric Gahn, the pharmacist Pehr Christopher Schulzen, and Carl Wilhelm Scheele.

In July 1775 the printer Henric Fougt personally delivered the first 35 copies to the Collegium Medicum. One copy was given to the court bookbinder Schneidler to be bound for the king. Other bound copies were presented to those who had in one way or another contributed to the new pharmacopoeia, who, besides members of the Collegium, included Linnaeus, Johan Gottschalk Wallerius, Torbern Bergman, Jonas Sidrén and Scheele. Scheele's copy with a handwritten dedication from Collegium Medicum is preserved in the Astra Draco historical book collection in Lund.

The *Pharmacopoea Svecica* was well-received both within the country and abroad. A German translation appeared in Leipzig as early as 1776 under the title of *Schwedische Pharmacie oder Apotheker-Buch,* a translation that was severely criticized by Scheele in the form of a letter to David Schulz von Schulzenheim published in *Stockholms Lärda Tidningar* 1778. The anonymous translator had insufficient knowledge in both Latin and in chemistry, and Scheele, who himself had contributed to the pharmacopoeia, had reason to reveal the translator's profound ignorance publicly.

The present interleaved copy is noteworthy as it is heavily annotated throughout, in the text, in the margins, on the inside covers, on the free endpapers and on the blank inserted leaves. The bulk of the handwritten text is considerably greater than the printed text in the book. About 150 pages are filled with running commentaries in Swedish, providing additional notes on the various drugs, their composition, use and effect on different diseases, colour, taste, etc. One section of 10 pages contains 40 compositions under the heading of *Charlataneria Bergii* (Peter Jonas Bergius was professor of pharmacy and natural history and one of the main contributors to the *Pharmacopoea Svecica*). The hand is evidently that of an experienced pharmacist or physician, whose identity remains to be unveiled.

Anders Grape, 'Linné, Abraham Bäck och Pharmacopoea Svecica av år 1775', in *SLÅ*, XXIX, (1946), pp. 1-34; Grape, 'Scheele, Schulzenheim och 1775 års svenska farmakopé,' in *Lychnos* 1946/47, pp. 262-72; Ahlberg, pp. 395-400; Hjelt, III, pp. 491-500; Gustaf Drake, 'Linné och Pharmacopoea Svecica Ed.1, in *SLÅ*, IV (1921), pp. 1-14; Waller 7409.

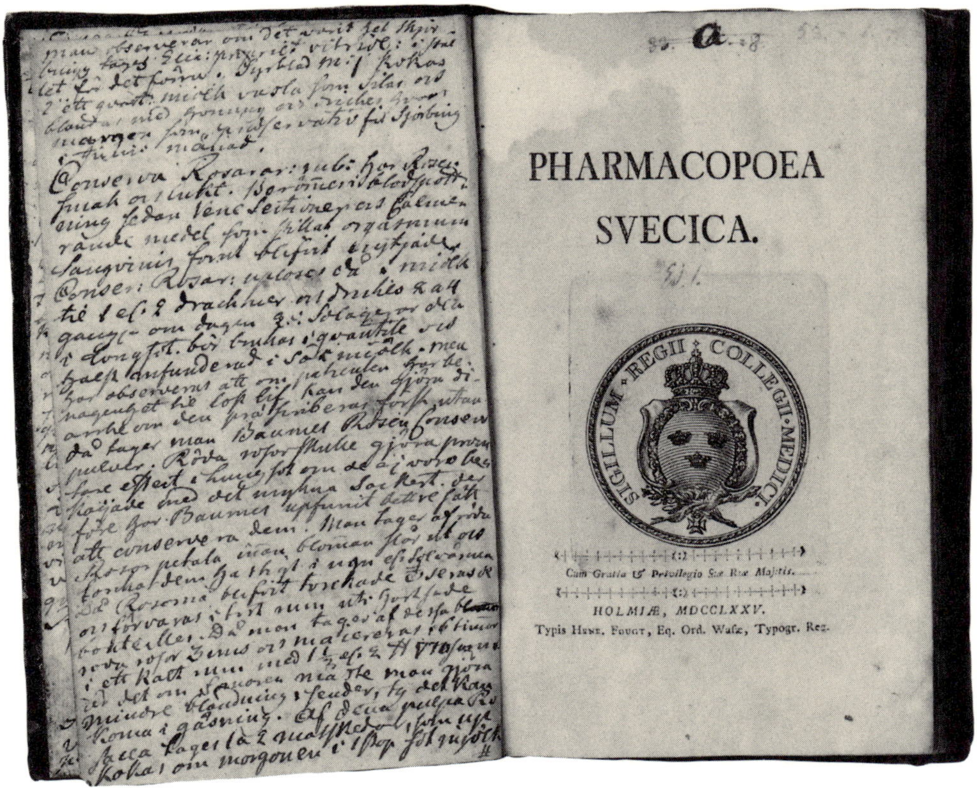
PHARMACOPOEA
SVECICA.
SIGILLUM · REGII · COLLEGII · MEDICI ·
Cum Gratia & Privilegio Sæ Ræ Majestis.
HOLMIÆ, MDCCLXXV.
Typis Henr. Fougt, Eq. Ord. Wasæ, Typogr. Reg.

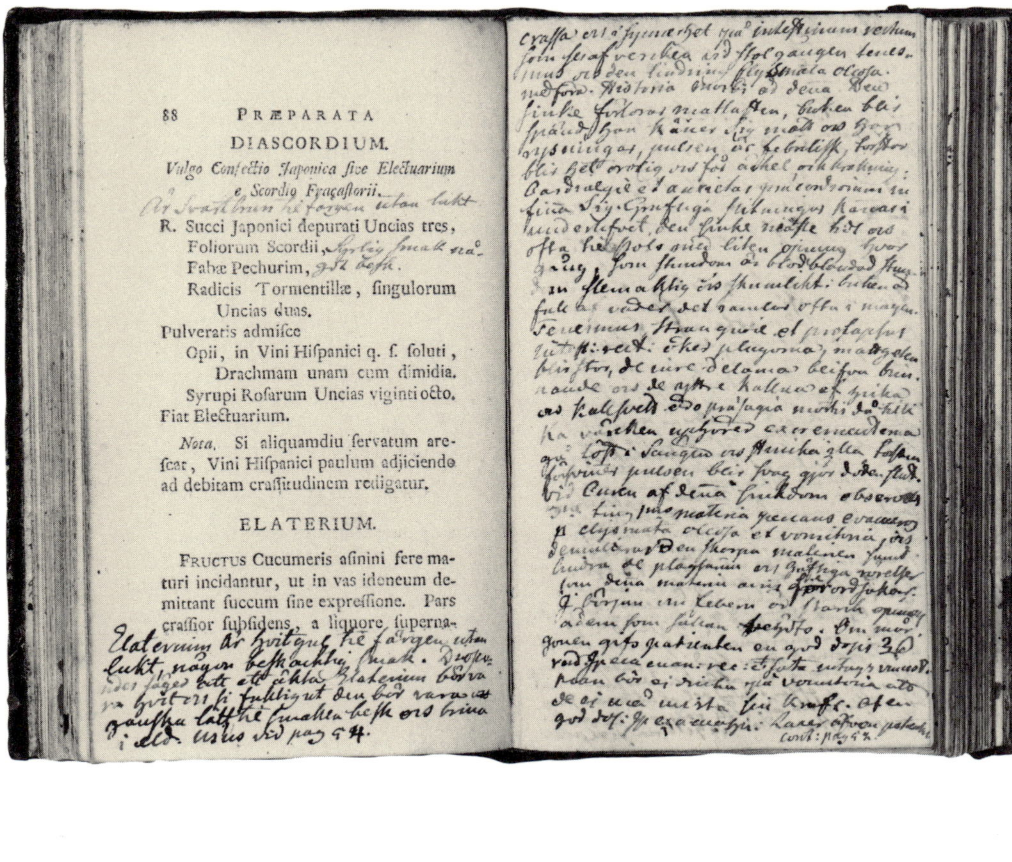
88 PRÆPARATA
DIASCORDIUM.
Vulgo Confectio Japonica sive Electuarium e Scordio Fracastorii.
R. Succi Japonici depurati Uncias tres,
Foliorum Scordii,
Fabæ Pechurim,
Radicis Tormentillæ, singulorum Uncias duas.
Pulveratis admisce
Opii, in Vini Hispanici q. s. soluti, Drachmam unam cum dimidia.
Syrupi Rosarum Uncias viginti octo.
Fiat Electuarium.
Nota. Si aliquamdiu servatum arescat, Vini Hispanici paulum adjiciendo ad debitam crassitudinem redigatur.
ELATERIUM.
Fructus Cucumeris asinini fere maturi incidantur, ut in vas idoneum demittant succum sine expressione. Pars crassior subsidens, a liquore, superna-

A milestone in the history of chemistry

SCHEELE, Carl Wilhelm (1742–1786)

Chemische Abhandlung von der Luft und dem Feuer. Nebst einem Vorbericht von Torbern Bergman.
Uppsala, printed by Johan Edman for Magnus Swederus, Uppsala, and Siegfried Lebrecht Crusius, Leipzig, 1777.

Octavo – *leaf*: 215 *x* 140 *mm. Pp.* [2] *title with engraved vignette,* [4] Vorrede, 1-16 [Vorbericht], 1-155, [1] *adverts. One folding engraved plate. Entirely uncut in contemporary blank boards, handwritten spine title. This copy does not have the rarely seen inserted half-title leaf, which was apparently added after publication. For a detailed bibliographical description see Rolf Du Rietz in* SWIM, *Part* 1:13, *and* TEXT 1974:4, *pp.* 217-225.
From the C.D. Carlsson Collection.

A wonderful copy of the rare first edition of one of the most famous and important books in the history of chemistry and one of the great Swedish contributions to scientific world literature.

The present copy is uncut in its original wrappers as issued and has inside its front cover an antiquarian bookseller's annotations in French, from which it may be presumed that C.D. Carlsson purchased the book in Paris. It is a copy without the later inserted half-title, which gives the name of the printer 'Upsala,/Gedruckt bey Johan Edman, 1777', not mentioned in the main-title impressum or in any colophon. It may therefore be assumed to be one of the copies for the continental market distributed from Crusius in Leipzig, who shared the edition with Swederus in Uppsala.

Carl Wilhelm Scheele was born on the 19th of December 1742, at Stralsund, the main town in Pomerania, then a part of Sweden. Like his oldest brother, Johann Martin, he became interested in pharmacy and 'experimentation' at an early age. At the age of fourteen, after finishing school, Carl Wilhelm went to Gothenburg and became an apprentice to Martin Bauch of the Unicorn Apothecary Shop, succeeding his elder brother, who had died before reaching the age of twenty. Bauch played an important role in Scheele's career, giving him opportunity for extensive laboratory work and providing him with chemistry books to read. Kunckel's *Laboratorium chymicum,* Lemery's *Cours de Chymie* and Caspar Neumann's *Prælectiones chemicæ* were available in Bauch's pharmacy and these works were much admired and used by Scheele throughout his life. He undertook to repeat the numerous experiments in these extensive books, copies of various editions of which are to be found in our historical collection. When Bauch's pharmacy was sold in 1765, Scheele left Gothenburg for Malmö and was employed by Peter Magnus Kjellström of the Eagle Apothecary Shop. Kjellström fully understood Scheele's preference for experimental work and allowed him to work in his laboratory.

In the nearby university at Lund, Scheele became acquainted with the pharmacist Anders Jahan Retzius, later famous professor of natural history, father of Anders and grandfather to Gustav, both great names in the history of science. Scheele and Retzius became life-long friends. It was in a paper by Retzius on 'Experiments on Tartar and its Acid' (*Om Vinsten och dess Syra*), published in 1770, that Scheele's name appeared for the first time, the work being actually a result of their joint labour. In 1768, Scheele moved to Stockholm to serve at the Golden Raven apothecary shop, but was here allowed only to prepare prescriptions, which is why he moved to Uppsala after two years. Whilst in Stockholm, Scheele met Johan Gottlieb Gahn, an assistant to professor Torbern Bergman at Uppsala. Gahn introduced Scheele to Bergman, who was impressed by his knowledge and advised him to investigate pyrolusite (manganese dioxide) – a research which led to the discovery of chlorine in 1774 – and thereafter did everything in his power to bring Scheele's work before the scientific world. The two scientists soon formed a friendship that was not ended until Bergman died in 1784. There is no doubt that Scheele was the greatest scientist, indeed a genius, Bergman more of an extraordinarily talented investigator.

In February 1775, during a meeting at which the king was present, Scheele was elected a member of the Swedish Academy of Science, an unprecedented honour for an apothecary's assistant, and in the same year he moved to the small out-of-the-way town of Köping to manage the apothecary shop of the widow of Hindrich Pascher Pohl. There he came to stay for the rest of his life. On his deathbed he was married to

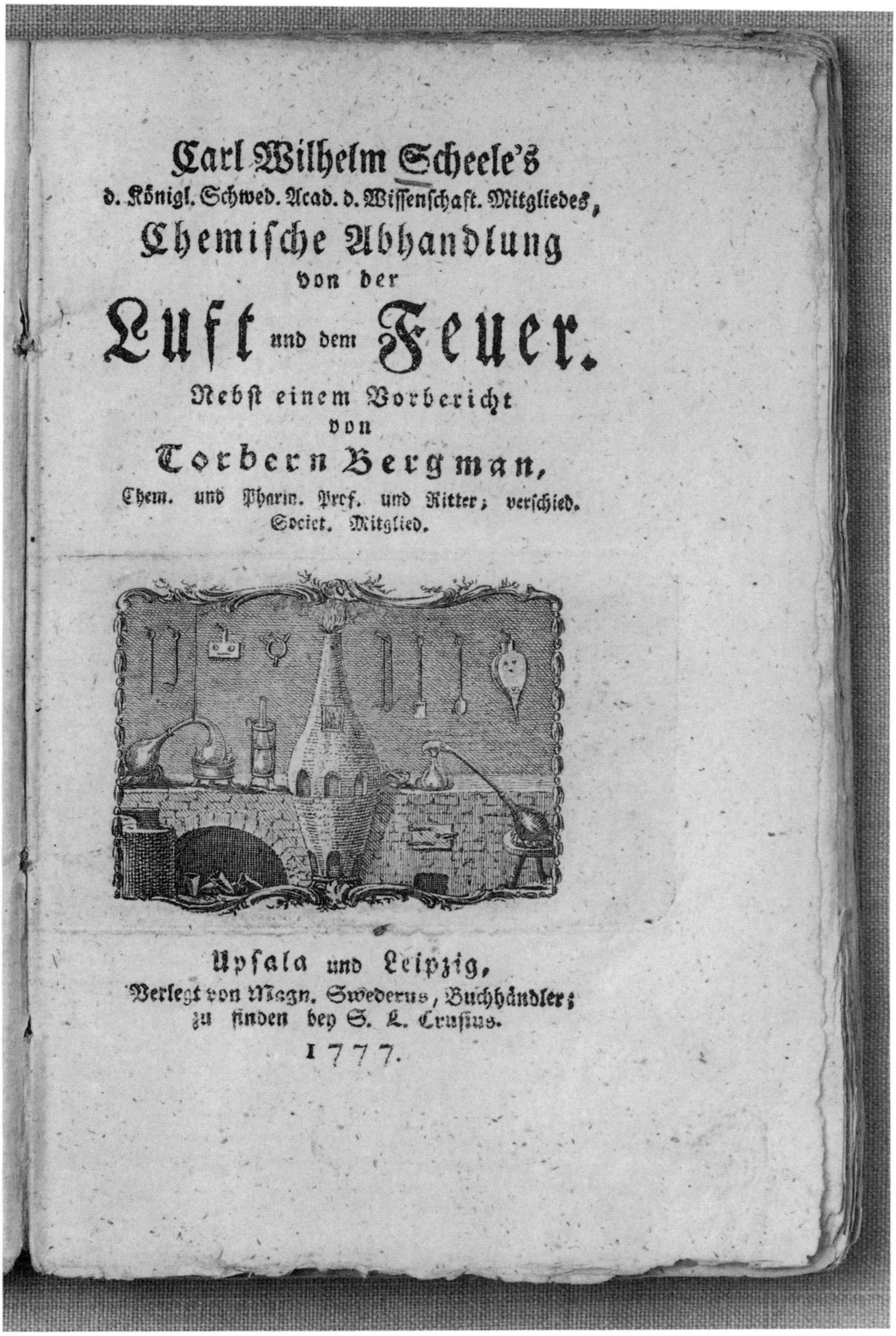
Carl Wilhelm Scheele's
d. Königl. Schwed. Acad. d. Wissenschaft. Mitgliedes,
Chemische Abhandlung
von der
Luft und dem Feuer.
Nebst einem Vorbericht
von
Torbern Bergman,
Chem. und Pharm. Prof. und Ritter; verschied.
Societ. Mitglied.

Upsala und Leipzig,
Verlegt von Magn. Swederus, Buchhändler;
zu finden bey S. L. Crusius.
1777.

his predecessor's widow in order to ensure that the apothecary's privilege should remain with her. He left Köping only once, for a few days, to travel to Stockholm, where he took his long-postponed pharmacist's examination and swore the pharmacist's oath in November 1777. In the same year he had an offer from Frederick the Great in Berlin to be Marggraf's successor with a proposed salary of 1200 *Reichstalers*, but in spite of offers of happier and lucrative posts Scheele remained at Köping the rest of his life. It was there, during the last ten years of his life, 'that he attained the zenith of scientific eminence; it was then that he reached the climax of his European fame as the most expert, the most deep thinking, and the most untiring single-handed experimenter the world has ever known' (John Geddes M'Intosh).

Scheele's researches were extraordinarily extensive in their range of subjects, and his skill in experimentation was remarkable. Yet all his work was done under the most unfavourable conditions, and in the course of a very short life. Few, if any, chemists have discovered more new substances than Scheele. He considered himself mainly an apothecary, commenting 'I am doing my research work only as a sideline so as not to neglect my duties in the apothecary shop'. Of his many papers, published in the Transactions of the Swedish Academy of Science, almost each one announced a discovery of fundamental importance. His very numerous experiments, estimated to 15-20 000 in number, are found in his manuscript notes.

Scheele's most important discovery was oxygen, and his priority is established by his laboratory notes and letters. The manuscript of *Chemische Abhandlung von der Luft und dem Feuer* was sent to the printer, Swederus in Uppsala, on December 22, 1775, but the printing of the work was delayed for nearly two years, partly because Torbern Bergman did not deliver his promised preface until 1 July 1777. The book was published in the following month. By then oxygen was already known, and some of the observations in the book had been published by others. On August 1, 1774 Joseph Priestley informed Lavoisier and other scientists of his discovery of a new remarkable gas, and that date was long accepted as the 'birthday' of oxygen. Now it is known from Scheele's laboratory notes that the discovery was made at least two years before Priestley's. Even the notion that Priestley should have published it earlier is negated when it is noted that Bergman published a summary of Scheele's discovery of oxygen in *Nova Acta Regiae Societatis Upsaliensis*, vol. II. 1775, p. 159 and pp. 232-4, many months before Priestley revealed his discovery (*Experiments and Observations on Different Kinds of Air*, vol. II, 1775). Scheele blamed Swederus for the delay in the publication of the book. In letters to Gahn and to Bergman Scheele said in 1776: 'It will be said I have drawn from their papers and only altered them somewhat. For all this I have Swederus to thank'.

It has been said that at the time it was published, there was no chemistry book in existence which contained a greater number of new and important facts. Scheele demonstrated by numerous simple but brilliant experiments that air was composed of two different gases, 'fire air' (oxygen), indispensable to combustion and breathing, and 'foul air' (nitrogen). The book also contains the first systematic experiment on radiant heat and announces the photo-sensitive nature of silver chloride. He established that violet light has a stronger blackening effect on silver chloride than the rest of the spectrum – a discovery which led to the invention of photography.

The amazing number, quality, and variety of experiments performed by Scheele are astonishing. His accomplishments were gargantuan. Besides being the first discoverer of oxygen, Scheele discovered or identified nitrogen, chlorine, glycerin, manganese, baryta and copper arsenite (Scheele's green), as well as a number of inorganic acids: arsenic, tungstic, molybdic, hydrofluoric – and a number of organic acids: lactic, gallic, pyrogallic, oxalic, citric, tartaric, malic, mucic and uric. He produced oxide of arsenic and the highly poisonous arsenic hydride, which he appears to have handled rather carelessly. The intricate problem with the colouring principle of Prussian blue was one of the most difficult of Scheele's career, and it took eighteen years for him to reach his goal: the discovery of prussic acid. He reported in a letter to Retzius that this acidum berolinense (hydrocyanic acid) had 'a peculiar but not disagreeable smell, a taste somewhat approaching sweet, and is warm in the mouth, at the same time exciting coughing'. 'It is difficult', says Partington, 'to understand how he escaped with his life'.

There is no true portrait of Scheele. The earliest and probably most resemblant, as verified by some of his friends, adorns a commemorative medallion issued by the Swedish Academy of Science in 1790, four years after Scheele's death. The portraitist had, however, never seen the eminent apothecary of Köping and there were immediately grumblings about the likeness, which have persisted to this day.

The portrait most commonly seen, reproduced worldwide in books, is the one taken from a miniature painting on an ivory medallion now owned by the Swedish Pharmaceutical Society and on exhibit in their museum. It is nevertheless most unlikely that it represents Scheele. It was in the possession of the concert-singer Angelica Brüggemann (b.1813), whose maternal grandfather was Carl Wilhelm's elder brother, Friedrich Christoph Scheele (1741–1820). She used to display it as a portrait of her esteemed great-uncle in his mid-twenties, that is to say in the 1760s, when he would have been an apothecary's apprentice in Malmö. However, experts have since determined that the clothing of the young gentleman in the picture is more likely to be from

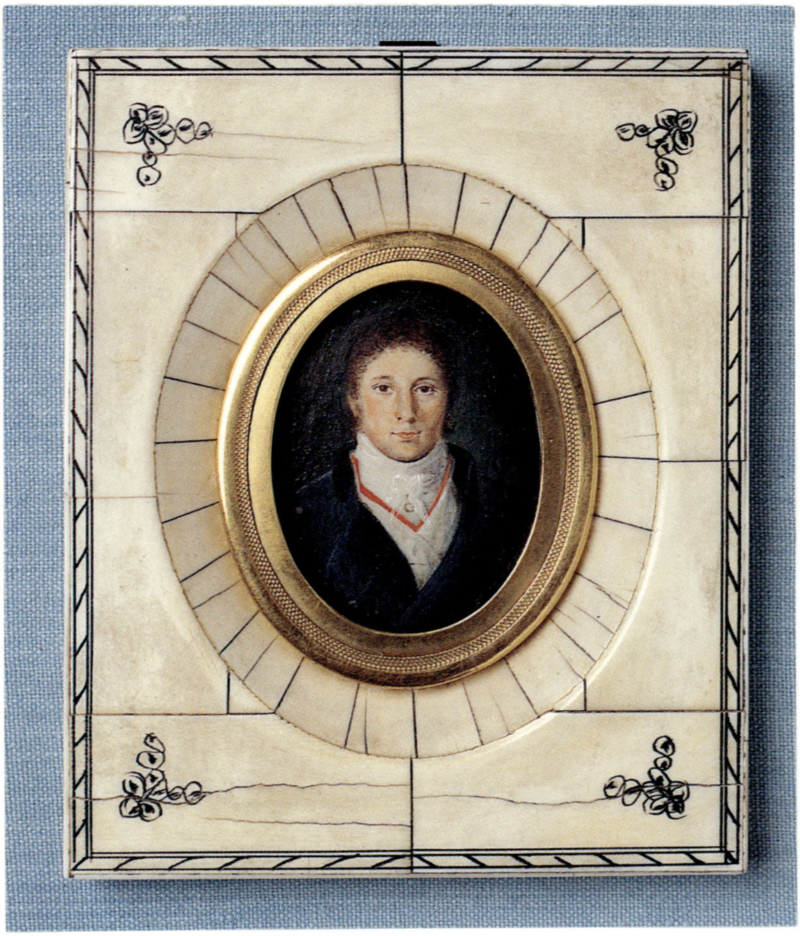

the 1810s rather than from the 1760s, thus invalidating Angelica's claim. In the 1930s the medallion was acquired by the Swedish Pharmaceutical Society. It had been inherited by Angelica Brüggemann's niece, whose widower sold it.

The sensational portrait of the great scientist had been noticed already in 1886 by professor Wilhelm Rollmann in Stralsund, who had a photograph made of it. The pharmacologist Friedrich Flückiger obtained a copy of this photograph, which later found its way to the famous pharmacognosist W.O.A. Tschirch, who had the portrait reproduced in an article, of which he sent an offprint to the then chairman of the Swedish Pharmaceutical Society, Stellan Gullström, who, with the help of the pharmacist John Quist of Trelleborg, managed to find the owner of the medallion in Berlin-Schöneburg. Already in 1901, the famous polar explorer A.E. Nordenskiöld, himself a great authority on Scheele, had managed to track the medallion, but had been unable to afford the exorbitant sum asked for it by its then owner, the marine painter Hermann Brüggemann, Angelica's younger brother.

Therefore, this sensational find, long supposed to represent Carl Wilhelm Scheele, must join the ranks of the many busts, statues, engravings, lithographs and paintings that have been freely produced by various artists, none of which is authentic. During the 1942 bicentennial celebration of Scheele's birth the portrait adorned a Swedish postage stamp (5 and 10 öre), issued in a number of no less than 72 400 000 copies, which must be a kind of world record for spreading a dubious portrait of such a prominent person.

Horblit, *One Hundred Books Famous in Science*, 92; Dibner, *Heralds of Science*, 41; Partington, III, 143-50; Lars Ohlon in *Swedish Men of Science*, 141-50; Partington, 'The Discovery of Oxygen', in *Journal of Chemical Education*, 39 (1962), pp 123-5; Cowen & Helfand, 116; Eder, *History of Photography*, 96-8; Haskell F. Norman Library, 1905; S. Gullström, *Carl Wilhelm Scheele. Einige historische Einzelheiten aus seinem Leben . . . und etwas über das Suchen nach seinem Porträt.* 1934; Lauritz Gentz, 'Hur såg C.W. Scheele ut?', in *Svensk Farmaceutisk Tidskrift*, 17 (1958), pp. 373-94, 405-21; Waller 11225.

RYDBÄCK, Eric Olof (1732–1795)

Confiscated and burnt

Det Svenska Apotheket, eller Svensk Öfversättning af den, utaf Kongl. Collegio Medico senast utgifne Pharmacopoea Svecica. Linköping, Biörckegrens Enka, 1780.

Octavo – *leaf*: 155 *x* 100 *mm. Pp.* 96 (*all printed*). *Modern half calf, gilt spine. This copy formerly belonged to the Royal Pharmaceutical Institute, now in the Scheele-room, Biomedical Library, Faculty of Pharmacy, Uppsala University.*

One of the great rarities in Swedish pharmaceutical literature. The printing of this Swedish translation of the *Pharmacopoea Svecica Editio Altera emendata* (1779) was never completed. Only six sheets, signatures A-F[8] (96 pages) were printed before publication was disrupted. The book was printed in Linköping at Biörckegren's widow, who here used roman types, a novelty in printing Swedish text at that time, introduced from England by Henric Fougt, who had used Roman in printing the original Latin edition of the *Pharmacopoea Svecica.*

In the year 1780 Eric Rydbäck, the municipal physician of Vadstena, began to publish his own translation into Swedish of the second edition of the Latin *Pharmacopoea Svecica.* This endeavour would certainly have been welcomed by many, but when the *Apotekare Societeten* (The Swedish Pharmaceutical Society) got wind of Rydbäck's work, they filed a complaint to the Collegium Medicum, claiming that the author in his preface was slanderous to the Society and had even made insinuating comments about the Collegium itself. The Collegium Medicum, moreover, regarded the translation as erroneous in many respects and made a written demand to the Crown that the enterprise be forbidden. The provincial governor of Linköping was asked to seize the work. He, however, contacted the municipal physician of Vadstena and suggested an amicable settlement which turned out to be agreeable to both parties. Rydbäck announced that he was willing to part with all printed sheets thus far produced for 50 'Riksdaler', and moreover promised to have no further dealings with the translation of the pharmacopoea.

Three of the members of the Collegium Medicum together with the *Apotekare Societeten* jointly produced the desired amount and redeemed the printed copies. In 1782 the *Apotekare Societeten* had a large part of the edition burnt in presence of Collegium Medicum officials. However, a number of copies were saved in the archives of the *Apotekare Societeten.* Some were apparently donated to other libraries, and a few must somehow have found their way to book collecting circles.

A note originally made by the pharmacist Pehr Christopher Schulzen (1736–1822) outlining the history of the prohibition and the burning of the book is found in all copies we have been able to examine. Schulzen was at the time commissioned by the Society to collect biographical notes on Swedish pharmacists and his notes and papers were given to the Society after his death. That the present copy belonged to the Pharmaceutical Institute cannot escape notice as their large blue library stamp covers one fourth of the title page. It has been rebound without piety in modern half calf and somewhat cut down. Of special interest is, however, that besides Schulzen's note, dated 1782, on a leaf at the front, it also has ten leaves bound in at the end with a handwritten continuation of the text that was never printed, and moreover three leaves (six pages) with notes on the faults that caused the prohibition, signed by P.C. Schulzen. There are some fifty such adverse remarks with corrections, one of which refers to page 23, where Rydbäck has added a formula for *Aqva Abietis* (Gran-vatten) not found in the Latin *Pharmacopoea Svecica,* but which he incorporated for its common and beneficial use.

Eric Rydbäck was born in the parish of Ringarum in Östergötland. He studied at the University of Uppsala and defended a zoological dissertation under Linnaeus, *Pandora Insectorum* (1758), dealing with the host plants of various insects, for which Rydbäck himself engraved a plate depicting insects (this plate is known to exist in a very few copies only and is one of the rarest treasures for any collector of Linnaeus' dissertations). He also wrote a wonderful little treatise on the use of cultivation, *Tal om Planterings Nytta och Nödvändighet* (1762). His interest was not limited to natural history, and after having received his M.D. in 1765 he settled in Vadstena, where he had been appointed municipal physician and later also served as inspector of the Medevi Spa. He died at Vadstena in 1795.

Waller 9371.

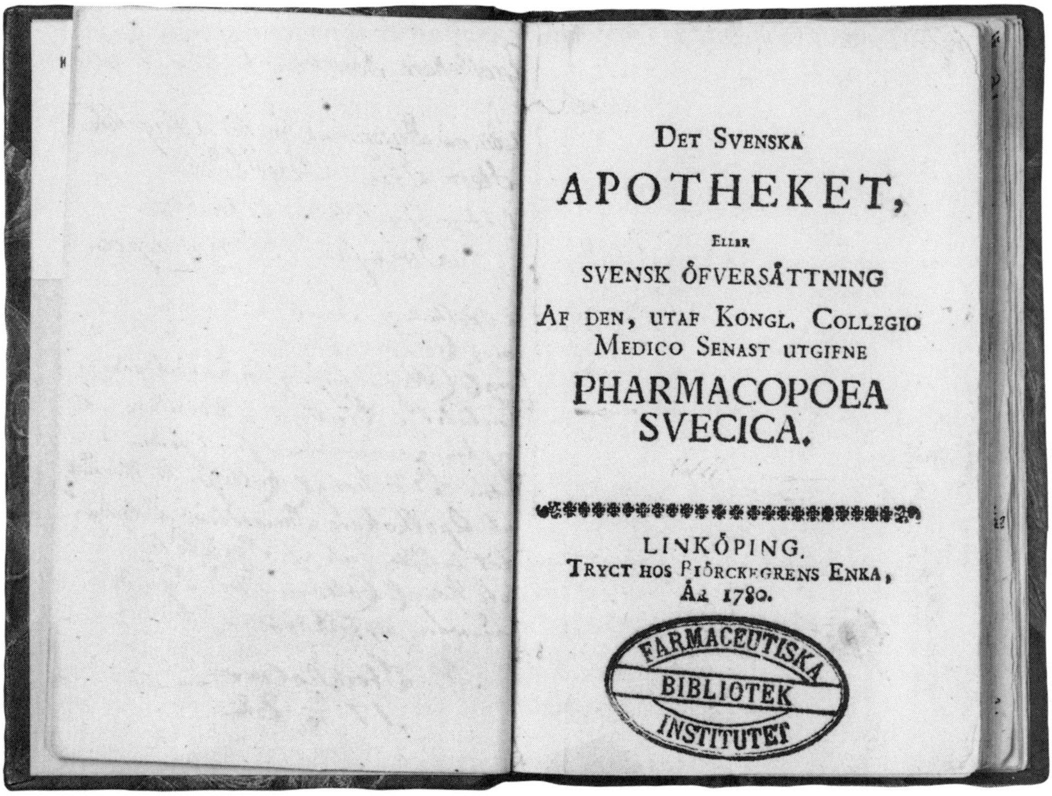
DET SVENSKA
APOTHEKET,
ELLER
SVENSK ÖFVERSÄTTNING
AF DEN, UTAF KONGL. COLLEGIO MEDICO SENAST UTGIFNE
PHARMACOPOEA SVECICA.
LINKÖPING.
TRYCT HOS BIÖRCKEGRENS ENKA,
ÅR 1780.
FARMACEUTISKA
BIBLIOTEK
INSTITUTET

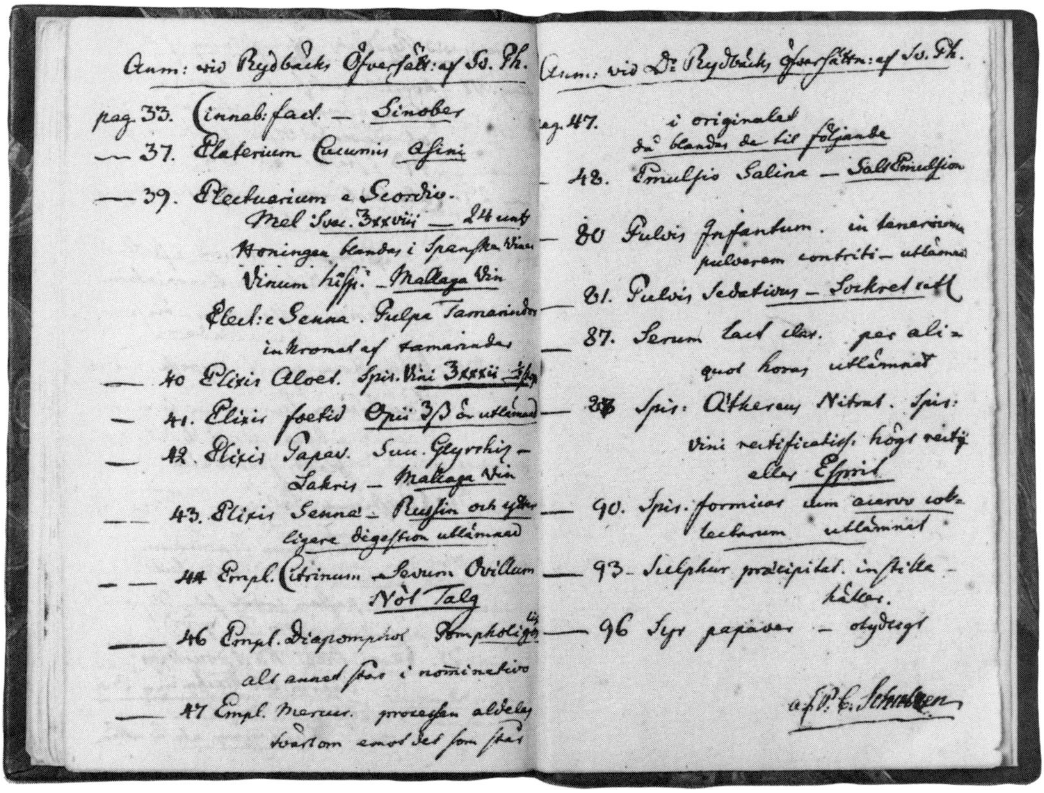
Anm: vid Rydbäcks Öfversätt: af Sv. Ph.
Anm: vid Dr Rydbäcks öfversättn: af Sv. Ph.
pag. 33. Cinnab: fact. — Sinober
— 37. Elaterium Cucumis asini
— 39. Electuarium e Scordio.
— 40 Elixir Aloet.
— 41. Elixir foetid
— 43. Elixir Sennae
— 44 Empl. Citrinum Sevum Ovillum Nöt Talg
— 46 Empl. Diapomphol
— 47 Empl. Mercur.
pag. 47. i originalet
— 48. Emulsio Salina — Salt Emulsion
— 80 Pulvis Infantum.
— 81. Pulvis Sedativus — Sockret
— 87. Serum lact
— 90. Spir. formicar
— 93. Sulphur praecipitat.
— 96 Syr papaver

Four hundred and four Chinese drugs

CHINESE DRUGS. Manuscript.

Namn ock Beskrifning på En Samling Chinesiska Droguer. 1sta Bandet Från No. 1 Till ock med No. 202; 2dra Bandet från No. 203 till ock med No. 404.
(Canton, China [?], second half of the eighteenth century).

Folio – *leaf: 370 x 240 mm. Paper watermarked* J WHATMAN, *with crowned shield. Volume* I: *20 unnumbered leaves; volume* II: *20 unnumbered leaves. Two volumes covered in Chinese silk brocade with a honeycomb pattern of small hexagons, each with a red swastika against a yellow background. The two volumes comprise 78 pages with text in Swedish and with the Chinese characters written with a brush in black ink. Pages and columns ruled in red.*

This interesting and neatly written manuscript describes a collection of 404 Chinese drugs and may have been written down at the trading station of the Swedish East India Company in Canton. The hand is reminiscent of other documents from the period of the East India Company, and is most likely that of a clerk assisted by a native scribe, who has written the plant names in Chinese characters with a brush. The manuscript is so far unrecorded. It bears no date and is not signed. The left hand page gives in columns the number of the canister storing the drug, the name of the plant in Chinese followed by the name in Swedish phonetic transcription, and what part of the plant is used, e.g. the root, the stem, the flower, the seed, the juice, etc. On the right hand page, a description is given in Swedish of which disease or ailment can be treated by the drug and sometimes also how the drug is prepared. The fluent Chinese hand and the covers in Chinese silk brocade indicate that the manuscript was probably produced in China.

Neither Latin nor Swedish plant names are given, just the Chinese name in Chinese characters with 'Swedish' transcription. The detailed description for which ailment the drug is used may be the work of someone experienced in Chinese healing art, but seems more likely to be a translation from Chinese with the help of an interpreter or some missionary versed in the Chinese language; maybe made for a Swedish physician in service of the Company, who often gives his personal comments. There is no provenance but it is no doubt the same Chinese *Materia Medica* manuscript in two folio volumes, which was a gift in 1831 from Carl Wilhelm Bonté of the *Hvita Björn* pharmacy in Stockholm, who for a few months in 1829 had served as librarian for the Swedish Pharmaceutical Society. He died in 1832 at the early age of 35.

Swedish trade with China was opened in 1732. Linnaeus, always anxious to enrich his collections of natural history objects with exotic specimens, never neglected to instruct the captains or chaplains and physicians accompanying the ships bound for East India to collect samples for him. The most important collection of Chinese plants that he received was from his pupil Pehr Osbeck. It is also known that the Director of the Swedish East India Company at Gothenburg, Magnus von Lagerström (1696–1759), who supplied his friend Linnaeus with exotic plants, had received a collection from China of about 1000 drugs as well as a copy of the great Chinese Materia Medica, *Pen tsáo kang mu*, in 36 volumes.

The drug contained in Canister No. 1 is the famous *Gin-Seng*, here called '*Genn-Schamm*' with the following long description of its use and preparation:

> 'Ett Stärkande Medicament för alla de Noblare delarne invärtes; denne som är den Chinesiska anses som den yppersta i hela Werlden, säges wäxa på ett enda ställe som är belägit långt Norr ut ifrån Pekin, wid namn Leeu-toan, ock brukas för Svag mage ock de som beswäras af kräkningar, ande-täppa och starka knipningar i underlifwet; Likaledes då mattighet och öfverflödiga Svettningar inträffa. – Tillredes och nyttjas af Chineserne på följande sätt: Rothen sönderskiäres i helt tunna Skifwor, lägges i en Större The-kopp fyld med friskt godt kiällewatten å hwilken de lägga ett Lock som ofwanuppå har en liten iholighet. Denna koppen sättes antingen ensam på en sackta eld, eller i en liten panna fyld med watn som upkokas hwarigenom rothen i koppen småningom uplöses, och för at weta rätta tiden då alt detta är färdigt ock skal tagas från Elden, lägges några risgryn i holigheten på Locket med watn derå ock när dessa grynen af hettan äro så mycket uplöste, at de kunna ätas, wet man at dryckens kraft är lagom, hwilken nyttjas som annat The watn om mårnarna ock giör den stora wärkan de förwänta. – Manderiner ock annat förmöget folck som äro något till åren nyttja denna dryck nästan dageligen. – At denne roten i många hänseender är ett ståteligit medicament, derpå är aldeles inget tvifvel men troligit är att man för at nyttja denna roten med samma förmohn som Chinesen bör wara lika så widskieppelig, ty ingen siukdom kan nämnas som icke de tro med denna roten kan botas, ja de anse den ofta såsom den där kan återkalla menniskian till lifwet.'

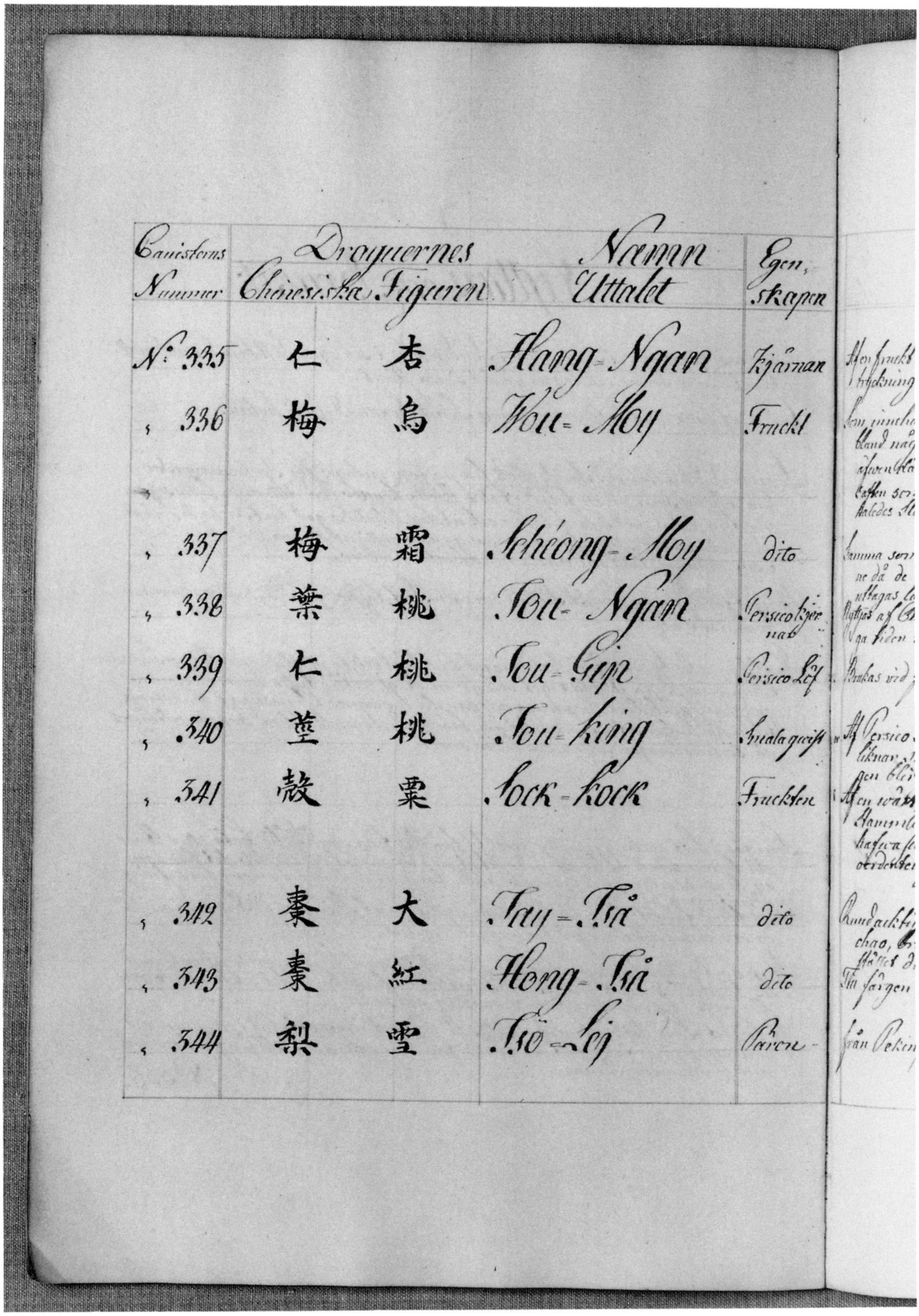

Canistrens Nummer	Droguernes Chinesiska Figuren		Namn Uttalet	Egenskapen
N:o 335	仁	杏	Hang-Ngan	Kjärnan
„ 336	梅	烏	Wou-Moy	Frucht
„ 337	梅	霜	Schéong-Moy	dito
„ 338	藥	桃	Tou-Ngan	Persico kjärnan
„ 339	仁	桃	Tou-Gin	Persico Löf
„ 340	莖	桃	Tou-king	Smala qvist
„ 341	殼	粟	Sock-kock	Fruckten
„ 342	棗	大	Tay-Tså	dito
„ 343	棗	紅	Hong-Tså	dito
„ 344	梨	雪	Sio-Lej	Päron

HAPPE, Andreas Friedrich (1733–1802)

A gigantic one-man work with 595 hand-coloured plates

Botanica Pharmaceutica exhibens plantas officinales quarum nomina in Dispensatoriis recensentur cum iconibus, ab auctore aere incisis, et vivo colore expressis; adjectis nominibus tam pharmaceuticis, quam e systemate Linnei depromtis. Centuria I. (-VI).
Berlin, 1788 (1785– ?1806).

Folio – *leaf*: 358 *x* 230 *mm. Six* 'Centuries' (*each containing one hundred plates*) *bound in two volumes. Contemporary half calf. All the title pages with engraved vignette depicting a botanist in a charming landscape scene with a river.*

Centuria I: *Pp.* [2] *title,* [4] *Dedication to Wilhelm* II, *pp.* 1-50. *Engr. frontispiece and plates* 1-100.

Centuria II: *Pp.* [2], 51-88. *Engr. frontispiece and plates* 101-200.

Centuria III: *Pp.* [2], 89-118, [2] *index to* III. *Engr. frontispiece and plates* 201-300.

Centuria IV: *Pp.* [2], 119-148. *Engr. frontispiece and plates* 301-400.

Centuria V: *Pp.* [2], 149-178. *Engr. frontispiece and plates* 401-500.

Centuria VI: (*without title leaf and frontispiece*): *Pp.* 179-204, *plates* 501-595.

This copy formerly belonged to the Royal Pharmaceutical Institute, now in the Scheele-room, Biomedical Library, Faculty of Pharmacy, Uppsala University. The front fly-leaf in the second volume bears the signature of Carl Juhlin-Dannfelt (1823–1904) *and the date* 1840.

This work was originally issued in parts (Heft 1-78), the first appearing in January, 1785, and the last in 1806 (cf. Nissen), that is after the author's death. The present edition, with the date 1788 on all titles, has the wording in the title changed from '*in Dispensatoriis Brandengurgico*' to '*in Dispensatoriis*'; the number of the volumes 'CENTURIA I (-V)' is not letterpress but in manuscript. The engraved title-vignette is the same for all title pages. There is no title-leaf nor frontispiece to *Centuria* VI. The frontispiece to *Centuria* IV is the same one as in *Centuria* I, showing a botanical artist in an ancient dress sitting in front of a giant plant in a pot, the sun rising in the background. The frontispiece to *Centuria* II represents the North with a walrus and *Centuria* V the South with a blackamoor placed in an exotic landscape. *Centuria* III has the title within a wreath of flowers.

Happe was born in Aschersleben and studied pharmacy in Berlin. In 1760 he received the title of *Medicin-Apotheker* through marriage. He also worked as a draughtsman and engraver for the Berlin Academy of Science and is known as a botanist and collector of natural history specimens. At his own expense he published a great number of colour plate books, depicting not only pharmaceutical plants, but also fungi, lichens, as well as insects and butterflies, works that are seldom found. Happe did not only draw the plates, but also executed the engraving and the hand-colouring himself. In the present copy the five frontispieces and the 595 plates are neatly coloured with many details added in manuscript. Some of the plates in *Centuria* II are original watercolours. Most of the plates have the name of the plant engraved, but for many the number and the plant's name are written by hand. Happe left many works unpublished. Recently a monumental collection of no less than 3814 folio plates in original watercolours turned up, bound in sixteen volumes, dated 1773-76 (Heribert Tenschert, *Katalog* XXXVII, 1996). Happe's publications were certainly issued in very limited editions; the *Botanica Pharmaceutica* was for lack of money not produced in more copies than shown on the subscription list of 71 names.

Nissen (p. 200) does not have anything favourable to say about Happe's botanical plates, nor does he sympathize with the excessive prices that collectors of the day are prepared to pay for his *Botanica Pharmaceutica*, a work referred to by Nissen as an inferior 'Machwerk . . . die mehr schlecht als recht gezeichnet, vielfach nach fremden Vorlagen kopiert' etc. Hunt (p. 424), however, finds Happe's charming drawings to be made with considerable care of botanical detail, and with a delicate eye for colour and line. 'If some designs are a little stiff, if the artist prove to be no Ehret or Redouté, he nevertheless communicates an appreciation of a very large variety of nature's forms, and at the same time simple statements now of value to the historical taxonomist'.

Nissen, BBI, 784; Hunt, 659 (note); Johnston, *Cleveland Herbals* 564; Pritzel, 3779; Hein/Schwarz, *Deutsche Apotheker-Biographie, Ergänzungsband* (1986), p. 173; Heribert Tenschert, *Katalog* 37, 1996.

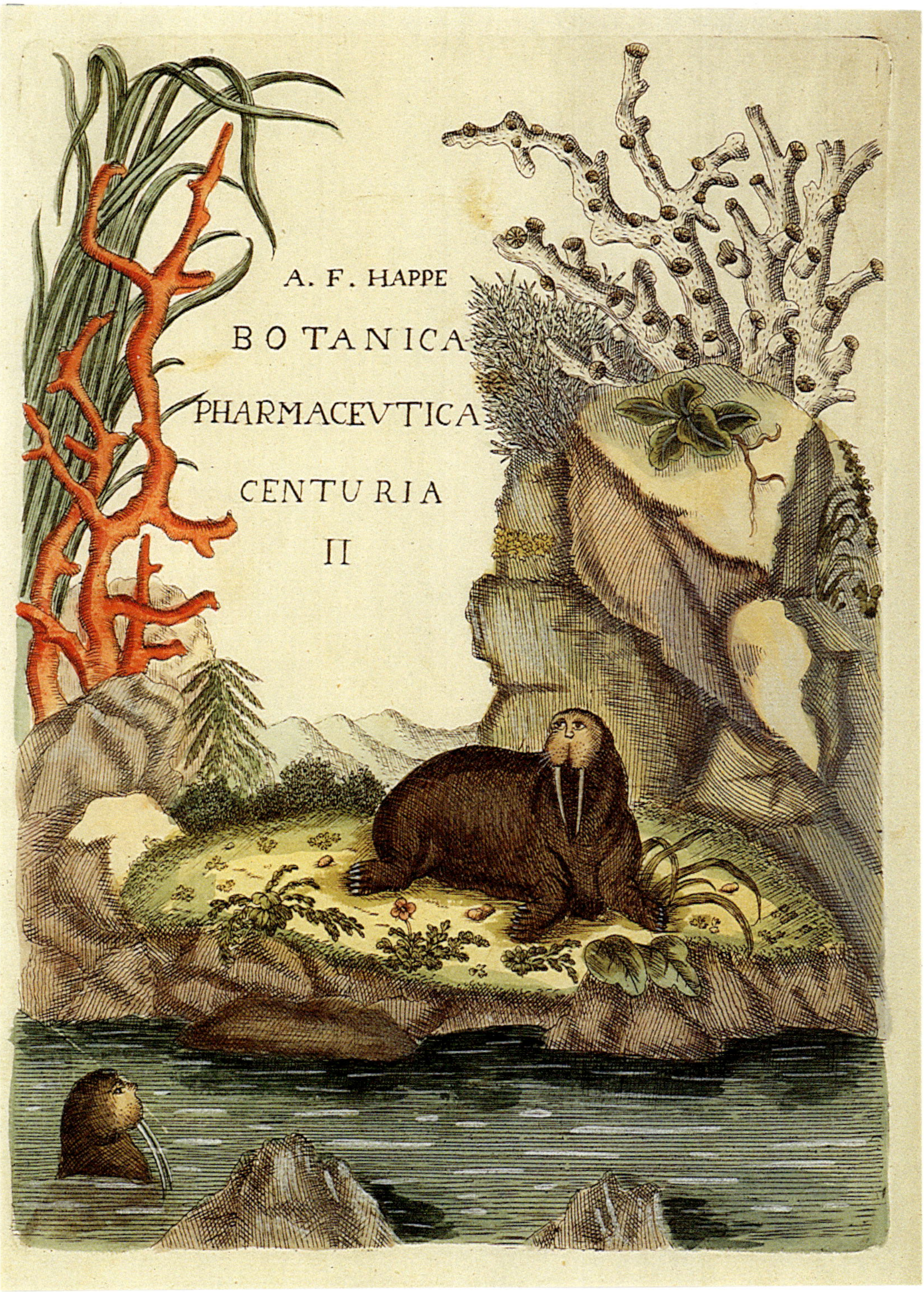
A. F. HAPPE
BOTANICA
PHARMACEVTICA
CENTURIA
II

The first American materia medica

SCHOEPF, Johan David (1752–1800)

Materia Medica Americana potissimum Regni Vegetabilis.
Erlangen, Johann Jakob Palm, 1787.

Octavo – *leaf*: 196 *x* 115 *mm. Pp.* xviii, 170. *From the collection of* Professor Thor Ekecrantz, *who had his books rebound in quasi-antique half calf of poor quality.*

First edition of the first full American *materia medica*, and one of the earliest works devoted to North American medical botany. Schoepf's *Materia Medica Americana* is considered to be not only the rarest work on American medicinal plants but also among the rarest and most significant books of medical Americana. The editors of the 'facsimile' reprint of 1903 in the *Bulletin of the Lloyd Library* were unable to find any copy of the book in America and relied for their 'facsimile' upon a transcript of a copy in Erlangen.

Schoepf was born in Wunsiedel, a small town in Bavaria. In 1776 he was given the doctor's degree in Erlangen, the title of his dissertation being *De medicamentorum mutatione in corpore humano*. Early in 1777 he left Germany as a field surgeon together with some thousand mercenaries sold by the Margrave of Ansbach as part of the 22 000 Hessian troops hired by the English Government for about three million pounds, to assist in the war against the North American colonies. The troops arrived at Staten Island in June, 1777. For six long years Schoepf attended to his duties as army surgeon. When the war ended in 1783, thousands of former enemies, especially the German soldiers in English service, remained in America. Others stayed for a while to explore the country and to study its resources and possibilities. One of these was Schoepf, who obtained permission to remain for the purpose of travel and study.

Schoepf's journey was only one of the successful botanical and medico-botanical exploring expeditions through North America which were undertaken by foreigners in the years following the Revolutionary War. He began his travels in the company of an Englishman named Hairs. From New York they crossed New Jersey to Philadelphia, thence they went via Bethlehem into the Alleghanies, to Pittsburg and to Kentucky. Then he started on his southern tour through Virginia, North and South Carolina to Charleston, where he remained for two months and then went to Florida. He visited the Bahama Islands, and in June 1784 he left for Europe and arrived in England after a thirty-day trip. He returned via Paris to his native Ansbach and there he began to prepare for the publication of his studies and observations made in America. His comprehensive work on the American *materia medica* is one of the prime sources for our knowledge of the natural sciences, medicine, and pharmacy in America at the close of the eighteenth century.

Medical botany had been cultivated in North America during early colonial time. Schoepf was astonished to find that physicians in America relied upon costly imported medicaments, when the New World afforded such an abundant native *materia medica* and also had learned many wrinkles in herbal therapy from the red man. Thus there was a basis of experience to build on. Schoepf's *Materia Medica Americana* is based largely on the observations made by the excellent American botanist Gotthilf Henry Ernest Muhlenberg and the works of Bartram, Clayton, Colden, Pehr Kalm, Catesby and others. In a letter written to Muhlenberg from Germany, April, 1786, Schoepf states that he has prepared a 'Materia Medica Americana' containing the descriptions of about 400 North American plants and continues: 'My lists make it certain that North America owns a rich indigenous materia medica in her plants and can find all she needs, apart from a few East Indian spices and plants, on her own soil . . . I almost may flatter myself in writing this little book to have rendered sufficient services to America to be pardoned for my assistance in combatting her.'

Besides his *Materia Medica Americana* Schoepf published a narrative of his journey, *Reise durch einige der mittlern und südlichen vereinigten nordamerikanischen Staaten nach Ost-Florida und den Bahama-Inseln*, in two volumes (Erlangen, 1788), and papers on mineralogy and fishes in North America. 'Among travelers in America it would be difficult to find his equal in combined breadth of interests, accuracy of observation and judgment, wit, and serene good temper' (DAB).

Garrison-Morton, 1837; E. Weil, *Catalogue* 26, item 115; Kremers & Urdang (1940), pp. 158-9; Haskell F. Norman Library, 1909; New York Academy of Medicine, *Exhibition Catalogue, Medical Americana* (1927), No. 57; (DAB) *Dictionary of American Biography*; Waller, 8675.

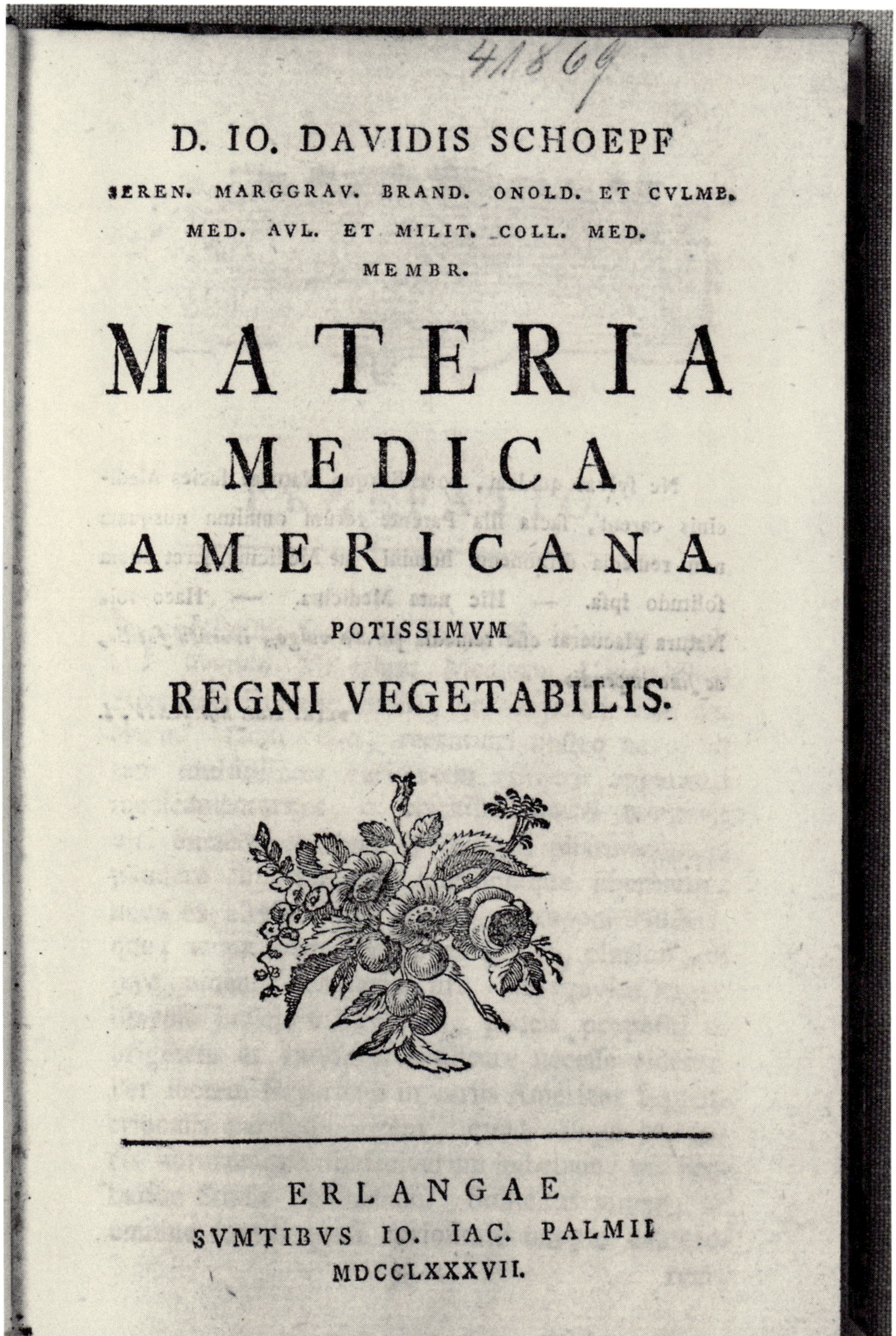

D. IO. DAVIDIS SCHOEPF

SEREN. MARGGRAV. BRAND. ONOLD. ET CVLMB. MED. AVL. ET MILIT. COLL. MED. MEMBR.

MATERIA MEDICA AMERICANA

POTISSIMVM

REGNI VEGETABILIS.

ERLANGAE
SVMTIBVS IO. IAC. PALMII
MDCCLXXXVII.

The first pharmaceutical periodicals

TROMMSDORFF, Johann Bartholomeus (1770–1837) editor.
Journal der Pharmacie für Aerzte und Apotheker. Volumes 1-26, 1794 to 1817 & Neues Journal der Pharmacie für Aerzte, Apotheker und Chemiker. Volumes 1-15 (of 27), 1817 to 1824.
Leipzig, S.L. Crusius & F.C.W. Vogel, 1794–1824.

Octavo – *leaf*: 170 x 103 *mm. This set lacks the last eleven volumes of the New Series* (1825–1834). *Each annual volume is divided into two parts with separate title leaves. Up to volume* 17 (1808) *they are bound together in one volume, but from then on each part is separately bound. Cumulative indexes are found in vols.* 15 *and* 26 *of the first series and in vols.* 7 *and* 27 *of the New Series. Engraved title vignettes and plates. Bound in fifty volumes, contemporary sprinkled boards and blue paper boards. Gift in* 1829 *from* Moses Söderström, *apothecary in Karlskrona, who translated Trommsdorff into Swedish.*

Almanach oder Taschen-Buch für Scheidekünstler und Apotheker. Volumes 1-50, 1780–1829. [From 1820 as J. B. Trommsdorffs Almanach oder Taschenbuch für Chemiker und Apotheker].
Weimar, Hoffmann, 1780–1829.

Small octavo – *leaf*: 126 x 84 *mm. A complete set of* 50 *volumes. Engraved title vignettes and plates. The first volume* (1780) *is in the third, revised edition* (1784), *and the third volume* (1782) *in the second, revised edition* (1783). *The second volume* (1781) *is present in both the first* (1781) *and the third edition* (1786). *Contemporary sprinkled boards, red sprinkled edges. From the* C.D. Carlsson Collection.

Johann Bartholomeus was the eldest son of nine children in the 'Schwanen Ring' pharmacy at Erfurt, owned by his father Wilhelm Bernhard Trommsdorff, who was professor of medicine at Erfurt. His father died two days before Johann's twelfth birthday. Financial difficulties soon arose, and Trommsdorff had to abandon plans for higher education and enter pharmacy. He served as an apprentice under his father's old friend, Wilhelm Heinrich Bucholz, Goethe's teacher in chemistry and botany, who was director of the 'Hof-Apotheke' in Weimar, and under Bucholz's employee, the chemist Johann Friedrich Göttling. After three years of apprenticeship in Weimar and three additional years as a journeyman he took over the family apothecary shop in Erfurt.

In 1795 Trommsdorff was appointed extraordinary, and in 1805 ordinary, professor of chemistry. In 1790 he began his long series of textbooks on pharmacy, among them the first textbook on pharmacognosy written in German, *Handbuch der pharmaceutischen Waarenkunde*, of which our library has the first edition of 1799, a volume of over 1000 pages. His numerous published works were exceptionally popular and went through many editions and translations. His institute, founded in 1795 at Erfurt, became the base for the modern education of pharmacists and played a major role in the training of the founding generation of German pharmaceutical industry.

Trommsdorff was a highly esteemed man, and well-known in public life. 'No other pharmacist and teacher of pharmacy can claim to have taught and effected so much by word, action and writing as Trommsdorff, this star of first magnitude among the pharmacists' (Johann Andreas Buchner).

Most of Trommsdorff's hundreds of articles and monographs on various chemical and pharmaceutical topics were published in his own 'Journal', the first pharmaceutical journal that was published continuously over a longer period of time, and which became the leading periodical dealing not only with pharmacy, but with chemistry, chemical technology, medicine and mineralogy as well. It was preceded by the *Almanach oder Taschenbuch für Scheidekünstler und Apotheker*, the very first journal exclusively devoted to pharmacy, edited by Trommsdorff's friend Göttling, and after his death by Christian Friedrich Bucholz (1803–1818) and from 1820 by Trommsdorff. From the C.D. Carlsson donation our library also has a long run of the *Berlinisches Jahrbuch der Pharmacie*, illustrated with hand-coloured botanical plates, from its first volume in 1795 up to 1828, published under varying titles. These important journals, the starting point of the formation of the international pharmaceutical professional press, are today of the greatest rarity.

Wolfgang Götz, *Bibliographie der Schriften von Johann Bartholomäus Trommsdorff* (Ver. der Intern. Gesellschaft für Geschichte der Pharmazie, N.F. vol. 34, 1985); Partington, III, pp. 587-9; DSB, XIII, pp. 465-6: Kremers & Urdang, p. 85; Waller 5213 (Journal, vol. 14 only).

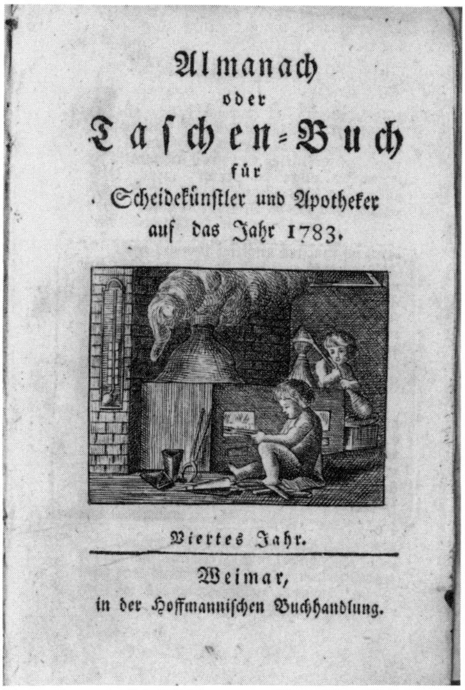

Almanach
oder
Taschen-Buch
für
Scheidekünstler und Apotheker
auf das Jahr 1783.

Viertes Jahr.

Weimar,
in der Hoffmannischen Buchhandlung.

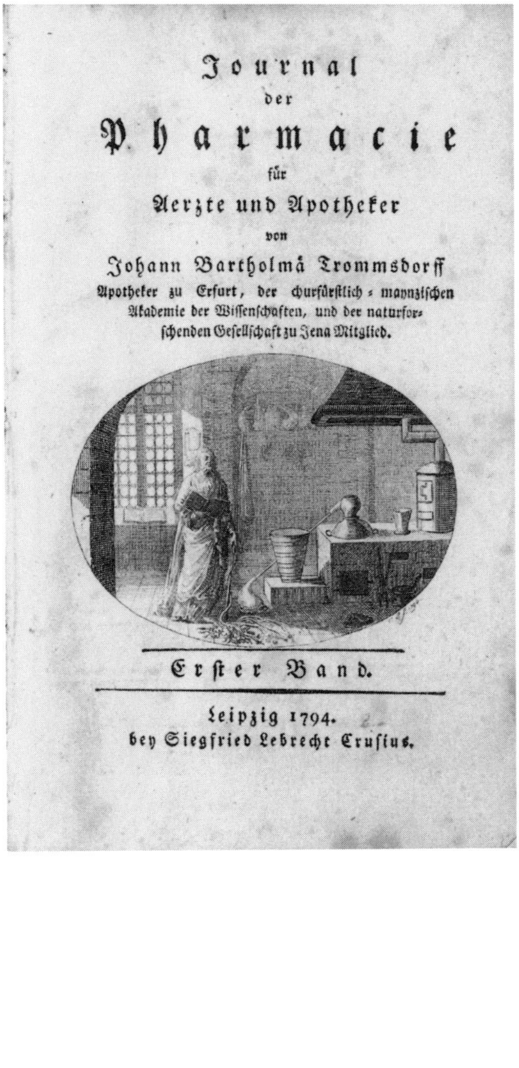

Journal
der
Pharmacie
für
Aerzte und Apotheker
von
Johann Bartholmä Trommsdorff
Apotheker zu Erfurt, der churfürstlich-maynzischen Akademie der Wissenschaften, und der naturforschenden Gesellschaft zu Jena Mitglied.

Erster Band.

Leipzig 1794.
bey Siegfried Lebrecht Crusius.

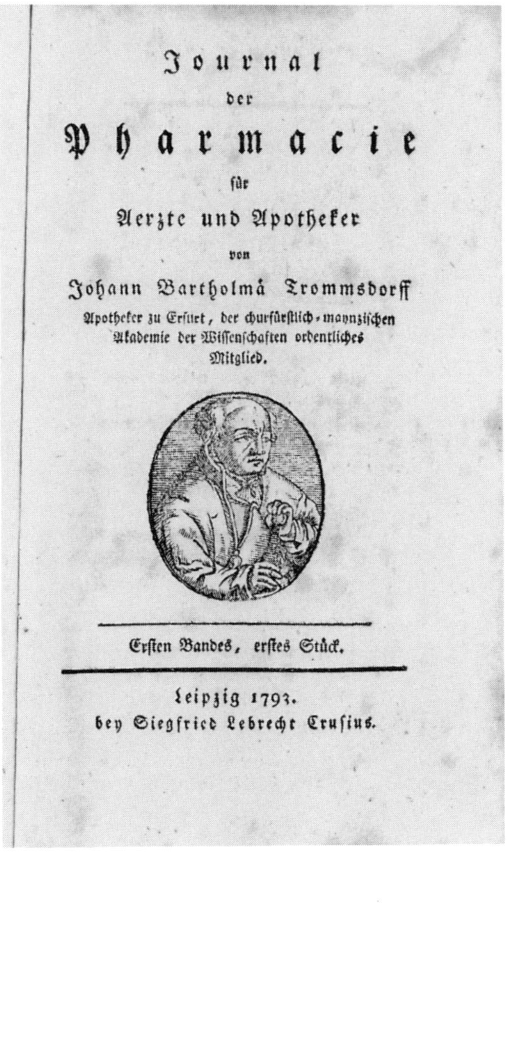

Journal
der
Pharmacie
für
Aerzte und Apotheker
von
Johann Bartholmä Trommsdorff
Apotheker zu Erfurt, der churfürstlich-maynzischen Akademie der Wissenschaften ordentliches Mitglied.

Ersten Bandes, erstes Stück.

Leipzig 1793.
bey Siegfried Lebrecht Crusius.

RIS, Hans Nicolaus (1780–1853)

Prince of Apothecaries

Res- och Lefvernes-Beskrifning.
Kristianstad, Schmidt & Comp. for the Author, 1835.

Octavo – *leaf*: 190 x 115 *mm. Pp.* [4], 235, [1]. *Cloth-backed boards. The original printed wrappers preserved, with list of contents printed on the back wrapper. Isidor Nordin's copy with two newspaper clippings with poems by Ris and a note that Ris died on the 2nd of November,* 1853, *of cholera 'å säteriet Stigen i Färglanda socken, Wahlbo härad'.*

First edition of this most noble, if ridiculously pretentious, work. The son of the preacher Thorbjörn Ris of Ramlösa, it was at an early age that Hans Nicolaus developed the qualities that later brought him to call himself 'the Swedish Cupid' and 'the Epicentre of Sex'. In 1795 he entered 'the territory of Esculapus' and was received as a pupil at the Helsingborg pharmacy *Lejonet* (the Lion). After a short period at the Ystad pharmacy *Svanen* (the Swan), he became an apothecary's apprentice in 1801. In 1805 he passed the Danish pharmacist's examination in Copenhagen and in 1806 became entitled to open a pharmacy in Skandeborg, though he never did. When he tried to become an apothecary in Sweden on the strength of his Danish examination, his request was curtly rejected.

Ris' 1802 move to Stockholm began a fifty-year period of wandering. After having worked at the pharmacy *Morianen* (the Blackamoor) for some months, he went to Copenhagen and from 1802 to 1815 travelled in Denmark, Germany, France and England. The Napoleonic wars were then raging, and Ris had many adventures. He was arrested several times as a suspected spy and bore witness to many memorable events. Amongst other things he saw Napoleon. Later, he was to claim that he had caused the great man's downfall, and when asked how, Ris answered: 'I let him rush blindly to his ruin'.

Ris returned to Sweden in 1815 and soon began to set his impressions on paper, mainly in the form of poems, which were published in small local newspapers. His goal, however, was to publish a description of his life and travels, and for this he required money. He now began his 'subscription round', which meant that for the following ten years he travelled around for some 2000 miles in Sweden recruiting subscribers. He would travel on horseback or in a chaise. He also brought a small, private menagerie with him, consisting of various breeds of dogs, a tame fox and a tame wolf, which was 'thin but docile' and which he fed with astrakhan apples. His appearance was, according to himself, noble despite a frostbitten nose, and he was bow-legged from riding. He spared no means when it came to getting new subscribers and never omitted a single manor. On arriving at a prospective subscriber's home and finding the master of the house to be away, Ris would eagerly emphazise the extremely important nature of his errand and could wait for weeks, during which time he would be well provided for. He never left until he had received some money, and even then might stay an extra week.

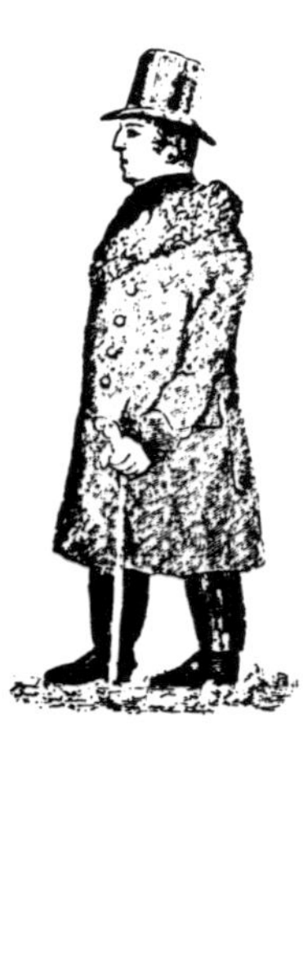

Finally the number of subscribers was sufficient and his book was published in Kristianstad in 1835, with a second edition following two years later. Ris' *Res- och Lefvernes-Beskrifning* is one of the most indigestible books ever published in the Swedish language, and in it he displays astounding powers of association, but as a document of its time and cultural history, it has not yet received the attention it deserves. Nonetheless, this unsurpassable collection of insanities, an absolutely preposterous work, has assured its author a place in posterity. Strindberg declared that 'no-one, with the possible exception of the author himself, has been able to read these 240 pages, of which each and every one is filled with silliness'.

After having been rejected by a Scanian matron, 'worthy of the title *Cleopatra of the North*' Ris on later travels was often accompanied by a very young girl, Augusta Adolfina Gerhardt, who for some reason had become quite attached to 'the Epicentre of Sex' and who came to be as famous as he was. In the 1840s, our 'Prince of Apothecaries' (Riksapotekare), as he now called himself, periodically lived in Stockholm, where he gained repute for riding in the lead during the mounting of the guard.

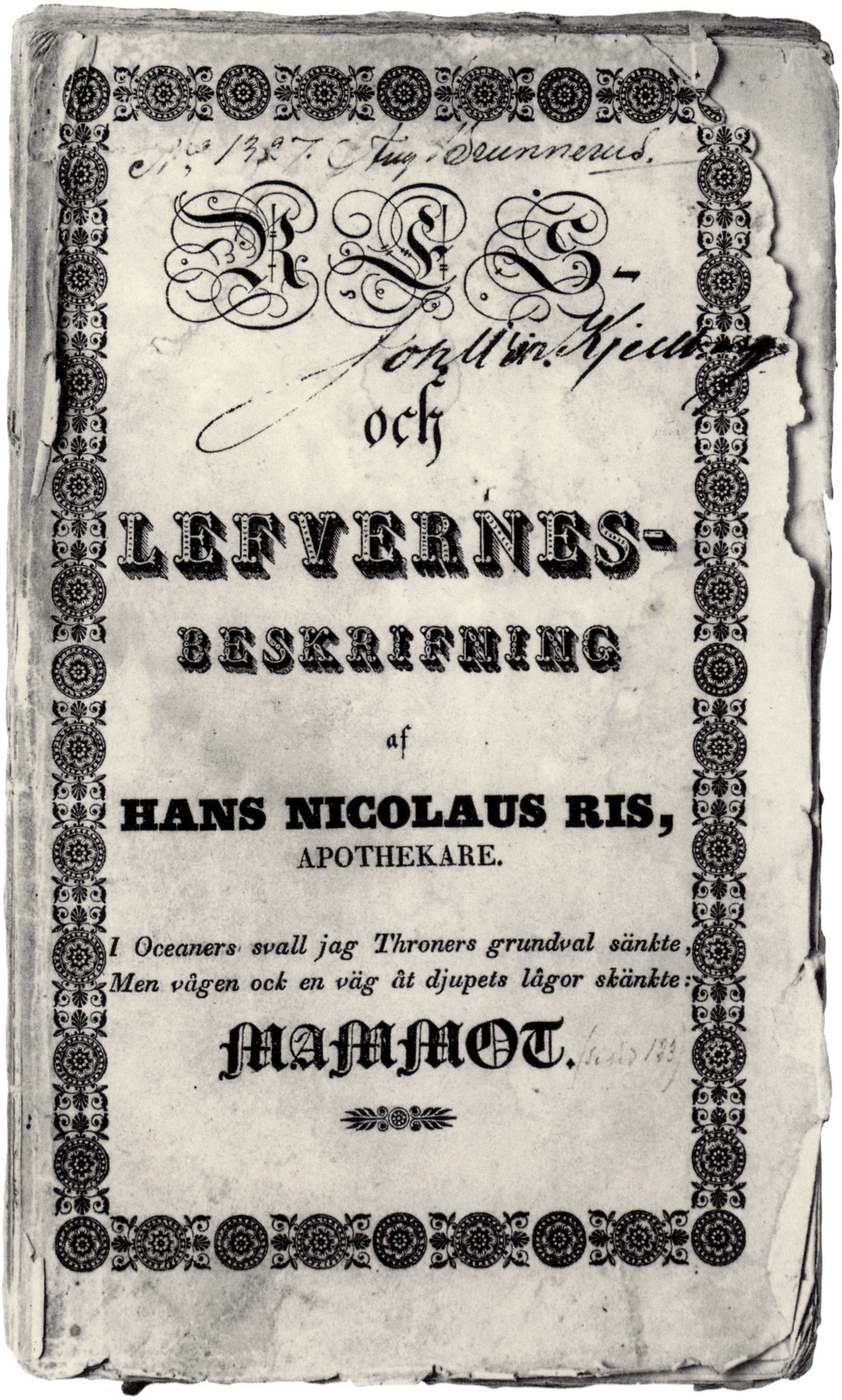
RES-

och

LEFVERNES-

BESKRIFNING

af

HANS NICOLAUS RIS,

APOTHEKARE.

I Oceaners svall jag Throners grundval sänkte,
Men vågen ock en väg åt djupets lågor skänkte:

MAMMOT.

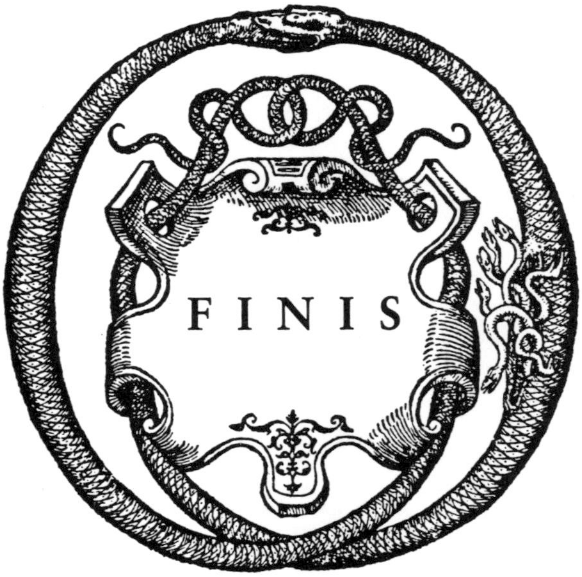

The Ouroboros,
or tail-eating serpent

Books corresponding to the Bibliotheca Walleriana

(different editions within brackets)

Aken, Hus- och Rese-Apotheque	Skara, 1746	No. 252
Albertus Magnus, De secretis mulierum, Augsburg, 1489	[Other editions]	4 & 5
Albertus Magnus, Heimlichkeit dess Weiblichen geschlecht, 1592	[Frankfurt, 1595]	318
Bock, Kreütterbuch, 1580	[Strassburg, 1552]	11463
Bossler, Dialogus oder gesprech, 1521	N.p., n.d.	19424
Brunfels, Von allerhandt Apoteckischen Confectionen	Frankfurt, 1552	1563
Brunschwig, Hauss apoteck, Augsburg, 1538	[Augsburg, 1539]	1582
Carrichter, Neuaffgerichtete Stadt- und Landt-Apotheke	Nuremberg, 1677	1786
Charas, Nouvelles Experiences sur la Vipere, 1669	[Paris, 1694]	11793
Cordus, Dispensatorium, Nuremberg, 1551	[Later editions]	2128-30
Croll, Basilica Chymica, Frankfurt, 1629	[Latin edition]	11107
Dioscorides, Pharmacorum Simplicium	Strassburg, 1529	2486
Ferber, Hortus Agerumensis	Stockholm, 1739	11506
Fioravanti, Del compendio dei secreti rationale, 1566	[Venice, 1560]	3050
Forordning om Medicis oc Apotecker	Copenhagen, 1672	3134
Fraundorffer, Tabula Smaragdina, 1726	[Nuremberg, 1713]	3236
Fuchs, New Kreüterbuch, 1543	[Latin edition, 1542]	11512
Gart der Gesundheit, Augsburg, 1534	[Earlier editions]	4932
Grim, Compendium Medico-chymicum	Augsburg, 1684	3747
Clusius [l'Écluse], Rariorum Plantarum Historia	Antwerp, 1601	11556
Linnaeus, Materia Medica	Stockholm, 1749	5907
Månsson, En myckit nyttigh Örta-Book	Stockholm, 1654	6231
Mattioli, Commentarii . . . Dioscoridis, Venice, 1570	[Venice, 1558]	6323
Medicinal-Ordningar 1699	Stockholm, 1699	5376
Mesue, Opera [& Grabadin] 1505, 1589.	[Other editions]	6523
Palmberg, Serta Florea Svecana eller Swenske Örtekrantz	Strängnäs, 1684	11698
Paracelsus, Sechster Theil . . . Basel, 1590	[Th. I-2, 10 only]	20080
Paracelsus, Bücher und Schrifften, I-II. Strassburg, 1603	[Strassburg, 1616]	20081
Paulli, Flora Danica	Copenhagen, 1648	11703
Paullini, Heilsame Dreck-Apotheke, Frankfurt, 1696	[Frankfurt, 1697]	7240
Petersen, Kongl. Rese-Apotheque	Stockholm, 1766	4203
Pharmacopoeia Augustana, 1573 and following editions	[Augsburg, 1734 only]	7385
Pharmacopoeia Holmiensis	Stockholm, 1686	7393
Pharmacopoea Persica	Paris, 1681	7403
Pharmacopoea Svecica	Stockholm, 1775	7404
Piso, Historia Naturalis Brasiliae, Leyden, 1648	[Amsterdam, 1658]	7472
Porta, Phytognomonica, Frankfurt, 1591	[Naples, 1588]	7568
Prevost, Dispensatorium, Lyon, 1505	[Lyon, 1517]	6859
Quiricus de Augustis, Lumen apothecarium, Venice, 1497	[Cremona, 1494]	23
Ricettario Fiorentino, 1550, 1567 and other editions	[Florence, 1567 only]	7941
Rosen von Rosenstein, Hus- och Rese-Apoteque	Stockholm, 1765	8191
Rydbäck, Det Svenska Apotheket	Linköping, 1780	9371
Ryff, New Kochbuch	Frankfurt, 1545	8356
Ryff, Reformierte Deutsche Apothek	Strassburg, 1573	8363
Scheele, Chemische Abhandlung von der Luft und dem Feuer	Uppsala, 1777	11225
Schoepf, Materia Medica Americana	Erlangen, 1787	8675
Schröder, Medicin-Chymische Apotheke, Nuremberg, 1686	[Latin edition, 1649]	8698
Serapion, Practica [and other authors], Lyon, 1525	[Venice, 1530]	8868
Thurneysser, Historia sive descriptio plantarum	Berlin, 1578	9578
Trommsdorff, Journal der Pharmacie, 1794–1824	[Volumes 14 and 20 only]	5213
Ulstadius, Coelum Philosophorum	Strassburg, 1536	9742
Underrättelse om Några ändringar	Stockholm, 1757, also facs.	5372

Important Donations, Gifts, Purchases and Provenances

Gift from Moses Söderström (1774–1857), Karlskrona, 1829:

Gift from Carl Wilhelm Bonté (1797–1832], 1831:

Purchase from the heirs of Isidor Nordin (1846–1906), 1907:

Purchase of the Carl Hyltén-Cavallius (1817–1853) Collection, 1910:

From the Thor Ekecrantz (1856–1939) donation, 1921:

Donation from the heirs of Ernst Matérn (1879–1954), 1955:

From the C.D. Carlsson (1875–1965) donation:

GIFT FROM AXEL KOCKUM (1869–1958):

GIFT FROM BERTIL BJURLING (1951):

GIFT FROM E. WISTRÖM:

FORMERLY IN THE LIBRARY OF THE ROYAL PHARMACEUTICAL INSTITUTE,
now in the Scheele-room, Biomedical Library, Faculty of Pharmacy, Uppsala University:

FROM THE LIBRARY OF THE FARMACEUTISKA FÖRENINGEN:

FROM THE LIBRARY OF CHRISTOPH WENZEL GRAF VON NOSTITZ (1643–1712)
[a lot of books from the Carlsson & Matérn collections bears his signature]

FROM THE LIBRARY OF ADAM HORN (1717–1778)

FROM THE VIBYHOLM LIBRARY, VIVECA TROLLE (1721–1806)

Principal Reference Works used and cited in this Catalogue

ADLUNG, A. & George URDANG. Grundriss der Geschichte der deutschen Pharmazie. Berlin, Julius Springer, 1935.

AHLBERG, Karl. Den svenska farmaciens historia. [*Includes a bibliography of Swedish pharmaceutical literature,* 1589–1908]. Stockholm, Wilhelm Bille, 1908.

ANDERSON, Frank J. An Illustrated History of the Herbals. New York, Columbia University Press, 1977.

ARBER, Agnes. Herbals, Their Origin and Evolution. A Chapter in the History of Botany 1470–1670. Third Edition, with an Introduction and Annotations by William T. Stearn. Cambridge University Press, 1986.

BALLHAUSEN, C.J. & Paul JOHANSEN. Thesaurus Librorum Danicorum 17. århundrede. Copenhagen, Rosenkilde & Bagger, 1990.

BENZING, Josef. Walther H. Ryff und sein literarisches Werk. Eine Bibliographie. Hamburg, Ernst Hauswedell, 1959.

BENZING, Josef. Die Drucke Jakob Cammerlanders zu Strassburg 1531–1548. Wien, Walter Krieg, 1963.

BIOGRAPHIE MÉDICALE. Tome Premier-Septième. A-Z. [Part of *Dictionnaire des Sciences Médicales*], Paris, C.L.F. Panckoucke, 1820-25.

BIRD, D.T. A Catalogue of Sixteenth-Century Medical Books in Edinburgh Libraries. Edinburgh, Royal College of Physicians of Edinburgh, 1982.

BLUNT, Wilfrid & Sandra RAPHAEL. The Illustrated Herbal. London, Thames and Hudson, 1979.

BLUNT, Wilfrid & William T. STEARN. The Art of Botanical Illustration. New Edition, revised and enlarged. Woodbridge, Suffolk, Antique Collectors' Club in association with The Royal Botanic Gardens, Kew, 1994.

BOERLIN, Paul H. Leonhard Thurneysser als Auftraggeber. Kunst im Dienste der Selbstdarstellung zwischen Humanismus und Barock. Basel, Birkhäuser, 1976.

BORBA DE MORAES, Rubens. Bibliographia Brasiliana. A bibliographical essay on rare books about Brazil published from 1504 to 1900 and works of Brazilian authors published abroad before the Independence of Brazil in 1822. Two Volumes. Amsterdam & Rio de Janeiro, Colibris Editora Ltda, 1958.

BRUZELIUS, A.J. Sveriges Apotekare-Historia ifrån Konung Gustaf I:s till närvarande tid. Ny Följd (1833–1878). See: Sacklén (–1833). Stockholm, 1878.

CASTIGLIONO, Arturo. A History of Medicine. Translated from the Italian and Edited by E.B. Krumbaar. Second Edition, revised and enlarged. New York, Alfr. A. Knopf, 1947.

CAVE, Richard & Geoffroy WAKEMAN. Typographia Naturalis. A history of nature printing. [Limited to 333 copies]. Wymondham, Brewhouse Press, 1967.

CHOULANT, Ludwig. Graphische Incunabeln für Naturgeschichte und Medicin. Enthaltend Geschichte und Bibliographie der ersten naturhistorischen und medicinischen Drucke des XV. und XVI. Jahrhunderts welche mit illustrierenden Abbildungen versehen sind. Leipzig, 1858. Reprint: München, 1924.

CHOULANT, Ludwig. Handbuch der Bücherkunde für die ältere Medicin zur Kenntniss der griechischen, lateinischen und arabischen Schriften im ärztliche Fache und zur bibliographischen Unterscheidung ihrer verschiedenen Ausgaben, Uebersetzungen und Erläuterungen. Zweite durchaus umgearbeitete und stark vermehrte Auflage. Leipzig, 1841. Reprint, n.d.

CLAIR, Colin. Christopher Plantin. London, Cassell & Comp., 1960.

COLE, F.J. A History of Comparative Anatomy. From Aristotle to the Eighteenth Century. London, Macmillan & Co., 1944.

COLE LIBRARY – Eales, Nellie B. The Cole Library of Early Medicine and Zoology. Catalogue of books and pamphlets. Part I, 1472 to 1800. Oxford, The Alden Press, 1969.

COLE, William A. Chemical Literature 1700–1860. A Bibliography with Annotations, Detailed Descriptions, Comparisons and Locations. London, Mansell Publ. Ltd., 1988.

Principal Reference Works used and cited in this Catalogue

COLLIJN, Isak. Sveriges Bibliografi 1600-talet. Uppsala, 1942-44.

COWEN, David L. & William H. HELFAND. Pharmacy. An Illustrated History. New York, Harry N. Abrams, 1990.

DAEMS, W.F. & L.J. VANDEWIELE. Noord- en Zuidnederlandse Stedelijke Pharmacopeeën. Mortsel-Antwerpen, Iticio, 1955.

DIBNER, Bern. Heralds of Science as represented by two hundred epochal books and pamphlets in the Dibner Library, Smithsonian Institution (1955). Revised Edition. Norwalk, Burndy Library, 1980.

DSB – Dictionary of Scientific Biography. Editior in Chief: Charles Coulston Gillispie. Fifteen Volumes plus Index. New York, Charles Scribner's, 1970-78.

DUNTHORNE, Gordon. Flower and Fruit Prints of the 18th and early 19th centuries. Their history, makers and uses, with a catalogue raisonné of the works in which they are found. Washington, by the Author, 1938.

DU RIETZ, Rolf E. 'Originaleditionen av Scheele's *Chemische Abhandlung* 1777: Ett 200-årsminne', in *Text: Svensk Tidskrift för Bibliografi*, 1974:4, pp. 217-25. Uppsala, Dahlia Books, 1977.

DURLING, Richard J. A Catalogue of Sixteenth Century Books in the National Library of Medicine. Bethesda, NLM, 1967.

DUVEEN, Denis I. Bibliotheca Alchemica et Chemica. An Annotated Catalogue of Printed Books on Alchemy, Chemistry and Cognate Subjects in the Library of Dennis I. Duveen. London, E. West, 1949.

EDER, Joseph Maria. History of Photography. Translated by Edward Epstean. New York, Columbia University Press, 1945.

ELGOOD, Cyril. A Medical History of Persia and Eastern Caliphate from the Earliest Times until the Year A.D. 1932. Cambridge Univ. Press, 1951.

ENCYCLOPEDIA BRITANNICA. A Dictionary of Arts, Sciences, Literature and General Information. Eleventh Edition. New York, 1910–1911.

ERIKSSON, Gunnar. Botanikens historia i Sverige intill år 1800 [Lychnos-Biblioteket 17:3]. Uppsala, Almqvist & Wiksell, 1969.

FABER DU FAUR, Curt von. German Baroque Literature. A Catalogue of the Collection in the Yale University Library. New Haven, Yale Univ. Press, 1958.

FAIRFAX MURRAY – Davies, Hugh Wm. Catalogue of a Collection of Early French Books in the Library of C. Fairfax Murray. London, The Holland Press, 1961.

FALCK, A. Die Arzneibücher (Pharmakopöen) vergleichend besprochen mit einem Verzeichnis der Arzneibücher. Leipzig, J.A. Barth, 1920.

FERCHL, Fritz. Chemisch-Pharmaceutisches Bio- und Bibliographikon. Mittenwald, Arthur Nemayer, 1937.

FERCHL, Fritz. Geschichte der Pharmazie in einer Stunde. Tübingen, Intern. Gesellschaft f. Geschichte d. Pharmazie, 1951.

FERGUSON, John. Bibliotheca Chemica. A Bibliography of books on Alchemy, Chemistry and Pharmaceutics. In Two Volumes. [Reprint of Bibliotheca Chemica. A Catalogue of the Alchemical, Chemical and Pharmaceutical Books in the Collection of the late James Young of Kelly and Durris, 1906]. London, Derek Verschoyle Publ., 1954.

FISCHER, Ernst. 'Zweihundert Jahre Naturselbstdruck' pp. 186-213, in *Gutenberg Jahrbuch*, Mainz, 1933.

FLÜCKIGER, Friedrich & Daniel HANBURY. Pharmacographia. A History of the Principal Drugs of Vegetable Origin, met with in Great Britain and British India. London, Macmillan & Co., 1874.

FORBES, R.J. Short History of the Art of Distillation from the Beginnings up to the death of Cellier Blumenthal. Leiden, E.J. Brill, 1948.

FRIES, Th. M. Linné. Lefnadsteckning. I-II. Stockholm, 1903 [& Personregister utarbetat av Hans Krook. Uppsala, 1956].

GARRISON, Fielding H. An Introduction to the History of Medicine. Fourth Edition (1929). Reprint. Philadelphia, W.-B. Saunders Company, n.d.

GARRISON-MORTON – Morton's Medical Bibliography. An Annotated Check list of Texts Illustrating the History of Medicine (Garrison and Morton). Edited by **Jeremy M. Norman.** Fifth Edition. Aldershot, Great Britain, Scolar Press, 1991.

GW – **Gesamtkatalog der Wiegendrucke.** Vols. I-IX (cont.). Leipzig, Berlin, Hiersemann & Akademie Verlag, 1925-81.

GNUDI, Martha Teach & Jerome Pierce WEBSTER. The Life and Times of Gaspare Tagliacozzi of Bologna 1545–1599. With a Documented Study of the Scientific and Cultural Life of Bologna in the Sixteenth Century. New York, Herbert Reichner, 1950.

GOLDSCHMIDT – **E.P. Goldschmidt & Co. Ltd.** London. *Catalogues.*

GREAT FLOWER BOOKS – **Sitwell, Sacheverell & Wilfrid Blunt.** Great Flower Books 1700–1900. New Edition. London, H.F.& G. Witherby, 1990.

GREENE/EGERTON – **Greene, Edward Lee.** Landmarks of Botanical History. Edited by Frank M. Egerton. In Two Volumes. Stanford University Press, 1983.

HAGGARD, Howard W. Devils, Drugs, and Doctors. The Story of the Science of Healing from Medicine-Man to Doctor. New York, Harper & Brothers, 1929.

HAIN – **Hain, L.** Repertorium Bibliographicum, in quo libri omnes ab arte typographica inventa usque ad annum MD. 4 vols. in two. Stuttgart & Paris, 1826-38.

HAMBERG, N.P. Svensk Pharmaceutisk Bibliografi (1522–1862). Stockholm, 1862. & Isidor Nordin. Svensk Farmaceutisk Bibliografi (1862–1892). Stockholm, 1893. Offprints: *Pharmaceutisk Tidskrift.*

HEBBE, P.M. Den Svenska Lantbrukslitteraturen. I. Från äldsta tid t.o.m. år 1800. II. Från 1801 till 1850. Bibliografisk Förteckning. Stockholm, Kungl. Lantbruksakad., 1939-45.

HEILMANN, Karl Eugen. Kräuterbücher in Bild und Geschichte. München, K. Kölbl, 1966.

HEIMANN – **Sandbergs Bokhandel. Rare Book Department,** Stockholm. *Catalogues,* compiled by Willy Heimann.

HENREY, Blanche. British Botanical and Horticultural Literature before 1800. Comprising a history and bibliography of botanical and horticultural books printed in England, Scotland, and Ireland from the earliest times until 1800. Three Volumes. London, Oxford Univ. Press, 1975.

HIRSCH – **Hirsch, August** (ed.) Biographisches Lexikon der hervorragenden Ärzte aller Zeiten und Völker. Vols. I-VI. Dritte, unveränderte Auflage. München, Urban & Schwarzenberg, 1962.

HJELT, Otto A.E. Svenska och Finska Apoteksväsendets Historia 1663–1812. (Offprint: Svenska och Finska Medicinalverkets Historia). Helsingfors, 1898.

HOPPE, Brigitte. Das Kräuterbuch des Hieronymus Bock. Wissenschaftshistorische Untersuchung, mit einem Verzeichnis sämtlicher Pflanzen des Werkes, der literarischen Quellen der Heilanzeigen und der Anwendungen der Pflanzen. Stuttgart, Hiersemann, 1969.

HORBLIT, Harrison D. One Hundred Books Famous in Science. Based on an Exhibition held at the Grolier Club. New York, The Grolier Club, 1964.

HUNGER, F.W.T. Clusius-Tentoonstelling in het Stedelijk Museum "De Lakenhal" te Leiden, October, 1926. Catalogus. Leyden, 1926.

HUNGER, F.W.T. Charles De L'Ecluse Nederlandsch Kruidkundige 1526–1609. I-II. The Hague, 1927-43.

HUNT – **Quimby, Jane & Allan Stevenson** (compilers). Catalogue of Botanical Books in the Collection of Rachel McMasters Miller Hunt. In Two Volumes. 1477–1800. Pittsburgh, Hunt Botanical Library, 1958-61.

HUSEMANN, Theodor. A Facsimile of the First Edition of the Pharmacopoeia Augustana. With Introductory Essays by Theodor Husemann. Madison, State Historical Society of Wisconsin, 1927.

ILLUSTRIERTER APOTHEKER-KALENDER. Berlin, Deutscher Apotheker-Verein, I. 1925 –1977.

INTERNATIONALEN GESELLSCHAFT FÜR GESCHICHTE DER PHARMAZIE e.V. NEUE FOLGE – Veröffentlichungen, Band 1-59. Stuttgart, Wissenschaftliche Verlagsanstalt, 1953-94.

JOHNSTON, Jr, Stanley H. The Cleveland Herbal, Botanical, and Horticultural Collections. A Descriptive Bibliography of Pre-1830 Works from the Libraries of the Holden Arboretum, the Cleveland Medical Library Association, and the Garden Center of Greater Cleveland. Kent, Ohio, Kent State University Press, 1992.

JUNK RARA – Junk, Wilhelm. Rara Historico-Naturalia et Mathematica. I-II + Supplementum: Die Historico-Bibliophilie. Berlin, 1900-13, 1926-36, 1939. Reprint.

KLEBS, Arnold C. Incunabula scientifica et medica [Reprint from OSIRIS, IV, pp. 1-359, Bruges, 1938]. Hildesheim, Georg Olms, 1963.

KREMERS, Edward & George URDANG. History of Pharmacy. A Guide and a Survey. Philadelphia, J.B. Lippincott Company, 1940.

KRIVATSY, Peter. A Catalogue of Seventeenth Century Printed Books in the National Library of Medicine. Bethesda, NLM, 1989.

KROK, Th. O.B.N. Bibliotheca Botanica Suecana – Svensk Botanisk Litteratur från äldsta tider t.o.m. 1918. Uppsala, Almqvist & Wiksell, 1925.

LA WALL, Charles H. The Curious Lore of Drugs and Medicines [= Four Thousand Years of Medicine]. Garden City, N.Y., Garden City Publ. Co., (1927).

LISNEY, Arthur A. A Bibliography of British Lepidoptera 1608–1799. London, The Chiswick Press, 1960.

LÖWEGREN, Yngve. Naturaliekabinett i Sverige under 1700-talet. Ett bidrag till zoologiens historia. (Lychnos-Biblioteket, 13). Lund, Lychnos, 1952.

LOWNES – Godine, David R. & Owen Gingerich (compilers). Renaissance Books of Science from the collection of Albert E. Lownes. Dartmouth College, Hanover, 1970.

MAJOR, Ralph H. A History of Medicine. Springfield, Illinois, Charles C. Thomas, 1954.

MELLON COLLECTION – Macphail, Ian (compiler). Alchemy and the Occult. A Catalogue of Books and Manuscripts from the Collection of Paul and Mary Mellon given to the Yale University Library. Printed Books 1472–1790 . In Two Volumes. New Haven, Yale University Press, 1968.

MEYER, Ernst H.F. Geschichte der Botanik. [Facsimile of the original edition, Königsberg, 1854-57]. With an Introductory Essay by Frans Verdorrn. In Four Volumes. Amsterdam, Asher & Co., 1965.

MOEHSEN, J.C.W. 'Leben Leonhard Thurneissers zum Thurn, Churfürstl. Brandenburgischen Leibarztes. Ein Beitrag zur Geschichte der Alchymie, wie auch der Wissenschaften und Künste in der Mark Brandenburg gegen Ende des sechszehnten Jahrhunderts'. Pp. 1-198 in *Beiträge zur Geschichte der Wissenschaften in der Mark Brandenburg von den ältesten Zeiten an bis zu Ende des sechszehnten Jahrhunderts.* Ed. by J.C.W. Moehsen. Berlin & Leipzig, 1783.

MORTIMER, Ruth. Italian 16th Century Books. Harvard College Library, Department of Printing and Graphic Arts. Cambridge, Massachusetts, Harvard University Press, 1974.

MORTIMER, Ruth. French 16th Century Books. Harvard College Library, Department of Printing and Graphic Arts. Cambridge, Massachusetts, Harvard University Press, 1964.

NEU, John. Chemical, Medical and Pharmaceutical Books Printed before 1800. In the Collections of the University of Wisconsin Libraries. Madison, University of Wisconsin, 1965.

NISSEN BBI – Nissen, Claus. Die botanische Buchillustration. Ihre Geschichte und Bibliographie. Zweite Auflage. Stuttgart, Anton Hiersemann, 1966.

NORMAN, Haskell F. One Hundred Books Famous in Medicine. Catalogue edited by Hope Mayo. New York, The Grolier Club, 1995.

NORMAN LIBRARY – Hook, Diana H. & Jeremy M. Norman. The Haskell F. Norman Library of Science and Medicine. Two Volumes. San Francisco, Jeremy Norman & Co., 1991.

OSLER – Bibliotheca Osleriana: A Catalogue of Books illustrating the History of Medicine and Science. Collected, arranged and annotated by Sir William Osler and bequeathed to McGill University. Oxford, Clarendon Press, 1929. Reprint: Montreal & London, McGill-Queen's University Press, 1969.

PARKINSON, Ethel & Audrey LUMB. Catalogue of Medical Books in Manchester University Library 1480–1700. Manchester University Press, 1972.

PARTINGTON, J. R. A History of Chemistry. In Four Volumes. London, Macmillan & Co., 1970 (1961)–1972.

PHARMACY THROUGH THE AGES. Published by FARMITALIA CARLO ERBA. Vol. I. From the Beginnings to Modern Times (1987); II. From Laboratory to Industry (1989); III. Ancient Drugs (1990); IV. New Frontier (1992). Parma, 1987-92.

PHILLIPPE, A. Geschichte der Apotheker bei den wichtigsten Völkern der Erde seit den ältesten Zeiten bis auf unsere Tage . . . Aus dem Französischen übersetzt und mit einer Zusammenstellung der Förderer der Pharmazie alter und neuer Zeit vermehrt, von Hermann Ludwig. Zweite Auflage. Jena, Friedrich Mauke, 1859.

PMM – Printing and The Mind of Man. A descriptive catalogue illustrating the impact of print on the evolution of the Western civilization during five centuries. Compiled and edited by **John Carter & Percy H. Muir.** London, 1967. [Second edition, revised and enlarged: Munich, Karl Pressler, 1983].

PRITZEL, G. A. Thesaurus Literaturae Botanicae (1871). Reprint: Milano, Görlich, 1950.

PULTENEY, Richard. A General View of the Writings of Linnaeus. The Second Edition, with Corrections, Considerable Additions, and Memoirs of the Author, by William George Maton. London, 1805.

QUIRICUS DE AUGUSTIS. Dlicht d'Apotekers (1515). The first prescription book printed in the Low Countries. Facsimile. With an introduction by D.A. Wittop Koning. Niewkoop, B. De Graaf, 1967.

READ, John. Prelude to Chemistry. An Outline of Alchemy its Literature and Relationships. London, 1939.

READ, John. Through Alchemy to Chemistry. A Procession of Ideas & Personalities. London, 1957.

READ, John. Humour and Humanism in Chemistry. London, 1947.

SACKLÉN, J. F. Sveriges Läkarehistoria, ifrån Konung Gustaf I:s till närvarande tid. Vols. I-III & Supplement; New Supplement (by Hilarion Wistrand). Nyköping, Stockholm, 1822-35, 1853.

SACKLÉN, J. F. Sveriges Apotekare-Historia, ifrån Konung Gustaf I:s till närvarande tid. Ett Bihang till Sveriges Läkare-Historia. Nyköping, 1833(for cont. see: **BRUZELIUS**).

SARTON, George. Introduction to the History of Science. Vols. I, II:1-2, III:1-2. In Five Volumes. Baltimore, Carnegie Inst. of Washington, 1927-48.

SCHELENZ, Hermann. Geschichte der Pharmazie. Berlin, Springer Verlag, 1904.

SCHMID, Alfred. Zwei seltene Kräuterbücher aus dem vierten Dezennium des sechzehnten Jahrhunderts. Nebst einem bibliographischen Verzeichnis aller bekannten frühen Ausgaben der Brunfelsschen Kräuterbücher als Anhang. Separatabdruck: *Schweizerischen Gutenberg-museum*, 1936, Nr. 3. Bern, 1936

SCHMID, Alfred. Ueber alte Kräuterbücher. Bern, Paul Haupt, 1939.

SCHNALKE, Thomas. Natur im Bild. Anatomie und Botanik in der Sammlung des Nürnberger Arztes Christoph Jacob Trew. Eine Ausstellung aus Anlass seines 300. Geburtstages 8. November – 10. Dezember 1995. Schriften der Universitätsbibliothek Erlangen-Nürnberg, 27. Erlangen, 1995.

SCHREIBER, Wilhelm Ludwig. Die Kräuterbücher des XV. und XVI. Jahrhunderts. Unveränderter Abdruck der Ausgabe von 1924 . . . Herausgegeben und mit einem Nachwort versehen von Reimar Walter Fuchs. Stuttgart, Anton Hiersemann, 1982.

SIGERIST, H. E. Hieronymus Brunschwig and His Work. New York, Ben Abramson, 1946.

SINKANKAS, John. Gemology. An Annotated Bibliography. In Two Volumes. Metuchen, N.J., The Scarecrow Press, 1993.

SOULSBY, B.H. (ed.) A Catalogue of the Works of Linnaeus (and publications more immediately relating thereto) preserved in the Libraries of the British Museum (Bloomsbury) and the British Museum (Natural History) (South Kensignton). Second Edition. London, 1933. An Index to the Authors (other than Linnaeus) mentioned in the Catalogue . . . , London, 1936.

STILLMAN, John Maxson. The Story of Alchemy and Early Chemistry [1924]. Reprint: New York, Dover Publ., 1960.

STILLWELL, Margaret Bingham. The Awakening Interest in Science during the First Century of Printing 1450–1550. An annotated checklist of first editions viewed from the angle of their subject content. New York, The Bibliographical Society of America, 1970.

STÜBLER, Eberhard. Leonhart Fuchs. Leben und Werk. (*Münchener Beiträge zur Geschichte und Literatur der Naturwissenschaften und Medizin.* Heft 13/14). München, 1928.

SBL – Svenskt Biografiskt Lexikon. Vols. 1-28 (incl. Pederby). Stockholm, 1918-94.

SUDHOFF, Karl. Bibliographia Paracelsica. Besprechungen der unter Hohenheims Namen 1527–1893 erschienenen Druckschrifften. Unveränderter Abdruck der 1894 Ausgabe. Graz, Akad. Druck- und Verlagsanstalt, 1958.

SWEDISH MEN OF SCIENCE 1650 – 1950. Edited and with an introduction by Sten Lindroth. Stockholm, The Swedish Institute, 1952.

SWIM. Swedish Imprints 1731–1833: A Retrospective National Bibliography. Uppsala, Dahlia Books, 1977–.

TAX. LIT. – Stafleu, Frans A. and Richard S. Cowan. Taxonomic literature. A selective guide to botanical publications and collections with dates, commentaries and types. Second Edition. Volumes I-VIII. Utrecht, Bohn, Scheltema & Hockema. The Hague, W. Junk Publ., 1976-88.

TELLE, Joachim (ed.) Pharmazie und der gemeine Mann. Hausarznei und Apotheke in der frühen Neuzeit. Ausstellungskataloge der Herzog August Bibliothek, Nr. 36. Zweite vermehrte Auflage. Wolfenbüttel, Herzog August Bibliothek, 1988.

THOMPSON, G.J.S. The Mystery and Art of the Apothecary. London, John Lane, 1929.

THORNDIKE, Lynn. A History of Magic and Experimental Science. Volumes I-VIII. New York, Columbia University Press, (1923)–1958.

TSCHIRCH, A. Die Pharmakopöe ein Spiegel ihrer Zeit. Zürich, Orell Füssli, 1904.

TSCHIRCH, A. (Ed.) Handbuch der Pharmacognosie. I-III and Index in Seven Volumes, Leipzig, 1909-27.

URDANG, George. 'The Development of Pharmacopoeias', pp. 577-603 in *Bulletin World Health Organization*, 1951, 4, Geneva, 1951.

URDANG, George. 'How Chemicals entered the Official Pharmacopoeias', pp. 303-14 in *Archives Internationales d'Histoire des Sciences*, 7, No. 26, 1954. Paris, 1954.

URDANG, George. Pharmacy's Part in Society. Third Edition. Madison, Wisconsin, American Institute of the History of Pharmacy, 1959.

VICAIRE, Georges. Bibliographie Gastronomique. Réimpression de l'édition de Paris, 1890. Genève, Slatkine Reprints, 1978.

VOLCKRINGER, Jean. Évolution et unification des formulaires et des pharmacopées. Paris, Paul Brandouy, 1953.

WALLER – Sallander, Hans. Bibliotheca Walleriana. The Books illustrating the History of Medicine and Science collected by Dr. Erik Waller and bequeathed to the Library of the Royal University of Uppsala. In Two Volumes. Stockholm, Almqvist & Wiksell, 1955.

WARING, Edward John. Bibliotheca Therapeutica, or Bibliography of Therapeutics, chiefly in reference to Articles of the Materia Medica, with numerous critical, historical, and therapeutical annotations, and an Appendix containing the Bibliography of British Mineral Waters. In Two Volumes. London, The New Sydenham Society, 1878-79.

Principal Reference Works used and cited in this Catalogue

WEIL – Catalogue of Books, Manuscripts, Photographs and Scientific Instruments Fully Described and Offered for Sale by Ernst Weil, 1943–1965. Original thirty-three catalogues with a biographical memoir and full author-title index. (Reprint in two volumes). Storrs-Mansfield, CT, Maurizio Martino Publ., 1995.

WELLCOME – A Catalogue of Printed Books in the Wellcome Historical Medical Library. Volumes I-IV. I: Books printed before 1641; II-IV: Books printed from 1641 to 1850, A-R (all publ.) London, Wellcome Institute for the History of Medicine, 1962-95.

WOOTTON, A.C. Chronciles of Pharmacy. Two Volumes. London, Macmillan and Co., 1910.

ZEKERT, Otto. Carl Wilhelm Scheele. Sein Leben und seine Werke. Mittenwald, 1931-35.

INDEX

including names of persons, all but the most trivial, and a few subjects, the latter in italic.
Authors and titles subject for articles are in bold face.

APOTEKARSOCIETETEN
SWEDISH PHARMACEUTICAL SOCIETY

This book of 224 pages with 130 illustrations
of which 17 are tipped in colour-plates
is printed on
Munken Cream, 150 gsm,
a woodfree uncoated paper, total chlorine free (tcf),
no bleaching agents added,
from Munkedal Paper Mill, Sweden.
The colour plates are printed on Arctic Art, 100 gsm,
a woodfree fully coated paper, high gloss, elementary chlorine free (ecf)
from Håfreström Paper Mill, Sweden.
Board paper is screen printed on grey Ingres, 130 gsm,
and endpapers on black Ingres, 130 gsm,
from Hahnemühle Büttenpapierfabrik,
Dassel, Germany.

Typeface: Sabon [Jan Tschichold]

Produced by
HAGELIN RARE BOOKS

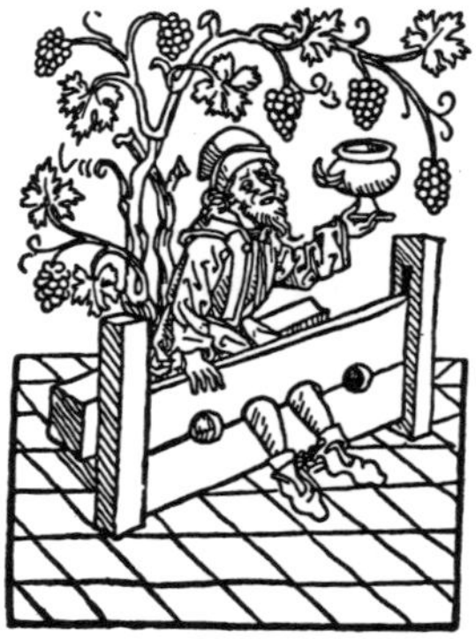